Springer Series in Statistics

Advisors:
P. Bickel, P. Diggle, S. Fienberg, U. Gather,
I. Olkin, S. Zeger

Springer Series in Statistics

(continued after index)

Paul W. Mielke, Jr.
Kenneth J. Berry

Permutation Methods
A Distance Function Approach

Second Edition

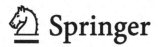 Springer

Paul W. Mielke, Jr.
Department of Statistics
Colorado State University
Fort Collins, CO 80523-1877
mielke@lamar.colostate.edu

Kenneth J. Berry
Department of Sociology
Colorado State University
Fort Collins, CO 80523-1784
berry@lamar.colostate.edu

ISBN 978-1-4419-2416-2   e-ISBN 978-0-387-69813-7

9 8 7 6 5 4 3 2 1

springer.com

To our families.

Preface to the Second Edition

Besides various corrections, additions, and deletions of material in the first edition, added emphasis has been placed on the geometrical framework of permutation methods. When ordinary Euclidean distance replaces commonly-used squared Euclidean distance as the underlying distance function, then concerns such as robustness all but vanish. This geometrical emphasis is primarily discussed and motivated in Chapters 1 and 2. Chapter 3 now addresses multiple binary choices and also includes a real data example that demonstrates an exceedingly strong association between heavy metal soil concentrations and academic achievement. Multiple binary choices are also placed in the randomized block framework of Chapter 4. Whereas the main addition to Chapter 5 is the generalization of MRPP regression analyses from univariate multiple linear regression in the first edition to multivariate multiple linear regression in the second edition, further clarification is made between the exchangeable random variable approach of MRPP regression analyses and the independent random variable approach of other analyses, such as the Cade–Richards regression analyses. Chapter 6 now includes an efficient approach due to L. Euler for obtaining exact goodness-of-fit P-values when equal probabilities occur. A resampling approach is now included for r-way contingency tables in Chapter 7, along with an investigation of log-linear analyses involving small sample sizes. While only a few minor changes occur in Chapter 8, a new Chapter 9 includes (1) a discrete analog of Fisher's continuous method for combining P-values, (2) a Monte Carlo investigation of Fisher's Z transformation, and (3) a new multivariate test for similarity between two samples. In addition to various other necessary additions to Appendix A and the subject index, an author index is also included.

Acknowledgments. The authors thank the American Meteorological Society for permission to reproduce excerpts from *Weather and Forecasting* and the *Journal of Applied Meteorology*, Sage Publications, Inc. to reproduce excerpts from *Educational and Psychological Measurement*, the American Educational Research Association for permission to reproduce excerpts from the *Journal of Educational and Behavioral Statistics*, Elsevier, Ltd. to reproduce excerpts from *Environmental Research*, and the editors and publishers to reproduce excerpts from *Psychological Reports* and *Perceptual and Motor Skills*.

The authors also wish to thank the following reviewers for their helpful comments: Brian S. Cade, U.S. Geological Survey; S. Rao Jammalamadaka, University of California, Santa Barbara; and Shin Ta Liu, Lynx Systems. At Springer–Verlag New York, Inc., we thank Executive Editor John Kimmel for guiding the project throughout, Senior Production Editor Jeffrey Taub, and copy editor Carla Spoon.

The authors are very appreciative of comments and corrections made by the following individuals, listed in alphabetical order: Bryan S. Cade, Kees Duineveld, Ryan Elmore, Phillip Good, S. Rao Jammalamadaka, Janis E. Johnston, Michael A. Long, and John S. Spear.

Paul W. Mielke, Jr.
Kenneth J. Berry

Preface to the First Edition

The introduction of permutation tests by R.A. Fisher relaxed the parametric structure requirement of a test statistic. For example, the structure of the test statistic is no longer required if the assumption of normality is removed. The between-object distance function of classical test statistics based on the assumption of normality is squared Euclidean distance. Because squared Euclidean distance is not a metric (i.e., the triangle inequality is not satisfied), it is not at all surprising that classical tests are severely affected by an extreme measurement of a single object. A major purpose of this book is to take advantage of the relaxation of the structure of a statistic allowed by permutation tests. While a variety of distance functions are valid for permutation tests, a natural choice possessing many desirable properties is ordinary (i.e., non-squared) Euclidean distance. Simulation studies show that permutation tests based on ordinary Euclidean distance are exceedingly robust in detecting location shifts of heavy-tailed distributions. These tests depend on a metric distance function and are reasonably powerful for a broad spectrum of univariate and multivariate distributions.

Least sum of absolute deviations (LAD) regression linked with a permutation test based on ordinary Euclidean distance yields a linear model analysis that controls for type I error. These Euclidean distance-based regression methods offer robust alternatives to the classical method of linear model analyses involving the assumption of normality and ordinary sum of least square deviations (OLS) regression linked with tests based on squared Euclidean distance. In addition, consideration is given to a number of permutation tests for (1) discrete and continuous goodness-of-fit,

(2) independence in multidimensional contingency tables, and (3) discrete and continuous multisample homogeneity. Examples indicate some favorable characteristics of seldom used tests.

Following a brief introduction in Chapter 1, Chapters 2, 3, and 4 provide the motivation and description of univariate and multivariate permutation tests based on distance functions for completely randomized and randomized block designs. Applications are provided. Chapter 5 describes the linear model methods based on the linkage between regression and permutation tests, along with recently developed linear and nonlinear model prediction techniques. Chapters 6, 7, and 8 include the goodness-of-fit, contingency table, and multisample homogeneity tests, respectively. Appendix A contains an annotated listing of the computer programs used in the book, organized by chapter.

Paul Mielke is indebted to the following former University of Minnesota faculty members: his advisor Richard B. McHugh for introducing him to permutation tests, Jacob E. Bearman and Eugene A. Johnson for motivating the examination of various problems from differing points of view, and also to Constance van Eeden and I. Richard Savage for motivating his interest in nonparametric methods. He wishes to thank two of his Colorado State University students, Benjamin S. Duran and Earl S. Johnson, for stimulating his long term interest in alternative permutation methods. Finally, he wishes to thank his Colorado State University colleagues Franklin A. Graybill, Lewis O. Grant, William M. Gray, Hariharan K. Iyer, David C. Bowden, Peter J. Brockwell, Yi-Ching Yao, Mohammed M. Siddiqui, Jagdish N. Srivastava, and James S. Williams, who have provided him with motivation and various suggestions pertaining to this topic over the years.

Kenneth Berry is indebted to the former University of Oregon faculty members Walter T. Martin, mentor and advisor, and William S. Robinson who first introduced him to nonparametric statistical methods. Colorado State University colleagues Jeffrey L. Eighmy, R. Brooke Jacobsen, Michael G. Lacy, and Thomas W. Martin were always there to listen, advise, and encourage.

Acknowledgments. The authors thank the American Meteorological Society for permission to reproduce excerpts from *Weather and Forecasting* and the *Journal of Applied Meteorology*, Sage Publications, Inc. to reproduce excerpts from *Educational and Psychological Measurement*, the American Psychological Association for permission to reproduce excerpts from *Psychological Bulletin*, the American Educational Research Association for permission to reproduce excerpts from the *Journal of Educational and Behavioral Statistics*, and the editors and publishers to reproduce excerpts from *Psychological Reports* and *Perceptual and Motor Skills*.

The authors also wish to thank the following reviewers for their helpful comments: Mayer Alvo, University of Ottawa; Bradley J. Biggerstaff, Centers for Disease Control and Prevention; Brian S. Cade,

U.S. Geological Survey; Hariharan K. Iyer, Colorado State University; Bryan F.J. Manly, WEST, Inc.; and Raymond K.W. Wong, Alberta Environment. At Springer–Verlag New York, Inc., we thank our editor, John Kimmel, for guiding the project throughout. We are grateful for the efforts of the production editor, Antonio D. Orrantia, and the copy editor, Hal Henglein. We wish to thank Roberta Mielke for reading the entire manuscript and correcting our errors. Finally, we alone are responsible for any shortcomings or inaccuracies.

Paul W. Mielke, Jr.
Kenneth J. Berry

Contents

1
Introduction

Many of the statistical methods routinely used in contemporary research are based on a compromise with the ideal (Bakeman et al., 1996). The ideal is represented by permutation tests, such as Fisher's exact test or the binomial test, which yield exact, as opposed to approximate, probability values (P-values). The compromise is represented by most statistical tests in common use, such as the t and F tests, where P-values depend on unsatisfied assumptions. In this book, an assortment of permutation tests is described for a wide variety of research applications. In addition, metric distance functions such as Euclidean distance are recommended to avoid distorted inferences resulting from nonmetric distance functions such as the squared Euclidean distance associated with the t and F tests.

Permutation tests were initiated by Fisher (1935) and further developed by Pitman (1937a, 1937b, 1938). Edgington (2007), Good (2000), Ludbrook and Dudley (1998), and Manly (1997) provide excellent histories of the development of permutation tests from Fisher (1935) to the present. An extensive bibliography is available from http://www.jiscmail.ac.uk/lists/exact-stats.html. Because permutation tests are computationally intensive, it took the advent of modern computing to make them practical and, thus, it is only recently that permutation tests have had much impact on the research literature. A number of recent books are devoted to the subject (Edgington, 2007; Good, 2000, 2006; Hubert, 1987; Lunneborg, 2000; Manly, 1997), and discussions now appear in several research methods textbooks (Howell, 2007; Marascuilo and McSweeney, 1977; Maxim, 1999; May et al., 1990; Siegel and Castellan, 1988). A substantial treatment of univariate and multivariate classical ranking techniques for one-sample, two-sample, and multi-sample inference problems is given by Hettmansperger and McKean (1998). In addition, many software packages also provide permutation tests, including S-Plus (MathSoft, Inc., Seattle, WA), Statistica (StatSoft, Inc., Tulsa, OK), SPSS (SPSS, Inc., Chicago, IL), SAS (SAS Institute, Inc., Cary, NC), Statistical Calculator (Mole Software, Belfast, Northern Ireland), Blossom Statistical Software (Fort Collins Ecological Science Center, Fort Collins, CO), and Resampling Stats (Resampling Stats, Inc., Arlington, VA). Perhaps the best-known package for exact permutation tests is StatXact (Cytel Software Corp., Cambridge, MA).

Permutation tests generally consist of three types: exact, resampling, and moment approximation tests. In an exact test, a suitable test statistic is computed on the observed data associated with a collection of objects, the data are permuted over all possible arrangements of the objects, and the test statistic is computed for each arrangement. The null hypothesis specified by randomization implies that each arrangement of objects is equally likely to occur. The proportion of arrangements with test statistic values as extreme or more extreme than the value of the test statistic computed on the original arrangement of the data is the exact P-value. The number of possible arrangements can become quite large even for small data sets. For example, an experimental design with 28 objects randomized into three treatments with 8, 9, and 11 objects in each treatment requires

$$\frac{28!}{8!\,9!\,11!} = 522,037,315,800$$

arrangements of the data. Therefore, alternative methods are often needed to approximate the exact P-value. Note that random sampling without replacement of $n \leq N$ objects from N objects consists of

$$\frac{N!}{(N-n)!}$$

equally-likely events, whereas random sampling with replacement of n objects from N objects (often termed "bootstrapping") consists of N^n equally-likely events.

One alternative is variously termed "resampling," "randomization," "approximate randomization," "sampled permutations," or "rerandomization," in which a relatively small subset of all possible permutations is examined, e.g., 1,000,000 of the 522,037,315,800 possible permutations. The usual method employed in resampling is to use a pseudorandom number generator to repeatedly shuffle (i.e., randomly order or permute) the observed sequence of N data points and to select a random subset of the $N!$ possible arrangements of the data, thereby ensuring equal probability of $1/N!$ for each arrangement. Thus, a shuffle is a random sample without replacement where $n = N$. The proportion of arrangements in the subset with test statistic values as extreme or more extreme than the value of the test statistic computed on the original arrangement of the data is the approximate P-value. Provided that the exact P-value is not too small and that the number of shuffles is large, resampling provides excellent approximations to exact P-values. Although some researchers contend that 5,000 to 10,000 resamplings are sufficient for statistical inference (e.g., Maxim, 1999), nearly every resampling application in this book is based on 1,000,000 resamplings (see Section 2.3.1). Caution should be exercised in choosing a shuffling algorithm because some widely-used algorithms are incorrect (Castellan, 1992; Rolfe, 2000).

A second alternative is the moment approximation approach, in which the lower moments of a continuous probability density function are equated to the corresponding exact moments of the discrete permutation distribution of the test statistic. The continuous probability density function is then integrated to obtain an approximate P-value. The moment approximation approach is very efficient for large data sets. Thus, it is an effective tool for evaluating independence of large sparse multidimensional contingency tables. Many of the example applications in this book are treated with both the resampling and the moment approximation approaches for comparison purposes. When feasible, the exact solution is also given. For very small data sets, only the exact P-value is provided.

Permutation tests are often termed "data-dependent" tests because all the information available for analysis is contained in the observed data set. Since the computed P-values are conditioned on the observed data, permutation tests require no assumptions about the populations from which the data have been sampled (Hayes, 1996a). Thus, permutation tests are distribution-free tests in that the tests do not assume distributional properties of the population (Bradley, 1968; Chen and Dunlap, 1993; Marascuilo and McSweeney, 1977). For a discussion and some limitations, see Hayes (1996b). With a parametric analysis, it is necessary to know the parent distribution (e.g., a normal distribution) and evaluate the data with respect to this known distribution. Conversely, a data-dependent permutation analysis generates a reference set of outcomes by way of randomization for a comparison with the observed outcome (May and Hunter, 1993). Since the randomization of objects is the basic assumption for permutation tests, any arrangement can be obtained by pairwise exchanges of the objects. Thus, the associated object measurements are termed "exchangeable." Hayes (1996b) provides an excellent discussion of exchangeability. For more rigorous presentations, see Draper et al. (1993), Lehmann (1986), and Lindley and Novick (1981).

Consider the small random sample of $N = 9$ objects displayed in Table 1.1. These nine objects represent a sample drawn from a population of school children where measurement x_1 is age in years, measurement x_2 is years of education, and measurement x_3 is gender, with 0 indicating male and 1 indicating female. Through a process of randomization, the first four cases are assigned to a treatment and the last five cases are the controls.

TABLE 1.1. Sample data of $N = 9$ objects with three measurements: age in years (x_1), years of education (x_2), and gender (x_3).

Object	x_1	x_2	x_3
1	7	1	1
2	8	2	0
3	10	4	1
4	8	3	0
5	9	3	1
6	10	5	0
7	14	8	1
8	14	7	1
9	17	11	0

Any permutation of the data randomly assigns each object to either a treatment or a control, with four treated objects and five control objects. What is important is that the three measurements on each object be coupled; that is, the objects are permuted, not the individual measurements. A permutation $x_1 = 7$, $x_2 = 11$, and $x_3 = 0$ for an object is impossible since none of the nine objects has these measurements; moreover, a seven-year-old with 11 years of education is incongruous. Thus, the objects are exchangeable, but the measurements x_1, x_2, and x_3 are coupled with each object and, consequently, are not individually exchangeable. The concept of coupling is particularly important for various regression analyses in Chapter 5. The response (i.e., dependent) variables and predictor (i.e., independent) variables correspond to specific objects in regression analyses. Consequently, the coupling of the response and predictor variables is intuitively a necessary property.

Let a distance function between objects I and J be denoted by $\Delta_{I,J}$. The distance function associated with classical parametric tests such as the two-sample t test is the squared Euclidean distance given by

$$\Delta_{I,J} = \left(x_I - x_J\right)^2,$$

where x_I and x_J are univariate measurements on objects I and J, respectively. This occurs because of the association of $\Delta_{I,J}$ with the variance of N objects given by

$$N \sum_{I=1}^{N} \left(x_I - \bar{x}\right)^2 = \sum_{I<J} \left(x_I - x_J\right)^2,$$

where

$$\bar{x} = \sum_{I=1}^{N} \frac{x_I}{N}$$

and $\sum_{I<J}$ is the sum of all $\binom{N}{2}$ I and J values where $1 \le I < J \le N$. If a parametric assumption such as normality is removed, then there is no theoretical justification for a distance function such as squared Euclidean distance. A distance function is a metric if it satisfies the three properties given by (1) $\Delta_{I,J} \ge 0$ and $\Delta_{I,I} = 0$, (2) $\Delta_{I,J} = \Delta_{J,I}$ (i.e., symmetry), and (3) $\Delta_{I,J} \le \Delta_{I,K} + \Delta_{K,J}$ (i.e., the triangle inequality). Consider the class of distance functions given by

$$\Delta_{I,J} = \left[\sum_{h=1}^{r} |x_{hI} - x_{hJ}|^p \right]^{v/p},$$

where x_{hI} and x_{hJ} are the hth coordinates of observations I and J in an r-dimensional space. The Minkowski (1891) family of metrics occurs when $v = 1$ and $p \ge 1$. When $v = 1$ and $p = 1$, $\Delta_{I,J}$ is a city-block metric. If $v > 0$, $r \ge 2$, and $p = 2$, then $\Delta_{I,J}$ is rotationally invariant (Mielke, 1987). When $v = 1$ and $p = 2$, $\Delta_{I,J}$ is the metric known as Euclidean distance. If $v = 2$ and $p = 2$, then $\Delta_{I,J}$ is squared Euclidean distance, which is not a metric since the triangle inequality is not satisfied. As demonstrated in this book, tests based on squared Euclidean distance possess counterintuitive properties. On the contrary, permutation tests based on Euclidean distance are shown to have highly intuitive properties (see Section 2.9).

The commonly-used one-sample t test based on n independent 1-dimensional values $(x_1, ..., x_n)$ from a normal population with mean μ and variance σ^2 demonstrates the strange nature of tests based on squared Euclidean distance. To test the null hypothesis that the mean is μ, consider the one-sample t-test statistic given by

$$t = \frac{(\bar{x} - \mu)\, n^{1/2}}{s},$$

where

$$\bar{x} = \frac{x_1 + \cdots + x_n}{n}$$

and

$$s^2 = \frac{(x_1 - \bar{x})^2 + \cdots + (x_n - \bar{x})^2}{n - 1}.$$

To represent the one-sample t-test statistic in a Euclidean framework, Fisher (1915) considered the n 1-dimensional values as a point in a conceptual n-dimensional Euclidean space. Also let $\mathbf{x} = (x_1, ..., x_n)$, $\bar{\mathbf{x}} = (\bar{x}, ..., \bar{x})$, and $\boldsymbol{\mu} = (\mu, ..., \mu)$ represent three points in this conceptual n-dimensional Euclidean space. The Euclidean distance between $\mathbf{x}$ and $\bar{\mathbf{x}}$ is

$$D(\mathbf{x}, \bar{\mathbf{x}}) = \left[(x_1 - \bar{x})^2 + \cdots + (x_n - \bar{x})^2 \right]^{1/2}$$

and the Euclidean distance between $\bar{\mathbf{x}}$ and $\boldsymbol{\mu}$ is

$$D(\bar{\mathbf{x}}, \boldsymbol{\mu}) = \left[n(\bar{x} - \mu)^2 \right]^{1/2}.$$

Then the relation between statistic t and the distances $D(\mathbf{x}, \bar{\mathbf{x}})$ and $D(\bar{\mathbf{x}}, \boldsymbol{\mu})$ of orthogonal line segments is given by

$$|t| = \frac{D\left(\bar{\mathbf{x}}, \boldsymbol{\mu}\right)}{D\left(\mathbf{x}, \bar{\mathbf{x}}\right)}\left(n-1\right)^{1/2}.$$

However, while the raw data $(x_1, ..., x_n)$ consist of n values in a 1-dimensional Euclidean data space, this same data in the one-sample t-test statistic is represented as a point in an artificial n-dimensional Euclidean analysis space that does not geometrically correspond to the 1-dimensional data space in question (Mielke, 1986). Section 2.2 includes (1) a discussion of this same geometric problem strictly in terms of distance functions and (2) further motivation that the data and analysis spaces should be congruent. Section 4.4 presents an alternative one-sample permutation test where the data and analysis spaces are congruent, i.e., both the data and analysis spaces are precisely the same 1-dimensional Euclidean space and, accordingly, satisfy the *congruence principle* (Mielke, 1984, 1985, 1986, 1991; Mielke and Berry, 1983, 2000a; Mielke et al., 1982). Consequently, any test based on squared Euclidean distance does not satisfy the congruence principle. In fact, many classical rank tests based on squared Euclidean distance are derivable from the Fisher (1915) artificial data representation (Hettmansperger and McKean, 1998, see pp. 4–12, 69–75, 145–151).

The lack of robustness induced by the present distance function paradigm using statistical methods based on nonmetric squared Euclidean distance is all but eliminated by using statistical methods based on metric Euclidean distance (see Sections 2.9 and 2.11). The improved robustness property of statistical methods based on Euclidean distance rather than squared Euclidean distance is a consequence of employing median rather than mean based statistical methods, respectively (see Section 2.2).

Chapters 2, 3, 4, and 5 describe permutation methods in which the distance functions are explicitly defined. Chapters 6, 7, 8, and 9 describe permutation methods where the distance functions are often implicit.

Chapter 2: Multiresponse permutation procedures (MRPP) are introduced in Chapter 2 as a permutation generalization of a one-way analysis of variance (ANOVA). Simple examples are provided to show the relationship between MRPP and statistics of the classical parametric techniques. A general version of MRPP is given along with exact and approximate methods for obtaining P-values. Various special-purpose versions of MRPP are then obtained either from alterations of constants or from the distance function of the MRPP statistic. Applications of MRPP utilizing an excess group and/or truncated distance functions are described. The permutation methods yield a multitude of statistical techniques that are very difficult either to obtain or to justify with a parametric approach. Properties of MRPP are demonstrated either analytically or via simulation. A simple argument, illustrated with examples, establishes why parametric tests based on the classical likelihood-ratio test associated with normality assumptions (e.g., one-way ANOVA, linear model methods based on least squares, Hotelling T^2 tests, etc.) cannot accommodate even one extreme measurement. Permutation tests based on ordinary Euclidean distance, involving observed values rather than rank-order statistics, are shown to be exceedingly stable (i.e., very robust) relative to a few extreme values. Different distance functions are shown to differ drastically in their ability to detect location differences in symmetric distributions, varying from being exceedingly peaked with very heavy tails to being essentially uniform. Finally, alternative multivariate tests depending on Euclidean distance are shown to be vastly superior to classical normality-based methods such as Hotelling's T^2 and closely related tests, e.g., Bartlett–Nanda–Pillai, Lawley–Hotelling, Roy maximum root, and Wilks λ multivariate tests. A surprising result of these studies is that the normality-based tests perform very poorly for cases involving location shifts parallel to the major axis of correlated data even when the normality assumptions of these tests are satisfied (such tests do very well for cases involving location shifts parallel to the minor axis of the correlated data).

Chapter 3: Additional applications of MRPP are given in Chapter 3. These applications include (1) multivariate autoregressive pattern detection, including the permutation version of the Durbin–Watson test for serial correlation; (2) asymmetric two-way contingency table analyses, including the permutation version of the Goodman–Kruskal τ measures; (3) multiple binary choices; (4) measures of agreement for various levels of measurement; (5) permutation analyses of cyclic data as alternatives to a group of parametric methods based on normal distributions involving circles, spheres, and hyperspheres; (6) generalized versions of the Wald–Wolfowitz runs test involving two or more groups plus an excess group; (7) alternative techniques based on rank-order statistics, which include all multisample linear rank tests such as the Kruskal–Wallis test; and (8) MRPP analyses based on real data establish beyond any reasonable doubt that heavy metal soil contamination has severely reduced the academic performance of fourth grade students. Many examples and simulation studies are included in Chapter 3 to describe the associations between the previous and new permutation approaches for specific analyses.

Chapter 4: Multivariate randomized block permutation procedures (MRBP) are introduced in Chapter 4 as a permutation generalization of randomized blocks ANOVA. Then, a general version of MRBP is given along with exact and approximate methods for obtaining P-values, including methods of analysis when unbalanced randomized block structures are encountered. Special cases involving rank and binary transformations are described, including Friedman's two-way ANOVA ($v = 2$), extensions of both Spearman's footrule ($v = 1$) and Spearman's rho ($v = 2$), Cochran's Q test along with a closely-related matrix occupancy problem, and multiple binary category choices. One-sample and matched-pair designs, including a wide variety of univariate and multivariate tests, are described. Simulated comparisons are made for a variety of univariate rank tests. An example suggests that another class of multivariate matched-pair tests has substantial advantageous discrimination properties over the permutation version of Hotelling's matched-pair T^2 test. The remainder of Chapter 4 is concerned with recent extensions of Cohen's kappa agreement measure to various levels of measurement. These extensions are commonly used in the various aspects of psychological and educational measurement problems. Specific attention is placed on multiple observers, independent groups of observers, agreement with a standard, and tests of significance.

Chapter 5: Chapter 5 describes permutation-based methods for multivariate multiple regression analysis, prediction, and agreement. As in the previous chapters, correspondence between the data and analysis geometries is emphasized. Following some historical comments and also a simple comparison between ordinary least (sum of) squared deviations (OLS) and least (sum of) absolute deviations (LAD) regressions, descriptions of permutation-based regression analyses are presented. MRPP analyses of both LAD and least sum (of) Euclidean distances (LSED) regression residuals are described for various balanced and unbalanced experimental designs. The MRPP analyses of LAD and LSED regression residuals have the desired property associated with permutation tests that type I statistical error is controlled, regardless of the distribution governing the residuals. The only restriction on the MRPP analyses of LAD and LSED regression is that alternative hypotheses must involve group differences. Comparisons are made among MRPP, Cade–Richards, and classical OLS regression analyses. An MRPP technique for finding confidence intervals of regression parameters is described. A simulation study of prediction model validation is discussed that involves drop-one cross-validation and OLS versus LAD regression comparisons for various conditions such as sample size, population agreement, inclusion of redundant predictors, and different severities of data contamination. In closing, some techniques and applications of linear and nonlinear multivariate multiple regression models for prediction are given.

Chapter 6: Discrete and continuous data goodness-of-fit techniques are discussed in Chapter 6. The discrete data goodness-of-fit techniques include Fisher's exact test (provided the number of distinct frequency configurations is not too large) and nonasymptotic tests based on both resampling and Pearson type III approximations, the latter confined to the Pearson χ^2 and Zelterman statistics. Each of these tests accommodates for expected cell frequencies based on parameters estimated from the observed data. If equal cell probabilities are in question, then efficient exact tests are described for fairly large data sets that depend on a partitioning scheme due to L. Euler. The continuous data goodness-of-fit techniques include the Smirnov matching, Kolmogorov empirical cumulative distribution function, Kendall–Sherman coverage, and Greenwood–Moran coverage tests. Although a serious deficiency is emphasized with the Smirnov matching test, the other tests are described and compared using simulation. Since the structures of the Kolmogorov test and the tests based on coverages (Kendall–Sherman and Greenwood–Moran) are considerably different, the simulated comparisons suggest types of alternatives where each of these tests yields substantial improvements in power.

Chapter 7: Chapter 7 discusses exact and nonasymptotic analyses associated with multidimensional contingency tables. After deriving the hypergeometric distribution conditioned on fixed marginals for multidimensional contingency tables, Fisher's exact test for independence is extended to multidimensional tables, and an efficient exhaustive enumeration algorithm is described for implementing these tests. Then, approximate nonasymptotic resampling and Pearson type III tests for independence of multidimensional contingency table categories are presented. For large sparse multidimensional contingency tables, a P-value comparison study indicates that the nonasymptotic Pearson χ^2 and nonasymptotic Zelterman P-values based on three exact moments are often very close to the exact Pearson χ^2 and exact Zelterman P-values, respectively. A concern involving log-linear analyses of sparse contingency tables is demonstrated. In order to identify the causes for rejecting independence, exact interaction tests for $2 \times 2 \times 2$ and $2 \times 2 \times 2 \times 2$ tables are discussed along with the obvious extensions. Finally, relationships between the Pearson χ^2 and Goodman–Kruskal τ statistics are investigated.

Chapter 8: Tests for homogeneity between two or more samples are described for discrete categorical and univariate continuous data in Chapter 8. For discrete categorical data, the MRPP test of Chapter 3 (see Section 3.2) is compared to the Pearson χ^2 and Zelterman tests of Chapter 7. An example analysis indicates that the P-values of these tests may be exceedingly different. For the univariate continuous data, the generalized runs test described in Chapter 3, the Kolmogorov–Smirnov test based on empirical cumulative distribution functions, and tests based on empirical coverages are discussed. Although each of these tests is able to discriminate small nontrivial differences with adequate sample sizes, examples indicate that these tests may be powerful competitors to almost any test for specific types of alternatives. Since the structures of these tests are substantially different, the latter statement is not surprising.

Chapter 9: Three distinct topics are contained in Chapter 9. The first topic is a comparison of the classical continuous method due to R.A. Fisher and a recent discrete method for combining P-values based on small data sets. Since the difference in the combined P-values based on the Fisher continuous and discrete methods is not trivial, this comparison impacts areas in statistics such as meta-analysis. The second topic is a simulation study that seriously questions the utility of the Fisher Z transformation for the sample correlation coefficient. Finally, the third topic presents a multivariate resampling permutation test based on distance functions for

comparing the similarity between two populations with corresponding unordered disjoint categories.

Appendix A: Appendix A contains a listing of all computer programs
used in the book. The programs are written in FORTRAN–77 and are
organized by chapter. Each program listing contains a brief description of
its function, input options, and output. The remaining material consists of
a list of references, an author index, and a subject index.

2
Description of MRPP

Multiresponse permutation procedures (MRPP) constitute a class of permutation methods for distinguishing possible differences among two or more groups in one or more dimensions. Consider samples of independent and identically distributed univariate random variables of sizes $n_1, ..., n_g$, namely, $(y_{11}, ..., y_{n_1 1}), ..., (y_{1g}, ..., y_{n_g g})$, drawn from g specified populations with cumulative distribution functions $F_1(x), ..., F_g(x)$, respectively. For simplicity, suppose that population i is normal with mean μ_i and variance σ^2 $(i = 1, ..., g)$. This is the standard one-way classification model with g groups. The classical test of a null hypothesis of no group differences tests $H_0: \mu_1 = \cdots = \mu_g$ versus $H_1: \mu_i \neq \mu_j$ for some $i \neq j$ using the F statistic given by

$$F = \frac{MS_{Between}}{MS_{Within}},$$

where

$$MS_{Between} = MS_{Treatment} = \frac{1}{g-1} SS_{Between},$$

$$SS_{Between} = \sum_{i=1}^{g} n_i (\bar{y}_i - \bar{y})^2,$$

$$MS_{Within} = MS_{Error} = \frac{1}{N-g} SS_{Within},$$

$$SS_{Within} = \sum_{i=1}^{g} \sum_{j=1}^{n_i} (y_{ji} - \bar{y}_i)^2,$$

$$SS_{Total} = SS_{Between} + SS_{Within} = \sum_{i=1}^{g} \sum_{j=1}^{n_i} (y_{ji} - \bar{y})^2,$$

$$\bar{y}_i = \frac{1}{n_i} \sum_{j=1}^{n_i} y_{ji},$$

for $i = 1, ..., g,$

$$\bar{y} = \frac{1}{N} \sum_{i=1}^{g} \sum_{j=1}^{n_i} y_{ji},$$

and

$$N = \sum_{i=1}^{g} n_i.$$

Under H_0, the distribution of F is Snedecor's F distribution with $g - 1$ degrees-of-freedom (df) in the numerator and $N - g$ df in the denominator. However, if any of the g populations is not normal, then the distribution of statistic F no longer follows Snedecor's F distribution. Nevertheless, the F statistic itself is still a meaningful measure of how consistent or inconsistent the data are with H_0. It compares the between-group variability with the within-group variability in the samples, and if the between-group variability is "much larger" than the within-group variability, then this can be interpreted as evidence against H_0. The critical value of F for rejecting H_0 depends on the distribution of F under the null hypothesis that the distributions of the g populations are identical, say $F_0(x)$.

An ingenious permutation method proposed by Pitman (1938) considers the conditional distribution of F given the N order statistics $x_{1,N} \leq \cdots \leq x_{N,N}$ of the combined data set. Under the null hypothesis that $F_i(x) = F_0(x)$ for $i = 1, ..., g$, each of the

$$M = \frac{N!}{\displaystyle\prod_{i=1}^{g} n_i!}$$

possible assignments of $y_{11}, ..., y_{n_g g}$ to the g groups with n_i values in the ith group $(i = 1, ..., g)$ occurs with equal probability. Thus, the conditional distribution of F given $x_{1,N} \leq \cdots \leq x_{N,N}$ does not depend on $F_0(x)$ and can be explicitly calculated by enumerating the M assignments and calculating the value of F corresponding to each assignment; i.e., a reference distribution of M equally-likely values of F. If F_o is the calculated value of F associated with the observed data for the g samples, the significance probability under H_0 is the proportion of the M values of F comprising the reference distribution equal to or greater than F_o. This procedure yields a conditionally exact significance test that is distribution-free; i.e., that does not depend on $F_0(x)$. This approach was initially proposed by Fisher (1935) in the context of randomized experiments, and later by Pitman (1938) in general, and is often termed the "Fisher–Pitman permutation test" for comparing g independent groups.

The MRPP are based on this concept, and an alternative representation of the F statistic is given by

$$F = \frac{2SS_{Total} - (N - g)\delta}{(g - 1)\delta},$$

where

$$\delta = \sum_{i=1}^{g} C_i \xi_i,$$

$$C_i = \frac{n_i - 1}{N - g},$$

$$\xi_i = \binom{n_i}{2}^{-1} \sum_{j<k} (y_{ji} - y_{ki})^2,$$

$n_i \geq 2$, and $\sum_{j<k}$ denotes the sum over $1 \leq j < k \leq n_i$ for $i = 1, ..., g$ (Berry and Mielke, 1983b). Since SS_{Total} is invariant under all M assignments of the N total values to the g groups, δ may be used as a test statistic, which is equivalent to F. Because large values of F correspond to small values of δ, the P-value of this test is

$$P(\delta \leq \delta_o \,|\, x_{1,N} \leq \cdots \leq x_{N,N}),$$

where δ_o is the observed value of δ that corresponds to F_o. This is equivalent to computing the proportion of the $N!$ permutations of $y_{11}, ..., y_{n_g g}$ that yields a value of δ equal to or less than δ_o. Thus, the Fisher–Pitman permutation test may utilize δ instead of F.

Given that data values are points in a data space, the statistic δ is based on "interpoint" distances of data values belonging to the same group. In fact, $\xi_i = 2s_i^2$, where s_i^2 is the sample variance; thus ξ_i is a measure of dispersion of the values $y_{1i}, ..., y_{n_i i}$ for $i = 1, ..., g$. If the values within distinct groups are relatively close to one another, then δ will be small. This feature may be described by saying that the within-group data values exhibit *clumping* or *clustering*. The P-value will be small if the observed data exhibit clumping relative to all possible permutations of the data values.

In summary, δ is a natural statistic to use when testing H_0 against alternatives in which the distributions $F_1(x), ..., F_g(x)$ differ with respect to location, i.e., are separated. Furthermore, variations of δ lead to natural and meaningful generalizations that are nontrivial to attain otherwise. Since the key ingredient of δ is the interpoint squared distance $(x_i - x_j)^2$, generalizations may be obtained by replacing $(x_i - x_j)^2$ by any symmetric distance function $\Delta_{i,j}$ that provides a meaningful measure of separation between x_i and x_j. An intuitively simple distance function is $|x_i - x_j|$. Any measure of separation $\Delta(s,t)$ satisfying $\Delta(s,t) \geq 0$, $\Delta(s,s) = 0$, and $\Delta(s,t) = \Delta(t,s)$ may be used, although for geometric reasons it would be desirable for $\Delta(s,t)$ also to obey the triangle inequality of a metric, i.e., $\Delta(s,t) \leq \Delta(s,u) + \Delta(t,u)$.

Another major advantage of using δ rather than F is the fact that it generalizes to multivariate data. If s and t are r-dimensional points and $\Delta(s,t)$ is a measure of separation in the r-dimensional space, then δ is automatically defined and measures the overall amount of clumping or clustering that exists within the g groups. These considerations predispose the use of δ, the MRPP statistic, as a test of H_0 in this more general setting.

2.1   General Formulation of MRPP

Let $\Omega = \{\omega_1, ..., \omega_N\}$ be a finite sample of objects that is representative of some target population in question. Let $x_I' = (x_{1I}, ..., x_{rI})$ denote r response measurements (i.e., r dimensions) for object ω_I ($I = 1, ..., N$), and let $S_1, ..., S_{g+1}$ designate an exhaustive partitioning of the N objects comprising Ω into $g+1$ disjoint groups. Also, let $\Delta_{I,J}$ be a symmetric distance function value of the response measurements associated with objects ω_I and ω_J. The MRPP statistic is given by

$$\delta = \sum_{i=1}^{g} C_i \xi_i,$$

where $C_i > 0$ is a classified group weight ($i = 1, ..., g$), $\sum_{i=1}^{g} C_i = 1$,

$$\xi_i = \binom{n_i}{2}^{-1} \sum_{I<J} \Delta_{I,J} \Psi_i(\omega_I) \Psi_i(\omega_J)$$

is the average distance function value for all distinct pairs of objects in group S_i ($i = 1, ..., g$), $n_i \geq 2$ is the number of a priori objects classified in group S_i ($i = 1, ..., g$), $K = \sum_{i=1}^{g} n_i$, $n_{g+1} = N - K \geq 0$ is the number of remaining (unclassified) objects in the "excess" group S_{g+1} (an empty group in many applications), $\sum_{I<J}$ is the sum over all I and J such that $1 \leq I < J \leq N$, and $\Psi_i(\cdot)$ is an indicator function given by

$$\Psi_i(\omega_I) = \begin{cases} 1 & \text{if } \omega_I \in S_i, \\ 0 & \text{otherwise.} \end{cases}$$

The null hypothesis (H_0) states that equal probabilities are assigned to each of the

$$M = \frac{N!}{\displaystyle\prod_{i=1}^{g+1} n_i!}$$

possible allocations of the N objects in Ω to the $g+1$ groups $(S_1, ..., S_{g+1})$. Consequently, the collection of r response measurements yields N r-dimensional exchangeable random variables under H_0. The δ statistic compares the within-group clumping of response measurements against the model specified by random allocation under H_0. The initial presentations and theoretical developments of MRPP are given in Brockwell et al. (1982), Brown (1982), Denker and Puri (1988), Mielke (1978, 1979, 1984, 1986), Mielke et al. (1976, 1981a, 1981b, 1982), O'Reilly and Mielke (1980), and Robinson (1983). Applications of MRPP in various disciplines include ecology (Biondini et al., 1988a, 1988b; Zimmerman et al., 1985), meteorology (Mielke, 1985; Mielke et al., 1982; Wong et al., 1983), forestry (Pellicane et al., 1989; Reich et al., 1991), anthropology (Berry et al., 1983), geology (Orlowski et al., 1993, 1995), and education (Mielke et al., 2005a; also see Section 3.7).

It should be emphasized that an excess group (S_{g+1}) is not merely a mathematical manipulation. The ability to include an excess group in an analysis can be very important. For example, the inclusion of an excess group was essential to an environmental analysis that involved the geographical concentration of lead in an urban area (Mielke et al., 1983) and influenced the removal of lead from gasoline. Examples utilizing an excess group are contained in Section 2.5.

2.1.1 Univariate Example of MRPP

The central concepts underlying the MRPP statistic, δ, can be illustrated very simply. Consider a comparison between two mutually exclusive groups of objects, S_1 and S_2, where a single measured response, x, has been obtained from each object. For this example, $r = 1$ dimension, $g = 2$ disjoint groups, and $N = 5$ with $n_1 = 2$, $n_2 = 3$, and $n_{g+1} = 0$. Since the excess group is empty, $K = N$. Let $C_1 = n_1/N$ and $C_2 = n_2/N$ so that the two groups are weighted in proportion to their sizes. Suppose that the $n_1 = 2$ observed response measurements for S_1 are $\{2, 5\}$ and the $n_2 = 3$ observed response measurements for S_2 are $\{4, 7, 8\}$. Figure 2.1 displays these measurements, where the responses of the $n_1 = 2$ objects in group S_1 are plotted as open circles ($\circ$) and the responses of the $n_2 = 3$ objects in group S_2 are plotted as filled circles ($\bullet$).

Table 2.1 contains an enumeration of the $M = 5!/2!\,3! = 10$ permutations of the response measurements with the observed measurements listed as the first permutation. To illustrate the calculations, consider the first

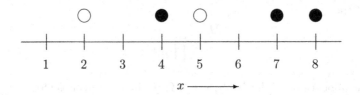

FIGURE 2.1. Plot of five data points.

TABLE 2.1. All possible permutations, ξ_1, ξ_2, and δ values for a data set with $r = 1$, $g = 2$, $n_1 = 2$, $n_2 = 3$, and $v = 1$.

Number	Permutation	ξ_1	ξ_2	δ
1	2,5–4,7,8	3.0000	2.6667	2.8000
2	2,4–5,7,8	2.0000	2.0000	2.0000
3	2,7–4,5,8	5.0000	2.6667	3.6000
4	2,8–4,5,7	6.0000	2.0000	3.6000
5	4,5–2,7,8	1.0000	4.0000	2.8000
6	4,7–2,5,8	3.0000	4.0000	3.6000
7	4,8–2,5,7	4.0000	3.3333	3.6000
8	5,7–2,4,8	2.0000	4.0000	3.2000
9	5,8–2,4,7	3.0000	3.3333	3.2000
10	7,8–2,4,5	1.0000	2.0000	1.6000

(i.e., observed) permutation $\{2,5$–$4,7,8\}$. Choose as the symmetric distance function between pairs of objects for this example

$$\Delta_{I,J} = |x_I - x_J|^v$$

with $v = 1$, i.e., Euclidean distance. For S_1 with $n_1 = 2$, $\Delta_{1,2} = |2 - 5| = 3$, and for S_2 with $n_2 = 3$, $\Delta_{3,4} = |4 - 7| = 3$, $\Delta_{3,5} = |4 - 8| = 4$, and $\Delta_{4,5} = |7 - 8| = 1$. Then,

$$\xi_1 = \binom{n_1}{2}^{-1} \Delta_{1,2} = \binom{2}{2}^{-1} 3 = 3.0000,$$

$$\xi_2 = \binom{n_2}{2}^{-1} (\Delta_{3,4} + \Delta_{3,5} + \Delta_{4,5}) = \binom{3}{2}^{-1} (3 + 4 + 1) = 2.6667,$$

and the observed test statistic

$$\delta_o = C_1\xi_1 + C_2\xi_2 = \left(\frac{2}{5}\right)(3.0000) + \left(\frac{3}{5}\right)(2.6667) = 2.8000.$$

The ξ_1, ξ_2, and δ values for each of the $M = 10$ permutations are listed in Table 2.1. Since four of the δ values (i.e., 2.0000, 2.8000, 2.8000, and

TABLE 2.2. All possible permutations, ξ_1, ξ_2, and δ values for a data set with $r = 1$, $g = 2$, $n_1 = 2$, $n_2 = 3$, and $v = 2$.

Number	Permutation	ξ_1	ξ_2	δ
1	2,5–4,7,8	9.0000	8.6667	8.8000
2	2,4–5,7,8	4.0000	4.6667	4.4000
3	2,7–4,5,8	25.0000	8.6667	15.2000
4	2,8–4,5,7	36.0000	4.6667	17.2000
5	4,5–2,7,8	1.0000	20.6667	12.8000
6	4,7–2,5,8	9.0000	18.0000	14.4000
7	4,8–2,5,7	16.0000	12.6667	14.0000
8	5,7–2,4,8	4.0000	18.6667	12.8000
9	5,8–2,4,7	9.0000	12.6667	11.2000
10	7,8–2,4,5	1.0000	4.6667	3.2000

1.6000) are less than or equal to the observed δ value of 2.8000, the exact P-value is $4/10 = 0.40$.

Now, consider the same data set, but define the symmetric distance function between pairs of objects to be

$$\Delta_{I,J} = |x_I - x_J|^v$$

with $v = 2$, i.e., squared Euclidean distance. Table 2.2 lists the $M = 10$ permutations of the response measurements with the first permutation containing the observed measurements. Consider the first permutation $\{2,5-4,7,8\}$. For S_1 with $n_1 = 2$, $\Delta_{1,2} = |2 - 5|^2 = 9$, and for S_2 with $n_2 = 3$, $\Delta_{3,4} = |4 - 7|^2 = 9$, $\Delta_{3,5} = |4 - 8|^2 = 16$, and $\Delta_{4,5} = |7 - 8|^2 = 1$. Then,

$$\xi_1 = \binom{n_1}{2}^{-1} \Delta_{1,2} = \binom{2}{2}^{-1} 9 = 9.0000,$$

$$\xi_2 = \binom{n_2}{2}^{-1} (\Delta_{3,4} + \Delta_{3,5} + \Delta_{4,5}) = \binom{2}{2}^{-1} (9 + 16 + 1) = 8.6667,$$

and the observed test statistic

$$\delta_o = C_1 \xi_1 + C_2 \xi_2 = \left(\frac{2}{5}\right)(9.0000) + \left(\frac{3}{5}\right)(8.6667) = 8.8000.$$

The ξ_1, ξ_2, and δ values for each of the $M = 10$ permutations are listed in Table 2.2. Since three of the δ values (i.e., 4.4000, 8.8000, and 3.2000) are less than or equal to the observed δ value of 8.8000, the exact P-value is $3/10 = 0.30$ with $v = 2$, compared with the exact P-value of 0.40 when $v = 1$. The dependence of the generalized MRPP distance function $\Delta_{I,J} = |x_I - x_J|^v$ on the value of v is discussed in more detail in Sections 2.2, 2.8, 2.9, and 2.10.

2.1.2 Bivariate Example of MRPP

Again consider a comparison between two mutually exclusive groups of objects, S_1 and S_2, where two measured responses, x_1 and x_2, have been obtained from each object. For this example, $r = 2$ dimensions, $g = 2$ groups, and $N = 7$ with $n_1 = 3$, $n_2 = 4$, and $n_{g+1} = 0$. Again, let $C_1 = n_1/N$ and $C_2 = n_2/N$ so that the two groups are weighted in proportion to their sizes. The data for this example (Mielke et al., 1981a) are given in Table 2.3 and displayed in Figure 2.2. Figure 2.2 shows how these responses could be represented in a two-dimensional diagram where the responses of the $n_1 = 3$ objects in group S_1 are plotted as open circles (o) and labeled as ω_1, ω_2, and ω_3, and the responses of the $n_2 = 4$ objects in group S_2 are plotted as filled circles (•) and labeled as ω_4, ω_5, ω_6, and ω_7. Although a visual impression suggests that the $g = 2$ groups are separated in the two-dimensional space, a more rigorous and objective characterization of this separation is needed before a quantitative evaluation or inference can be made. A classical approach would involve using the two-sample Hotelling (1931) T^2 test, which has the disadvantage of requiring the assumption that the response measurements of the two groups are distributed as the multivariate normal distribution with equal variances and covariances. Since these conditions are never met in practice, it is desirable to consider methods that do not require such assumptions, e.g., permutation procedures.

The symmetric distance function between pairs of objects for this example is given by

$$\Delta_{I,J} = \sum_{h=1}^{2} \left[(x_{hI} - x_{hJ})^2 \right]^{1/2},$$

which is Euclidean distance. For group S_1 with $n_1 = 3$,

$$\Delta_{1,2} = \left[(4-3)^2 + (5-4)^2 \right]^{1/2} = 1.4142,$$

$$\Delta_{1,3} = \left[(4-4)^2 + (5-3)^2 \right]^{1/2} = 2.0000,$$

and

$$\Delta_{2,3} = \left[(3-4)^2 + (4-3)^2 \right]^{1/2} = 1.4142.$$

For group S_2 with $n_2 = 4$,

$$\Delta_{4,5} = \left[(2-2)^2 + (3-2)^2 \right]^{1/2} = 1.0000,$$

$$\Delta_{4,6} = \left[(2-3)^2 + (3-2)^2 \right]^{1/2} = 1.4142,$$

$$\Delta_{4,7} = \left[(2-3)^2 + (3-1)^2 \right]^{1/2} = 2.2361,$$

$$\Delta_{5,6} = \left[(2-3)^2 + (2-2)^2 \right]^{1/2} = 1.0000,$$

$$\Delta_{5,7} = \left[(2-3)^2 + (2-1)^2 \right]^{1/2} = 1.4142,$$

TABLE 2.3. Example data set with $r = 2$, $g = 2$, $n_1 = 3$, and $n_2 = 4$.

Group	Object	Values x_1	x_2
S_1	ω_1	4	5
S_1	ω_2	3	4
S_1	ω_3	4	3
S_2	ω_4	2	3
S_2	ω_5	2	2
S_2	ω_6	3	2
S_2	ω_7	3	1

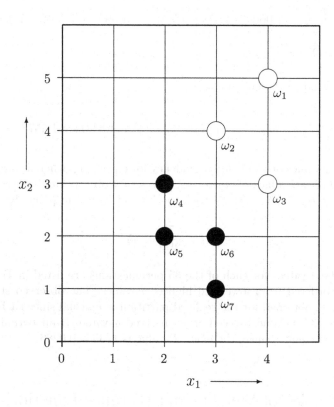

FIGURE 2.2. Scatter diagram of the data in Table 2.3.

and

$$\Delta_{6,7} = \left[(3-3)^2 + (2-1)^2\right]^{1/2} = 1.0000.$$

Then,

$$\xi_1 = \binom{n_1}{2}^{-1} (\Delta_{1,2} + \Delta_{1,3} + \Delta_{2,3})$$

$$= \binom{3}{2}^{-1} (1.4142 + 2.0000 + 1.4142)$$

$$= 1.6095$$

$$\xi_2 = \binom{n_2}{2}^{-1} (\Delta_{4,5} + \Delta_{4,6} + \Delta_{4,7} + \Delta_{5,6} + \Delta_{5,7} + \Delta_{6,7})$$

$$= \binom{4}{2}^{-1} (1.0000 + 1.4142 + 2.2361 + 1.0000 + 1.4142 + 1.0000)$$

$$= 1.3441,$$

and the weighted mean is given by

$$\delta = C_1 \xi_1 + C_2 \xi_2 = \left(\frac{3}{7}\right)(1.6095) + \left(\frac{4}{7}\right)(1.3441) = 1.4578.$$

Smaller values of δ indicate a tendency for clustering, whereas larger values of δ indicate a lack of clustering. The $N = 7$ objects can be partitioned into $g = 2$ groups, S_1 and S_2, with $n_1 = 3$ and $n_2 = 4$ in precisely

$$M = \frac{7!}{3!\,4!} = 35$$

ways. The δ values for each of the 35 permutations are listed in Table 2.4 and are ordered from lowest to highest δ values. The observed statistic, $\delta = 1.4578$, obtained for the realized partition is unusual since each of the remaining 34 δ values exceeds the observed δ value. If all permutations occur with equal chance, the exact P-value is $1/35 = 0.0286$.

2.2   Choice of Weights and Distance Functions

The choice of the classified group weights $(C_1, ..., C_g)$ and the symmetric distance function $\Delta_{I,J}$ specifies the structure of MRPP. Although $C_i = n_i/K$ is the suggested group weight since it is associated with efficient

TABLE 2.4. Ordered values of δ for groups S_1 and S_2 with fixed sizes of $n_1 = 3$ and $n_2 = 4$.

Rank	Value	Rank	Value
1	1.4578	19	2.1381
2	1.5421	20	2.1480
3	1.6939	21	2.1591
4	1.7505	22	2.1646
5	1.8389	23	2.1709
6	1.8547	24	2.1740
7	1.8935	25	2.1769
8	1.9898	26	2.1891
9	1.9915	27	2.1939
10	1.9988	28	2.2025
11	2.0060	29	2.2169
12	2.0157	30	2.2258
13	2.0176	31	2.2280
14	2.0522	32	2.2470
15	2.0575	33	2.2518
16	2.0829	34	2.2812
17	2.0944	35	2.2935
18	2.1158		

versions of MRPP $(i = 1, ..., g)$, other choices such as

$$C_i = \frac{n_i - 1}{K - g},$$

$$C_i = \frac{1}{g},$$

and

$$C_i = \frac{n_i(n_i - 1)}{\displaystyle\sum_{j=1}^{g} n_j(n_j - 1)}$$

have also been considered (Mielke, 1984). A discussion of the choices of C_i, along with additional comments pertaining to the initial papers on MRPP, is given at the end of Section 2.3. In most applications of MRPP, the symmetric distance function is given by

$$\Delta_{I,J} = \begin{cases} d_{I,J} & \text{if } d_{I,J} \leq B, \\ B & \text{otherwise,} \end{cases}$$

where

$$d_{I,J} = \left[\sum_{h=1}^{r} (x_{hI} - x_{hJ})^2 \right]^{v/2},$$

$B > 0$ is a specified truncation constant, and $v > 0$ is a specified power constant. Note that $\Delta_{I,J}$ is ordinary Euclidean distance if B is ∞ and $v = 1$. The choice of B is purely subjective since its use includes the detection of multiple clumping among objects of a single group. When multiple clumping exists, a small B mitigates the between-clump distances and emphasizes the within-clump distances (Mielke, 1991). As indicated in the examples of Sections 2.6 and 2.7, the value of B approximates the clump diameters in question.

Incidentally, let

$$d_{I,Q} = \left[\sum_{h=1}^{r} (x_{hI} - \theta_h)^2 \right]^{v/2}$$

denote the distance function value between an arbitrary r-dimensional point $(\theta_1, ..., \theta_r)$ and $(x_{1I}, ..., x_{rI})$, the Ith of N observed r-dimensional points, for $I = 1, ..., N$. If $(\theta_1, ..., \theta_r)$ is the r-dimensional point that minimizes

$$\sum_{I=1}^{N} d_{I,Q},$$

then $(\theta_1, ..., \theta_r)$ is either the r-dimensional median or mean when $v = 1$ or 2, respectively. A variety of distinct r-dimensional medians is discussed by Small (1990).

Even though $v = 2$ yields a nonmetric distance function since the triangle inequality is not satisfied (Mielke, 1986), the choice of $v = 2$ is associated with many commonly-used statistical methods such as the two-sample t test and all analysis-of-variance procedures derived from least squares regression. Because a data space is almost always a Euclidean space ($v = 1$), a congruence between the data space and the analysis space of a statistical method based on $v = 1$ exists and, consequently, satisfies the congruence principle (Mielke, 1984, 1985, 1986, 1991; Mielke and Berry, 1983, 2000a; Mielke et al., 1982). Since the geometry of analyses involving methods based on $v = 2$ differs from the geometry of the data in question, simple examples have shown that statistical methods based on $v = 2$ yield peculiar counterintuitive results compared with statistical methods based on $v = 1$ (Mielke, 1985, 1986). The substantial effect of a single value among 109 nonseeded and 108 seeded values of a weather modification experiment on MRPP with $v = 2$ is demonstrated by Mielke (1985). If one extreme observation of 0.709 is present, then the MRPP P-values based on 217 values with $v = 1$ and $v = 2$ are 0.0257 and 0.0856, respectively. If the questioned value is removed, then the MRPP P-values based on 216 values with $v = 1$ and $v = 2$ are 0.0151 and 0.0158, respectively. Since investigators plot their data in a Euclidean space, the previous results imply that erroneous geometrically induced conclusions due to $v = 2$ (which has no theoretical justification in many applications) can be avoided by using $v = 1$ (see Section 2.9). As subsequently implied, the congruence principle's correspondence between the geometries of the data in question and analyses based on $v = 1$ allows intuition to play a major role in constructing special-purpose permutation methods. Another property is that MRPP is a median-based technique if $v = 1$, whereas MRPP is a mean-based technique if $v = 2$. For clarification, consider the pairwise sum of univariate $(r = 1)$ symmetric distance functions given by

$$\sum_{i<j} \Delta(x_i, x_j) = \sum_{i<j} |x_i - x_j|^v,$$

where $x_1, ..., x_m$ are univariate response variables and $\sum_{i<j}$ is the sum over all i and j such that $1 \le i < j \le m$. Let $x_{1,m} \le \cdots \le x_{m,m}$ be the order statistics associated with $x_1, ..., x_m$. If $v = 1$, then the inequality given by

$$\sum_{i=1}^{m} |m - 2i + 1| \, |x_{i,m} - \theta| \ge \sum_{i<j} |x_i - x_j|$$

holds for all θ; equality holds if θ is the median of $x_1, ..., x_m$. If $v = 2$, then the inequality given by

$$m \sum_{i=1}^{m} (x_i - \theta)^2 \ge \sum_{i<j} (x_i - x_j)^2$$

holds for all θ; equality holds if and only if θ is the mean of $x_1, ..., x_m$. Thus, permutation tests in the present context that depend on $v = 1$ are median-based techniques. These median-based permutation tests are entirely different from the simple median test due to Mood (1954). Consequently, the poor power performance of the Mood (1954) median test (Freidlin and Gastwirth, 2000) does not pertain to the present median-based techniques.

The univariate pth quantile value for $0 \le p \le 1$ is now defined since the univariate median is a special case when $p = 0.5$. If (1) the probability of the univariate values $\le w_p$ is at least p and (2) the probability of the univariate values $\ge w_p$ is at least $1 - p$, then w_p is a univariate pth quantile. Sample quantile values assume that the probability for each of the n univariate values comprising the sample is $1/n$. For example, the minimum, lower quartile, median, upper quartile, and maximum values are denoted by w_0, $w_{0.25}$, $w_{0.5}$, $w_{0.75}$, and w_1, respectively. If $F(x)$ is a cumulative distribution function of a continuous random variable, then $F(w_p) = p$.

Although classical methods utilize between-group distance functions, δ is based on within-group distance functions. When $n_{g+1} = 0$, consider the decomposition given by

$$D_t = D_b + D_w,$$

where

$$D_t = \sum_{I<J} \Delta_{I,J}$$

is the invariant total sum over all $\binom{N}{2}$ distance functions,

$$D_b = \sum_{i<j} \sum_{I_i=1}^{n_i} \sum_{I_j=1}^{n_j} \Delta_{I_i,I_j}$$

is the sum over all $\sum_{i<j} n_i n_j$ between-group distance functions, and

$$D_w = \sum_{i=1}^{g} \sum_{I_i<J_i} \Delta_{I_i,J_i}$$

is the sum over all $\sum_{i=1}^{g} \binom{n_i}{2}$ within-group distance functions. Since D_t is invariant for any partitioning of the N subjects into g groups with a priori sizes $n_1, ..., n_g$, D_b is completely specified by D_w and vice versa. The pragmatic choice of using within-group distance functions in δ is computational efficiency.

2.3 P-Value of an Observed δ

The P-value associated with an observed value of δ (say δ_o) is the probability under the null hypothesis (H_0) of observing a value of δ as extreme or more extreme than δ_o. Thus, depending on the question specified, an exact P-value may be expressed as

$$P(\delta \le \delta_o \,|\, H_0) = \frac{\text{number of } \delta \text{ values} \le \delta_o}{M}$$

or

$$P(\delta \ge \delta_o \,|\, H_0) = \frac{\text{number of } \delta \text{ values} \ge \delta_o}{M}.$$

Although an algorithm exists for computing exact MRPP P-values (Berry, 1982; Berry and Mielke, 1984), this approach becomes unreasonable when M exceeds, say, 10^9, e.g., $g = 3$, $N = 30$, and $n_1 = n_2 = n_3 = 10$ yield $M = 5.55 \times 10^{12}$, and $g = 2$, $N = 50$, and $n_1 = n_2 = 25$ yield $M = 1.26 \times 10^{14}$. When M is very large, P-value approximations may be used. Two are considered here: Monte Carlo resampling and Pearson type III moment approximations.

2.3.1   Monte Carlo Resampling Approximation

A single realization of a resampling approximation consists of a complete random reordering of the original N objects, i.e., each of $N!$ reorderings can occur with equal chance. Then, the resampling approximation is based on L independent realizations, with δ_j being the associated δ statistic with the jth of L realizations. Thus, the P-value associated with the resampling approximation is given by

$$P(\delta \le \delta_o \,|\, H_0) \doteq \frac{\text{number of } \delta_j \text{ values} \le \delta_o}{L},$$

where δ_o is the observed value of δ. Since each realization of δ requires a constant multiple of N^2 operations, a resampling P-value requires a constant multiple of LN^2 operations. If ζ denotes either the power of a test or a P-value, the precision of an estimated ζ is controlled by L. Thus, a confidence of 95% in the precision depends on two standard deviations of the estimated ζ given by

$$2 \left[\zeta(1-\zeta)/L \right]^{1/2}.$$

Since power comparisons often involve values of ζ close to 0.5, precision within one unit of the third decimal place requires that $L = 1{,}000{,}000$. Similarly, precision within one unit of the fifth decimal place, when a P-value is close to 0.001, requires that $L = 40{,}000{,}000$. It is commonly assumed that δ_o is one of the L simulated values in order to avoid a P-value $= 0.0$; however, getting a P-value $= 0.0$ in the previously-described approach simply means that a P-value $< 1/L$ probably holds for δ_o.

2.3.2 Pearson Type III Approximation

The Pearson type III P-value approximation depends on the exact mean, variance, and skewness of δ under H_0 given by

$$\mu = \frac{1}{M} \sum_{I=1}^{M} \delta_I,$$

$$\sigma^2 = \frac{1}{M} \sum_{I=1}^{M} (\delta_I - \mu)^2,$$

and

$$\gamma = \left[\frac{1}{M} \sum_{I=1}^{M} (\delta_I - \mu)^3 \right] / \sigma^3,$$

respectively. In particular, the standardized statistic given by

$$T = \frac{\delta - \mu}{\sigma}$$

is presumed to follow the Pearson type III distribution, a specific gamma distribution, with the density function given by

$$f(y) = \frac{(-2/\gamma)^{4/\gamma^2}}{\Gamma(4/\gamma^2)} \left[-(2+y\gamma)/\gamma \right]^{(4-\gamma^2)/\gamma^2} e^{-2(2+y\gamma)/\gamma^2}$$

when $-\infty < y < -2/\gamma$ and $\gamma < 0$, or

$$f(y) = \frac{(2/\gamma)^{4/\gamma^2}}{\Gamma(4/\gamma^2)} \left[(2+y\gamma)/\gamma \right]^{(4-\gamma^2)/\gamma^2} e^{-2(2+y\gamma)/\gamma^2}$$

when $-2/\gamma < y < \infty$ and $\gamma > 0$, or

$$f(y) = (2\pi)^{-1/2} e^{-y^2/2}$$

when $\gamma = 0$, i.e., the standard normal distribution. If

$$T_o = \frac{\delta_o - \mu}{\sigma},$$

then

$$P(\delta \leq \delta_o \,|\, H_0) \doteq \int_{-\infty}^{T_o} f(y)\,dy$$

and

$$P(\delta \geq \delta_o \,|\, H_0) \doteq \int_{T_o}^{\infty} f(y)\,dy$$

denote approximate P-values, which are evaluated numerically over an appropriate finite interval. The Pearson type III distribution is used to approximate the permutation distribution of T because it is completely specified by γ (the skewness of T) and it includes the normal and χ^2 distributions as special cases. Thus, these distributions are asymptotic limits of the permutation distribution for some situations. Efficient computational expressions for μ, σ^2, and γ under H_0 are given by

$$\mu = D(1),$$

$$\sigma^2 = 2 \left\{ \sum_{i=1}^{g} C_i^2 \left[n_i^{(2)} \right]^{-1} - \left[N^{(2)} \right]^{-1} \right\} \left[D(2) - 2D(2') + D(2'') \right]$$

$$+ 4 \left[\sum_{i=1}^{g} C_i^2 n_i^{-1} - N^{-1} \right] \left[D(2') - D(2'') \right],$$

$$\gamma = \left\{ E\left[\delta^3 \right] - 3\mu\sigma^2 - \mu^3 \right\} / \sigma^3 ,$$

and

$$E\left[\delta^3\right] = 4\sum_{i=1}^{g} C_i^3 \left[n_i^{(2)}\right]^{-2} D(3)$$

$$+ 8\sum_{i=1}^{g} C_i^3 n_i^{(3)} \left[n_i^{(2)}\right]^{-3} \left[3D\left(3'\right) + D\left(3^*\right)\right]$$

$$+ 8\sum_{i=1}^{g} C_i^3 n_i^{(4)} \left[n_i^{(2)}\right]^{-3} \left[3D\left(3^{**}\right) + D\left(3^{***}\right)\right]$$

$$+ 6\sum_{i=1}^{g} C_i^2 \left\{1 - C_i + C_i n_i^{(4)} \left[n_i^{(2)}\right]^{-2}\right\} \left[n_i^{(2)}\right]^{-1} D\left(3''\right)$$

$$+ 12\sum_{i=1}^{g} C_i^2 \left\{(1 - C_i)n_i^{(3)} + C_i n_i^{(5)} \left[n_i^{(2)}\right]^{-1}\right\} \left[n_i^{(2)}\right]^{-2} D\left(3'''\right)$$

$$+ \sum_{i=1}^{g} C_i \left\{(1 - C_i)(1 - 2C_i) + 3C_i(1 - C_i)n_i^{(4)} \left[n_i^{(2)}\right]^{-2}\right.$$

$$\left. + C_i^2 n_i^{(6)} \left[n_i^{(2)}\right]^{-3}\right\} D\left(3''''\right),$$

where

$$N^{(c)} = \frac{N!}{(N - c)!}$$

and the 12 symmetric function model parameters are given by

$$D(1) = \frac{1}{N^{(2)}} \sum \Delta_{J_1,J_2},$$

$$D(2) = \frac{1}{N^{(2)}} \sum \Delta_{J_1,J_2}^2,$$

$$D(2') = \frac{1}{N^{(3)}} \sum \Delta_{J_1,J_2} \Delta_{J_1,J_3},$$

$$D(2'') = \frac{1}{N^{(4)}} \sum \Delta_{J_1,J_2} \Delta_{J_3,J_4},$$

$$D(3) = \frac{1}{N^{(2)}} \sum \Delta_{J_1,J_2}^3,$$

$$D(3') = \frac{1}{N^{(3)}} \sum \Delta_{J_1,J_2}^2 \Delta_{J_1,J_3},$$

$$D(3'') = \frac{1}{N^{(4)}} \sum \Delta_{J_1,J_2}^2 \Delta_{J_3,J_4},$$

$$D(3''') = \frac{1}{N^{(5)}} \sum \Delta_{J_1,J_2} \Delta_{J_1,J_3} \Delta_{J_4,J_5},$$

$$D(3'''') = \frac{1}{N^{(6)}} \sum \Delta_{J_1,J_2} \Delta_{J_3,J_4} \Delta_{J_5,J_6}.$$

$$D(3^*) = \frac{1}{N^{(3)}} \sum \Delta_{J_1,J_2} \Delta_{J_1,J_3} \Delta_{J_2,J_3},$$

$$D(3^{**}) = \frac{1}{N^{(4)}} \sum \Delta_{J_1,J_2} \Delta_{J_1,J_3} \Delta_{J_2,J_4},$$

and

$$D(3^{***}) = \frac{1}{N^{(4)}} \sum \Delta_{J_1,J_2} \Delta_{J_1,J_3} \Delta_{J_1,J_4},$$

where J_1, J_2, J_3, J_4, J_5, and J_6 denote distinct integers from 1 to N, and the sums are over all permutations of the indices. The primes and asterisks are used merely to designate the 12 distinct symmetric function model parameters. An additional comment pertains to the combinations of symmetric function model parameters given by $D(2') - D(2'')$ and $D(2) - 2D(2') + D(2'')$ in σ^2. Although $D(2') - D(2'')$ may be positive, negative, or zero, $D(2) - 2D(2') + D(2'')$ is nonnegative since

$$4\left[D(2) - 2D(2') + D(2'')\right]$$

$$= \frac{1}{N^{(4)}} \sum \left(\Delta_{J_1,J_2} - \Delta_{J_1,J_3} - \Delta_{J_2,J_4} + \Delta_{J_3,J_4}\right)^2 \geq 0.$$

The following results provide efficient computations for obtaining the 12 symmetric function model parameters (Mielke et al., 1976). If $d_{hI} = \sum_{J=1}^{N} \Delta_{I,J}^h$ and $d_h = \sum_{I=1}^{N} d_{hI}$ for $h = 1$, 2, and 3, then

$$D(1) = d_1 / N^{(2)},$$

$$D(2) = d_2 / N^{(2)},$$

$$D(3) = d_3 / N^{(2)},$$

$$D(2') = \left(\sum_{I=1}^{N} d_{1I}^2 - d_2\right) \Big/ N^{(3)},$$

$$D(2'') = \left[d_1^2 - 4N^{(3)} D(2') - 2d_2\right] \Big/ N^{(4)},$$

$$D(3') = \left(\sum_{I=1}^{N} d_{1I} d_{2I} - d_3\right) \Big/ N^{(3)},$$

$$D(3'') = \left[d_1 d_2 - 4N^{(3)} D(3') - 2d_3\right] \Big/ N^{(4)},$$

$$D(3^*) = 6 \sum_{I<J<L} \Delta_{I,J} \Delta_{I,L} \Delta_{J,L} \Big/ N^{(3)},$$

$$D(3^{**}) = \left\{2 \sum_{I<J} \Delta_{I,J} d_{1I} d_{1J} - N^{(3)} \left[2D(3') + D(3^*)\right] - d_3\right\} \Big/ N^{(4)},$$

$$D(3^{***}) = \left[\sum_{I=1}^{N} d_{1I}^3 - 3N^{(3)}D(3') - d_3 \right] \Big/ N^{(4)},$$

$$D(3''') = \left\{ N^{(3)} \left[d_1 D(2') - 4D(3') - 2D(3^*) \right] \right.$$
$$\left. - 2N^{(4)} \left[2D(3^{**}) + D(3^{***}) \right] \right\} \Big/ N^{(5)},$$

and

$$D(3'''') = \left\{ N^{(4)} \left[d_1 D(2'') - 4D(3'') - 8D(3^{**}) \right] \right.$$
$$\left. - 8N^{(5)}D(3''') \right\} \Big/ N^{(6)},$$

where $\sum_{I<J<L}$ is the sum over all I, J, and L such that $1 \leq I < J < L \leq N$. Thus, the actual computations involve only a constant multiple of N^2 operations to obtain the model parameters associated with μ and σ^2 and a constant multiple of N^3 operations to obtain the model parameters associated with γ. A Pearson type III algorithm for approximating MRPP *P*-values is given in Berry and Mielke (1983a). Pearson type III *P*-values are reasonably accurate within the usual range of interest, $0.005 \leq P\text{-value} \leq 0.10$, as demonstrated in Sections 2.11, 3.2, 4.4, and 7.3. Also, an algorithm for approximating MRPP *P*-values based on four exact moments is described by Berry et al. (1986).

2.3.3 *Approximation Comparisons*

Pearson type III *P*-value approximations based on exact moments have three major advantages over resampling (also termed "simulated," "Monte Carlo," "rerandomized," or "bootstrap") *P*-value approximations in that (1) they avoid the possibility of an additional type I statistical error due to the simulation process (Berry and Mielke, 1983b), (2) quantitative *P*-value approximations are possible even when the *P*-values are very small, and (3) Pearson type III *P*-values provide good approximations for *r*-way contingency tables when resampling *P*-values may be difficult to obtain. A concern with resampling *P*-value approximations is the chance of type I error when *L* is small (Berry and Mielke, 1983b; Mielke and Berry, 1994; Mielke et al., 1981c). To mitigate type I error, *L* should be in the range from 100,000 to 1,000,000, provided the exact *P*-value is not too small. An advantage of the resampling approximation for large *L* is that resampling will produce accurate *P*-values for the entire range from 0.001 to 0.999. An additional advantage of the resampling approximation is that resampling provides approximate *P*-values for cases where the exact moments are unattainable, e.g., analysis of the ratio of two random variables. The number of operations associated with resampling and Pearson type III approximations are constant multiples of LN^2 and N^3, respectively. Thus, the execution time of a Pearson type III approximation is roughly N/L that of a resampling approximation (in most applications, N is much less than L).

2.3.4   Group Weights

In this section, choices of the classified group weights C_i for $i = 1, ..., g$ are considered. If $N = K$, then the efficient choice of $C_i = n_i/K$ forces σ^2 to be proportional to N^{-2} since the expression in σ^2 that is proportional to N^{-1} vanishes (Mielke, 1979). Furthermore,

$$C_i = \frac{n_i - 1}{K - g},$$

is an efficient choice of C_i since σ^2 is also forced to be proportional to N^{-2} when $N = K$. Even when $N = K$, σ^2 is proportional to N^{-1} for $C_i = 1/g$ and

$$C_i = \frac{n_i \left(n_i - 1 \right)}{\displaystyle\sum_{j=1}^{g} n_j \left(n_j - 1 \right)},$$

except when $n_1 = \cdots = n_g$, where σ^2 is proportional to N^{-2} (Mielke, 1978). In this context, the inefficient choice of

$$C_i = \frac{n_i \left(n_i - 1 \right)}{\displaystyle\sum_{j=1}^{g} n_j \left(n_j - 1 \right)}$$

was used in early MRPP papers by Mantel and Valand (1970) and Mielke et al. (1976). The differences between these two papers were (1) Mantel and Valand (1970) erroneously assumed that δ asymptotically approached the normal distribution whereas Mielke et al. (1976) adjusted for nonnormality with a crude beta of the first kind distribution approximation based on γ (Mielke, 1978), and (2) the distance function of Mielke et al. (1976) was the Euclidean metric given by

$$\Delta_{I,J} = \left[\sum_{i=1}^{r} (x_{iI} - x_{iJ})^2 \right]^{1/2},$$

whereas the distance function of Mantel and Valand (1970) was the city-block metric given by

$$\Delta_{I,J} = \sum_{i=1}^{r} |x_{iI} - x_{iJ}|,$$

which is not invariant to rotation (Mielke, 1987).

Two general asymptotic distributional properties of the MRPP statistic δ are important. First, asymptotic nonnormality of statistic δ occurs when N/K and NC_i/n_i ($i = 1, ..., g \geq 2$) converge to 1 as $N \to \infty$ (Brockwell et al., 1982). Second, a necessary condition for the asymptotic normality of statistic δ is that $D(2') - D(2'') > 0$ as $N \to \infty$ (O'Reilly and Mielke, 1980).

2.3.5 Within-Group Agreement Measure

It is sometimes of interest to have a measure of agreement among object measurements within the classified groups. Such a measure for this purpose is the within-group agreement measure given by

$$\Re = 1 - \frac{\delta}{\mu}.$$

$\Re$ is a chance-corrected measure of agreement since $E[\Re] = 0$ under H_0. Because μ is a constant under H_0, the permutation distributions of δ and $\Re$ are equivalent, namely,

$$P(\delta \leq \delta_o \,|\, H_0) = P\left(\Re \geq 1 - \frac{\delta_o}{\mu} \,\bigg|\, H_0\right).$$

The values of $\Re$ range from negative values to a maximum of 1 for the extreme case when all object measurements within each classified group are identical (i.e., $\delta = 0$). Since the mean of $\Re$ under H_0 is 0, homogeneity of within-classified-group object measurements is associated with $\Re > 0$, and heterogeneity of within-classified-group object measurements is associated with $\Re < 0$ (Berry and Mielke, 1992).[1] The distribution of $\Re$ is usually asymmetric, and the upper and lower bounds depend on both the nature of the data and the structure of δ. The degree of homogeneity or heterogeneity depends on the permutation distribution of $\Re$. If large values of $n_1, ..., n_g$ and N are involved, a very small value of $P(\delta \leq \delta_o \,|\, H_0)$ may be associated with a small positive observed value of $\Re$, say $\Re_o$. Similarly, a large $\Re_o$ may be associated with a relatively large value of $P(\delta \leq \delta_o \,|\, H_0)$ if small values of $n_1, ..., n_g$ and N are involved. Incidentally, the unbiased correlation ratio is a special case of $\Re$ when $r = 1$, $v = 2$, $C_i = (n_i - 1)/(K - g)$, and $K = N$ (Kelley, 1935).

As defined, $\Re$ is a recommended choice of effect size for many applications. For example, Endler and Mielke (2005) used $\Re$ (termed K) to

---

[1] Adapted and reprinted with permission of Sage Publications, Inc. from K.J. Berry and P.W. Mielke, Jr. A family of multivariate measures of association for nominal independent variables. *Educational and Psychological Measurement*, 1992, 52, 41–55. Copyright © 1992 by Sage Publications, Inc.

TABLE 2.5. Example data set 1.

Group S_1		Group S_2	
Case	Value	Case	Value
1	472.14	14	472.51
2	472.17	15	472.57
3	472.25	16	472.62
4	472.31	17	472.66
5	472.36	18	472.69
6	472.38	19	472.73
7	472.42	20	472.74
8	472.44	21	472.78
9	472.47	22	472.80
10	472.50	23	472.85
11	472.53	24	472.86
12	472.55	25	472.87
13	472.61	26	472.92

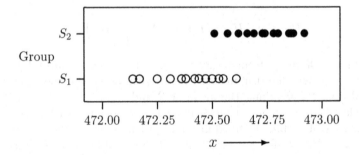

FIGURE 2.3. Plot of the data in Table 2.5.

demonstrate a variety of alternatives that MRPP with $v = 1$ could detect. Since many of the data sets encountered by Endler and Mielke (2005) were very large (i.e., $N > 500$), detection based on low P-values was possible with $\Re \doteq 0.01$.

2.4   Exact and Approximate P-Values

A large number of permutations makes it impractical to conduct an exact test, so an alternative procedure is essential. The following examples illustrate comparisons among exact, resampling, and Pearson type III P-values.

TABLE 2.6. Example data set 2.

Group S_1		Group S_2	
Case	Value	Case	Value
1	472.14	14	472.51
2	472.17	15	472.57
3	472.87	16	472.62
4	472.31	17	472.66
5	472.36	18	472.69
6	472.38	19	472.73
7	472.42	20	472.74
8	472.44	21	472.78
9	472.47	22	472.80
10	472.50	23	472.85
11	472.53	24	472.86
12	472.55	25	472.25
13	472.61	26	472.92

Consider the data set in Table 2.5 consisting of $N = 26$ objects in $g = 2$ groups with $n_1 = n_2 = 13$. For these example analyses, $r = 1$, $v = 1$, and

$$M = \frac{N!}{n_1!\,n_2!} = \frac{26!}{13!\,13!} = 10{,}400{,}600$$

permutations. For data set 1 given in Table 2.5 and displayed in Figure 2.3, with open circles (∘) and filled circles (•) denoting the values in groups S_1 and S_2, respectively, the observed δ is $\delta_o = 0.1596$ and the exact P-value of a δ value as extreme or more extreme than δ_o is $24/10{,}400{,}600 = 0.2308 \times 10^{-5}$. A resampling approximation with $L = 1{,}000{,}000$ yields $\delta_o = 0.1596$ and a P-value of 0.1000×10^{-5}. The Pearson type III approximation yields $\delta_o = 0.1596$, $\mu = 0.2566$, $\sigma^2 = 0.7247 \times 10^{-4}$, $\gamma = -2.2156$, and $T_o = -11.3981$, with a P-value of 0.8272×10^{-5}.

Data set 2 given in Table 2.6 and displayed in Figure 2.4 is a permutation of data set 1 in Table 2.5, with case 3 of group S_1 (472.25) interchanged with case 25 of group S_2 (472.87). In Figure 2.4, open circles (∘) and filled circles (•) denote the values in groups S_1 and S_2, respectively. For these data, the observed δ is $\delta_o = 0.2059$ and the exact P-value of a δ as extreme or more extreme than δ_o is $13{,}228/10{,}400{,}600 = 0.1272 \times 10^{-2}$. A resampling approximation with $L = 1{,}000{,}000$ yields $\delta_o = 0.2059$ and a P-value of 0.1305×10^{-2}. The Pearson type III approximation yields $\delta_o = 0.2059$, $\mu = 0.2566$, $\sigma^2 = 0.7247 \times 10^{-4}$, $\gamma = -2.2156$, and $T_o = -5.9614$, with a P-value of 0.1234×10^{-2}.

Data set 3 given in Table 2.7 and displayed in Figure 2.5 is a permutation of data se 2 in Table 2.6, with case 5 of group S_1 (472.36) interchanged with case 21 of group S_2 (472.78). In Figure 2.5, open circles (∘) and filled circles (•) denote the values in groups S_1 and S_2, respectively.

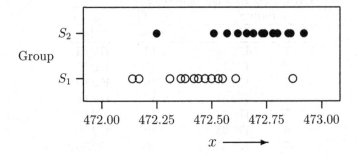

FIGURE 2.4. Plot of the data in Table 2.6.

TABLE 2.7. Example data set 3.

Group S_1		Group S_2	
Case	Value	Case	Value
1	472.14	14	472.51
2	472.17	15	472.57
3	472.87	16	472.62
4	472.31	17	472.66
5	472.78	18	472.69
6	472.38	19	472.73
7	472.42	20	472.74
8	472.44	21	472.36
9	472.47	22	472.80
10	472.50	23	472.85
11	472.53	24	472.86
12	472.55	25	472.25
13	472.61	26	472.92

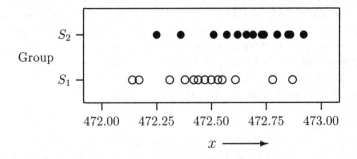

FIGURE 2.5. Plot of the data in Table 2.7.

For the data in Table 2.7, the observed δ is $\delta_o = 0.2346$ and the exact P-value of a δ as extreme or more extreme than δ_o is $306{,}570/10{,}400{,}600 = 0.2948 \times 10^{-1}$. A resampling approximation with $L = 1{,}000{,}000$ yields $\delta_o = 0.2346$ and a P-value of 0.2949×10^{-1}. The Pearson type III approximation yields $\delta_o = 0.2346$, $\mu = 0.2566$, $\sigma^2 = 0.7247 \times 10^{-4}$, $\gamma = -2.2156$, and $T_o = -2.5879$, with a P-value of 0.2880×10^{-1}.

Results close to the exact P-values can be obtained by using Pearson type III approximations or resampling approximations with large L. When the exact P-value is very small, e.g., less than 10^{-6}, the resampling P-value will usually be zero and the Pearson type III P-value will usually be conservative, i.e., larger than the exact P-value. For most applications, the resampling approximation with $100{,}000 \leq L \leq 1{,}000{,}000$ will require far more computation time than the Pearson type III approximation. Since the exact P-values are based on a discrete permutation distribution, the P-values obtained with the Pearson type III approximation are analogous to binomial distribution P-values approximated by a normal distribution. The computation of exact P-values is recommended when M is small.

A further application involving P-values is the classification of an additional object to one of the $g + 1$ disjoint groups $(S_1, ..., S_{g+1})$. Since δ is a measure of within-group object similarity and a P-value is the probability of δ being as small or smaller than an observed δ, the assignment of an additional object to a specified group should minimize the P-value relative to the $g + 1$ possible assignments. The selected group yields the smallest P-value obtained among the $g + 1$ P-values when the additional object is appended (if the additional object is classified in S_{g+1}, then it is an unclassified object). Consider the data in Table 2.7 where $g = 2$ and $n_1 = n_2 = 13$. Suppose an additional object has the value 472.82. Should the additional object be appended to S_1, S_2, or S_{g+1}? The exact, resampling approximation, and Pearson type III approximation P-values for S_1, S_2, and S_{g+1} are:

P-value	S_1	S_2	S_{g+1}
Exact	0.0635	0.0178	0.0342
Resampling	0.0633	0.0179	0.0341
Pearson type III	0.0643	0.0172	0.0362

Consequently, the additional object should be appended to S_2.

2.5 MRPP with an Excess Group

An example application of MRPP with an excess group when the distribution of δ is approximately normal involves an environmental study of lead concentrations in garden soils (Mielke et al., 1983). A perspective on lead in inner cities is described in Mielke (1999). The Mielke et al. (1983) study illustrates an analysis with one group, plus a substantial excess group. Undue exposure to lead is a public health problem, which, in the general population, is prevalent among children and is associated with degree of urbanization (Mahaffey et al., 1982). Although reduction of lead-based paint has been the prime focus for prevention of lead poisoning, about 40 to 45 percent of confirmed lead toxicity in the United States could not be attributed to lead paint. Mielke et al. (1983) investigated lead concentrations in garden soils and established that inner-city garden soils are consistently and heavily contaminated with lead and other heavy metals. The study was designed to survey and measure the distribution of soil lead and other heavy metals within metropolitan Baltimore, Maryland. Since vegetable garden cultivation creates many opportunities for contact between soils and humans, either directly via hand-to-mouth activities or indirectly via food chain linkages or contamination of the living space, attention was focused on vegetable garden soils. Soil samples were randomly collected from 422 locations within an area defined by a 30-mile radius from the intersection of Baltimore and Charles streets in downtown Baltimore. The prepared samples were analyzed for lead, cadmium, copper, nickel, zinc, and soil pH. Since soil pH was not anticipated as being associated with automobile pollution, its inclusion in the analysis served as a control for the heavy-metal pollution. Duplicates were prepared and run for all samples. One set of measurements based on the average of the duplicate samples was obtained for each of the 422 sites. The response measurements for each of the 422 soil samples are the (x, y) coordinates measured cartographically from the designated center of Baltimore. The MRPP analysis with $v = 1$ is consistent with the Euclidean geometry on which cartography is based, i.e., based on actual distances between observations. In order to investigate the geographic clustering of high soil-lead levels, the 422 soil samples were partitioned by the median value into two groups of 211 sites each. The MRPP test statistic is based on the average distance between all pairs of sites within the group with higher lead values. The excess group with lower lead values is treated as the remaining part of the finite population of 422 sites. Under the null hypothesis that the 211 sites of the group with higher lead values have the same chance of arising from any of the 422 sites, the distribution of the standardized MRPP test statistic is approximated by the standard normal distribution (O'Reilly and Mielke, 1980). The results of the 1983 study yielded the following P-values for lead, cadmium, copper, nickel, zinc, and soil pH.

Test	P-value
Lead	10^{-23}
Cadmium	10^{-18}
Copper	10^{-15}
Nickel	10^{-18}
Zinc	10^{-19}
Soil pH	0.39

To illustrate the MRPP analysis with an excess group, the lead data can be analyzed both with and without an excess group. The original data set consisted of $N = 562$ sites within a radius of 52 miles of the designated center of Baltimore. The lead data are illustrated in Figure 2.6, where lead values above and below the median are identified by open circles (o) and plus signs (+), respectively.

The data set analyzed in Mielke et al. (1983) was a restricted sample from the original data set and limited to a 30-mile radius. For the subsequent analyses involving soil lead, the full sample of $N = 562$ sites is considered. Consider an analysis with one classified group and an excess group, where the classified group consists of the sites with the higher soil-lead values and the excess group consists of the sites with the lower soil-lead values. Here, $N = 562, r = 2, v = 1, g = 1, n_1 = K = N/2 = 281$,

$$M = \frac{N!}{n_1! \, n_2!} = \frac{562!}{(281!)^2} = 0.5079 \times 10^{168},$$

$C_1 = 1, \delta = \xi_1, B$ is ∞,

$$N \left(\sum_{i=1}^{g} C_i^2 n_i^{-1} - N^{-1} \right) = 1,$$

$D\left(2'\right) - D\left(2''\right) = 36.8628, \mu = 11.5156, \sigma^2 = 0.2627, \gamma = -0.0247, \delta_o = 6.3636, T_o = -10.0527$, and the Pearson type III P-value is 0.2053×10^{-21}. Since the skewness value is very small ($\gamma = -0.0247$), the approximate $N(0,1)$ P-value is 0.4470×10^{-23}. In contrast to the analysis with $g = 1$ and an excess group, consider the same data set analyzed with two exhaustive groups, where the first group consists of the sites with the higher soil-lead values and the second group consists of the sites with the lower soil-lead values. Here, $N = 562, r = 2, v = 1, g = 2, n_1 = n_2 = N/2 = 281, K = N$, $C_1 = C_2 = 0.5, \delta = (\xi_1 + \xi_2)/2, B$ is ∞,

$$N \left(\sum_{i=1}^{g} C_i^2 n_i^{-1} - N^{-1} \right) = 0,$$

$D\left(2'\right) - D\left(2''\right) = 36.8628, \mu = 11.5156, \sigma^2 = 0.9690 \times 10^{-4}, \gamma = -1.6117$, the approximate distribution of T is neither $N(0,1)$ nor invariant since it depends on the data in question (Brockwell et al., 1982), $\delta_o = 10.9826$,

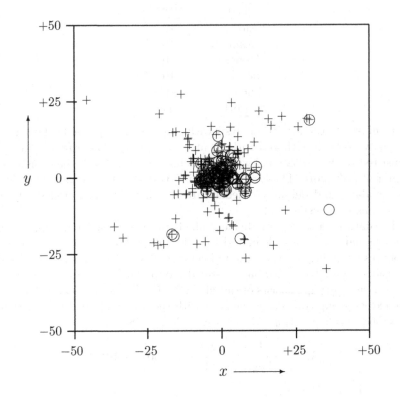

FIGURE 2.6. Plot of the Baltimore lead data.

$T_o = -54.1425$, and the Pearson type III P-value is 0.1581×10^{-28}. It should be noted that the omnibus test involving $g = 2$ and $v = 1$ detects changes in both location and scale (Mielke and Berry, 1994). Finally, if both

$$N \left(\sum_{i=1}^{g} C_i^2 n_i^{-1} - N^{-1} \right)$$

and $D\,(2') - D\,(2'')$ have finite positive values as $N \to \infty$, then the limiting distribution of $T = (\delta - \mu)/\sigma$ is $N(0,1)$ under H_0 (O'Reilly and Mielke, 1980).

The initial analysis addressed the question of whether the high-soil-lead group was more concentrated than the low-soil-lead group. The use of $g = 1$ with S_1 being the high-soil-lead group and the low-soil-lead group being an excess group corresponded directly with the goal of the study to identify geographical clumping in the high-soil-lead group. In addition, when the Mielke et al. (1983) paper was written, computer limitations prohibited an MRPP analysis with two groups for comparative purposes, i.e., computation of the exact skewness of the MRPP statistic when large group sizes were involved. Since the O'Reilly and Mielke (1980) results were known, the Mielke et al. (1983) analysis was based on a normal approximation, which only required computation of the exact mean and variance of the MRPP test statistic. Even though the MRPP analysis with two groups does not correspond in an intuitive manner to the goal of the study, the fact that the MRPP analysis with two groups may be more efficient is of interest, i.e., $\sigma^2 = 0.9690 \times 10^{-4}$ is much smaller for $g = 2$ than $\sigma^2 = 0.2627$ for $g = 1$ and an excess group. Although the anticipated efficiency of the two-group MRPP analysis is confirmed, an approach consistent with the identification of geographical clumping in the high-soil-lead group is a one-group MRPP analysis with an excess group.

The results can be clarified by considering the quantile distances from the bivariate medians of each group. An r-dimensional median is the r-dimensional point that minimizes the sum of the r-dimensional Euclidean distances from the median point to each of the N points in the r-dimensional space (Berry et al., 1984). The bivariate (x, y) median values of the sites with high and low lead values are $(-0.2928, 0.2711)$ and $(-3.6065, 0.1757)$, respectively. Note that the low-lead median site values are located a little over three miles west of the high-lead median site values. Selected quantile distances from the median site values for each group are listed in the following table. This is further illustrated in Figure 2.7, where the first quartile, second quartile (median), and third quartile lead amount values are plotted for the first 11 distance classes in miles from the center of Baltimore given by $[0, 1), [1, 2), ..., [10, 11)$.

Quantile	High lead	Low lead
0.00	0.559	1.237
0.05	0.834	2.498
0.10	1.054	3.225
0.25	2.133	4.442
0.50	3.986	7.888
0.75	5.299	12.775
0.90	7.000	22.698
0.95	8.690	28.990
1.00	37.992	49.072

Although the location shift between the two groups is only a little over three miles, the variability of the low-lead sites is vastly greater than the variability of the high-lead sites. Note that the excess group associated with $g = 1$ is the low-lead group associated with $g = 2$, i.e., the low-lead quantile values are the same.

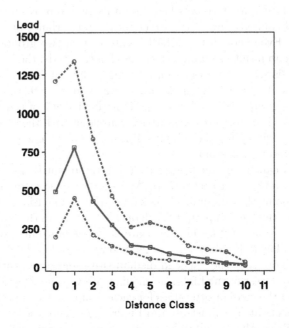

FIGURE 2.7. Plot of first, second, and third quartile lead amount values.

2.6   Detection of Multiple Clumping

If multiple clumping occurs for individual groups, e.g., locations of sugar maple trees occur in two or more clumps in a forest, then a truncated distance function, i.e., $B < \infty$ as defined in Section 2.2, provides a powerful tool for MRPP to detect multiple clumping (Mielke, 1991; Reich et al., 1991). Intuitively, truncation mitigates the influence of large distances between distinct clumps of a given group, e.g., locations of sugar maple trees. Consider the following set of data in Table 2.8 and displayed in Figure 2.8, which consists of 21 (x, y) coordinates of sugar maple trees and 23 (x, y) coordinates of white oak trees.

MRPP allows for an abundance of approaches to the analysis of a set of data. To illustrate a few of these approaches and for the purpose of comparison, six MRPP analyses of the sugar maple and white oak data contained in Table 2.8 are provided. The first two analyses consider the sugar maple trees as group S_1 and the white oak trees as an excess group, both with and without truncation. The second two analyses consider the white oak trees as group S_1 and the sugar maple trees as an excess group, both with and without truncation. The third two analyses consider the

TABLE 2.8. Data for multiple clumping example.

Sugar maple		White oak	
x	y	x	y
0.4	0.8	0.2	3.4
0.6	0.4	0.4	2.8
0.6	1.4	0.4	3.8
0.8	1.0	0.6	3.2
1.0	0.4	0.6	3.6
1.0	0.6	0.8	2.6
1.2	0.8	0.8	3.0
1.2	3.0	1.0	1.2
1.4	0.2	1.0	3.6
1.4	1.4	1.2	2.2
2.4	2.0	1.2	3.4
2.8	3.4	1.2	3.6
2.8	3.6	2.2	2.8
3.0	1.2	2.8	1.2
3.0	3.0	3.0	0.6
3.2	3.8	3.0	1.6
3.4	3.0	3.2	0.4
3.4	3.4	3.2	1.0
3.6	2.8	3.2	3.2
3.6	3.6	3.4	1.4
3.8	3.2	3.6	0.8
		3.6	1.2
		3.8	1.6

sugar maple trees and the white oak trees as $g = 2$ groups, i.e., S_1 and S_2 with no excess group, both with and without truncation.

For the first two MRPP analyses, consider the sugar maple trees as a single group and the white oak trees as an excess group. Note in Table 2.8 that the first 10 locations of the 21 sugar maple trees are positionally displaced from the second 11 locations. Figure 2.8 displays the sugar maple trees by open circles (○) and the white oak trees by filled circles (●). The displacement of the sugar maple trees in the lower-left quadrant of Figure 2.8 from the sugar maple trees in the upper-right quadrant of Figure 2.8 is readily apparent. The subjective choice of B depends on the analysis in question. Since the diameter of the sugar maple tree clumps is roughly 1.6 units, the present choice of B is 1.6 (the choice of B is intuitive and not optimal). Here, $N = 44$, $r = 2$, $v = 1$, $g = 1$, $n_1 = K = 21$, $C_1 = 1$, $\delta = \xi_1$, $B = 1.6$,

$$N \left(\sum_{i=1}^{g} C_i^2 n_i^{-1} - N^{-1} \right) = \frac{N}{n_1} - 1 = 1.0952,$$

TABLE 2.9. P-values for the Pearson type III and resampling approximations when $B = 1.6$ and B is ∞ for an MRPP one-group analysis with sugar maple trees as a single group and white oak trees as an excess group.

Truncation	Approximation	
constant	Pearson type III	Resampling
$B = 1.6$	0.1719×10^{-4}	0.3500×10^{-4}
B is ∞	0.2135	0.2140

$D(2') - D(2'') = -0.2880 \times 10^{-2}$, $\delta_o = 1.2799$, $\mu = 1.3915$, $\sigma^2 = 0.3072 \times 10^{-3}$, $\gamma = -0.7825$, $T_o = -6.3702$, and the Pearson type III P-value is 0.1719×10^{-4}. A resampling approximation with $L = 1,000,000$ yields $\delta_o = 1.2799$ and a P-value of 0.3500×10^{-4}. If B is ∞, then the differing values from the previous MRPP analysis are $D(2') - D(2'') = 0.3729 \times 10^{-1}$, $\delta_o = 2.1398$, $\mu = 2.2067$, $\sigma^2 = 0.7323 \times 10^{-2}$, $\gamma = -0.1770$, $T_o = -0.7822$, and the Pearson type III P-value is 0.2135. A resampling approximation with $L = 1,000,000$ yields $\delta_o = 2.1398$ and a P-value of 0.2140. The P-value results are summarized in Table 2.9. Although $B = 1.6$ yielded a much stronger test than when B is ∞, it is also interesting to note the influence of truncation on the values of $D(2') - D(2'')$, μ, σ^2, and γ. Since $D(2') - D(2'') > 0$ is a necessary condition for the distribution of δ to be approximately normal (O'Reilly and Mielke, 1980), the substantial skewness value ($\gamma = -0.7825$) when $B = 1.6$ is not surprising even in the presence of a sizeable excess group.

For the second two MRPP analyses of the data in Table 2.8 and Figure 2.8, consider the white oak trees as a single group and the sugar maple trees as an excess group. Note in Table 2.8 that the first 12 locations of the 23 white oak trees are positionally displaced from the second 11 locations. The displacement of the white oak trees in the upper-left quadrant of Figure 2.8 from the white oak trees in the lower-right quadrant of Figure 2.8 is readily apparent. The intuitive choice for B is again 1.6 units, for the previously stated reason. Here, $N = 44$, $r = 2$, $v = 1$, $g = 1$, $n_1 = K = 23$, $C_1 = 1$, $\delta = \xi_1$, $B = 1.6$,

$$N\left(\sum_{i=1}^{g} C_i^2 n_i^{-1} - N^{-1}\right) = \frac{N}{n_1} - 1 = 0.9130,$$

$D(2') - D(2'') = -0.2880 \times 10^{-2}$, $\delta_o = 1.2838$, $\mu = 1.3915$, $\sigma^2 = 0.2252 \times 10^{-3}$, $\gamma = -0.7137$, $T_o = -7.1750$, and the Pearson type III P-value is 0.2052×10^{-5}. A resampling approximation with $L = 1,000,000$ yields $\delta_o = 1.2838$ and a P-value of 0.2000×10^{-5}. If B is ∞, then the differing values from the previous MRPP analysis are $D(2') - D(2'') = 0.3729 \times 10^{-1}$, $\delta_o = 2.1006$, $\mu = 2.2067$, $\sigma^2 = 0.5917 \times 10^{-2}$, $\gamma = -0.1534$, $T_o = -1.3795$, and the Pearson type III P-value is 0.8707×10^{-1}. A resampling approximation

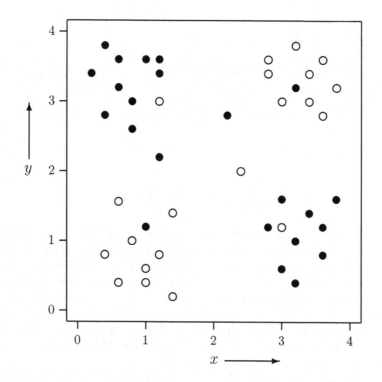

FIGURE 2.8. Plot of sugar maple (○) and white oak (●) trees.

with $L = 1{,}000{,}000$ yields $\delta_o = 2.1006$ and a P-value of 0.8776×10^{-1}. The P-value results are summarized in Table 2.10.

For the final two MRPP analyses of the data in Table 2.8 and Figure 2.8, consider the sugar maple trees and the white oak trees as two distinct groups with no excess group. Again, the intuitive choice for B is 1.6 units. Here $N = 44$, $r = 2$, $v = 1$, $g = 2$, $n_1 = 21$, $n_2 = 23$, $K = N$, $C_i = n_i/K$,

TABLE 2.10. P-values for the Pearson type III and resampling approximations when $B = 1.6$ and B is ∞ for the MRPP one-group analysis with white oak trees as a single group and sugar maple trees as an excess group.

Truncation	Approximation	
constant	Pearson type III	Resampling
$B = 1.6$	0.2052×10^{-5}	0.2000×10^{-5}
B is ∞	0.8707×10^{-1}	0.8776×10^{-1}

TABLE 2.11. P-values for the Pearson type III and resampling approximations when $B = 1.6$ and B is ∞ for the MRPP two-group analysis of sugar maple and white oak trees.

Truncation	Approximation	
constant	Pearson type III	Resampling
$B = 1.6$	0.7816×10^{-5}	0.2000×10^{-5}
B is ∞	0.2386×10^{-1}	0.2453×10^{-1}

$\delta = C_1\xi_1 + C_2\xi_2$, $B = 1.6$,

$$N \left(\sum_{i=1}^{g} C_i^2 n_i^{-1} - N^{-1} \right) = 0,$$

$D(2') - D(2'') = -0.2880 \times 10^{-2}$, $\delta_o = 1.2819$, $\mu = 1.3915$, $\sigma^2 = 0.1776 \times 10^{-3}$, $\gamma = -1.2267$, $T_o = -8.2222$, and the Pearson type III P-value is 0.7816×10^{-5}. A resampling approximation with $L = 1,000,000$ yields $\delta_o = 1.2819$ and a P-value of 0.2000×10^{-5}. If B is ∞, then the differing values from the previous MRPP analysis are $D(2') - D(2'') = 0.3729 \times 10^{-1}$, $\delta_o = 2.1193$, $\mu = 2.2067$, $\sigma^2 = 0.1080 \times 10^{-2}$, $\gamma = -1.7239$, $T_o = -2.6606$, and the Pearson type III P-value is 0.2386×10^{-1}. A resampling approximation with $L = 1,000,000$ yields $\delta_o = 2.1193$ and a P-value of 0.2453×10^{-1}. The P-value results are summarized in Table 2.11.

This example demonstrates the need for truncated distance functions to detect multiple clumping with MRPP. A related need for truncated distance functions involves the use of MRPP to detect overly regular position patterns of objects from random position patterns in an r-dimensional space (Mielke, 1991). Although it was anticipated that the MRPP analysis with two groups, no excess group, and truncation would yield the strongest result, the MRPP analysis with one group (white oak trees), an excess group (sugar maple trees), and truncation yielded a slightly stronger result. These analyses are complex, but they demonstrate useful techniques for distinguishing natural habitat patterns of plants and animals.

2.7   Detection of Evenly Spaced Location Patterns

If a collection of object locations appears to be evenly spaced in one or more dimensions, an investigator may wish to examine whether the pattern of locations differs from a random pattern. For example, a hydrologist wishes to know whether surface pebbles resulting from a hydraulic flume experiment are more evenly spaced than randomly placed pebbles. If a spatial pattern of objects is evenly spaced, then intuitively the ensemble of smaller object distances of nearest neighbors should be larger than the nearest neighbor distances of randomly placed objects. As an example, compare the evenly spaced pattern of 52 objects denoted by filled circles ($\bullet$) with the random pattern of 52 objects denoted by open circles ($\circ$) in Figure 2.9; the data of Figure 2.9 are given in Table 2.12.

An MRPP analysis examines whether the average between-object distance of nearest neighbors comprising the evenly spaced pattern of 52 objects is larger than the corresponding average of a random pattern of 52 objects if 52 objects had been randomly selected from the pooled collection of 104 objects. To mitigate the influence of large distances between objects that are not nearest neighbors, set the truncation constant $B = 0.6$ since 0.6 is the distance between nearest neighbors of the objects comprising the evenly spaced pattern. Thus, the MRPP analysis is based on $N = 104$, $r = 2$, $v = 1$, $g = 1$, $n_1 = K = 52$, $C_1 = 1$, $\delta = \xi_1$, $B = 0.6$, and

$$P\text{-value} = P\left(\delta \geq \delta_o \mid H_0\right),$$

where δ_o is the observed average between-object distance for all objects comprising the evenly spaced pattern. A resampling approximation with $L = 1{,}000{,}000$ yields $\delta_o = 0.6000$ and a P-value of 0.0000 since the exact P-value is extremely small. Because $\delta_o = 0.6000$, $\mu = 0.5902$, $\sigma^2 = 0.2068 \times 10^{-5}$, $\gamma = -0.4749$, and $T_o = 6.8019$, a Pearson type III approximation is not appropriate since $T_o > -2/\gamma = 4.2118$ (see Section 2.3).

2.8   Dependence of MRPP on v

To investigate the behavior of MRPP for univariate distributions with different values of $v > 0$ in the distance function

$$\Delta_{I,J} = |x_I - x_J|^v,$$

simulated power comparisons for a location alternative can be examined. In addition to the Laplace (i.e., double exponential), logistic, and normal distributions with probability density functions given by

$$f(x) = \tfrac{1}{2} e^{-|x|},$$
$$f(x) = e^x / \left(1 + e^x\right)^2,$$

and

$$f(x) = (2\pi)^{-1/2} e^{-x^2/2},$$

respectively, the family of Student t distributions, denoted by $t(m)$, is considered, with probability density function given by

$$f(x) = \left\{ \Gamma\left[(m+1)/2\right] \Big/ \left[(m\pi)^{1/2} \Gamma\left(m/2\right)\right] \right\} \left(1 + x^2/m\right)^{-(m+1)/2},$$

TABLE 2.12. Coordinates for 52 evenly spaced and 52 random objects.

Evenly spaced				Random			
x	y	x	y	x	y	x	y
0.18	0.20	2.26	0.20	1.95	1.06	0.64	3.42
0.18	0.80	2.26	0.80	0.28	0.45	1.57	3.74
0.18	1.40	2.26	1.40	2.27	0.13	3.86	1.99
0.18	2.00	2.26	2.00	3.36	1.71	0.80	1.69
0.18	2.60	2.26	2.60	1.25	0.66	2.14	1.60
0.18	3.20	2.26	3.20	3.32	2.31	0.95	3.57
0.18	3.80	2.26	3.80	3.18	2.20	3.83	3.65
0.70	0.50	2.78	0.50	0.30	3.06	0.42	2.08
0.70	1.10	2.78	1.10	3.96	1.40	1.29	2.42
0.70	1.70	2.78	1.70	3.37	2.29	3.15	2.36
0.70	2.30	2.78	2.30	1.53	0.27	0.69	3.43
0.70	2.90	2.78	2.90	2.52	1.63	2.25	2.15
0.70	3.50	2.78	3.50	2.86	0.98	1.66	1.61
1.22	0.20	3.30	0.20	3.48	1.72	0.15	2.50
1.22	0.80	3.30	0.80	3.42	0.91	3.05	1.62
1.22	1.40	3.30	1.40	3.62	1.03	3.32	3.37
1.22	2.00	3.30	2.00	3.38	0.40	0.51	1.00
1.22	2.60	3.30	2.60	2.17	3.24	1.38	2.24
1.22	3.20	3.30	3.20	2.59	1.32	3.22	2.23
1.22	3.80	3.30	3.80	0.85	3.15	2.32	2.58
1.74	0.50	3.82	0.50	3.02	2.74	3.45	3.80
1.74	1.10	3.82	1.10	3.95	0.74	2.55	2.84
1.74	1.70	3.82	1.70	2.50	2.16	2.76	0.26
1.74	2.30	3.82	2.30	1.76	1.05	0.30	1.08
1.74	2.90	3.82	2.90	3.53	1.93	2.67	1.71
1.74	3.50	3.82	3.50	1.12	1.12	2.52	0.68

where m is the degrees-of-freedom. Thus, $t(1)$ and $t(\infty)$ are the Cauchy and normal distributions, respectively. The family of symmetric kappa distributions characterized by parameter $\lambda > 0$ (Mielke, 1972; see Corollary 1), with probability density function

$$f(x) = \tfrac{1}{2}\lambda^{-1/\lambda}\left(1 + |x|^{\lambda}/\lambda\right)^{-(\lambda+1)/\lambda},$$

is also included. For convenience, a specific symmetric kappa distribution will be denoted by $SK(\lambda)$. Selected density functions of the symmetric kappa distribution are displayed in Figure 2.10.

The symmetric kappa distribution is exceedingly peaked at the origin with heavy tails when λ is very small and approaches a uniform distribution when λ is very large. The height of the symmetric kappa density function is minimized when $\lambda = e$, yielding the height of $\tfrac{1}{2}e^{-1/e} \doteq 0.3461$, approaches

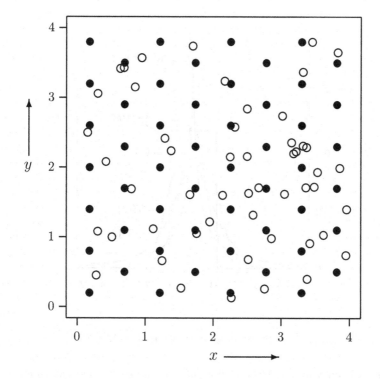

FIGURE 2.9. Evenly spaced ($\bullet$) and random ($\circ$) objects.

0.5 as λ approaches ∞, and becomes extremely large as λ approaches zero. For example, when $\lambda = 0.001$, the symmetric kappa distribution resembles a spike with long tails, where the height of the density function is $10^{3000}/2$, and when $\lambda = 100$, the symmetric kappa distribution resembles a loaf-like distribution with long tails, where the height of the density function is 0.4775. In general, the density function of the symmetric kappa distribution is spiked when $\lambda < 1$, peaked like a Laplace distribution when $\lambda = 1$, and rounded like a normal distribution when $\lambda > 1$. When λ is very large, the height of the symmetric kappa density function is about 0.5 for $-1 < x < +1$ and the height becomes very small for other values of x. Thus, the symmetric kappa distribution provides a family of distributions for comparing various choices of v. Incidentally, the rth moment of $|x|$ exists only when $r < \lambda$, and the symmetric kappa distribution with $\lambda = 2$, $SK(2)$, is $t(2)$.

For these power comparisons, two samples ($n_1 = n_2 = 20$) are considered with a location shift (LS) added to the values of the second sample. The values of LS for each distribution are given in Table 2.13. The values of LS in Table 2.13 were chosen to yield a full range of comparative power values

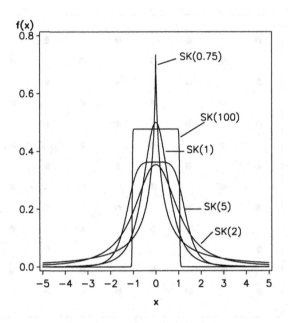

FIGURE 2.10. Selected symmetric kappa (SK) distributions.

for each distribution. The power for each case is based on 10,000 simulated tests where the $N = 40$ values are appropriately transformed real uniform numbers of $[0, 1)$ generated from a common seed using REAL FUNCTION UNI due to David Kahaner and George Marsaglia (Kahaner et al., 1988, pp. 410–411). Each simulated power value $(1 - \hat{\beta})$ presented in Table 2.14 is the proportion of the 10,000 P-values $\leq \alpha = 0.05$, where each P-value is based on the Pearson type III approximation. To demonstrate problems with the Pearson type III approximation when v is large and λ (of the symmetric kappa distribution) is small, corresponding simulated estimates of α ($\hat{\alpha}$) are presented in Table 2.15 with LS = 0.

The results in Table 2.14 demonstrate that the choice of v for detecting a location shift depends on the underlying distribution. In general, a small value of v is best for a location shift involving a peaked heavy-tailed distribution, whereas a large value of v is best for a location shift involving a loaf-shaped light-tailed distribution. Specifically, the highest power for the Laplace distribution occurs when $0.5 \leq v \leq 1.0$, and the highest power for the logistic distribution occurs when $1.0 \leq v \leq 1.5$. The highest powers for $t(1)$, $t(2)$, $t(3)$, $t(5)$, and $t(10)$ occur when $v = 0.25$, $v = 0.5$, $v = 1.0$, $v = 1.0$, and $v = 1.5$, respectively. The highest powers for $t(20)$, $t(50)$, and $t(\infty)$ all occur when $v = 2.0$. When $v = 0.25$, the highest power for $SK(\lambda)$ is attained when λ is 0.25, 0.5, and 1.0. Power is very poor when

TABLE 2.13. Values of the location shift (LS) for each distribution.

Distribution	LS
Laplace	1.00
logistic	1.25
$t(1)$, Cauchy	1.90
$t(2)$, $SK(2)$	1.40
$t(3)$	1.20
$t(5)$	0.90
$t(10)$	0.85
$t(20)$	0.80
$t(50)$	0.75
$t(\infty)$, normal	0.75
$SK(0.25)$	25.00
$SK(0.5)$	2.50
$SK(1)$	1.50
$SK(2.5)$	1.00
$SK(5)$	0.70
$SK(10)$	0.60
$SK(25)$	0.50
$SK(50)$	0.45
$SK(100)$	0.40

$v \geq 1.0$ for $SK(\lambda)$ with λ equal to 0.25 and 0.5. The highest power for $SK(2.5)$ and $SK(5)$ occurs when $v = 1.0$ and $v = 2.0$, respectively. Finally, $v = 6.0$ yields the highest power for $SK(\lambda)$ when λ is 10, 25, 50, and 100. It should be noted that the choices of v and λ are obviously far from being exhaustive in these analyses. The results in Table 2.15 indicate that $\hat{\alpha}$ is well below 0.05 for $t(1)$ when $v = 0.25$, $SK(0.25)$ when $v \geq 4.0$, SK(0.5) when $v \geq 2.0$, and $SK(1)$ when $v = 6.0$. Considering all 19 distributions, $v = 1$ provides the smallest overall differences between the nominal α value of 0.05 and the simulated $\hat{\alpha}$ values.

In summary, there most certainly is no single best choice of v, in terms of power considerations, for location shifts due to the dependence on specific distributions, where each simulation is based on a Pearson type III P-value approximation. Given that the underlying distribution is seldom known, the preference for $v = 1$ is intuitively based on the desired congruence between the data and analysis spaces (see Chapter 1 and Section 2.2). Since the simulated power and significance comparisons given in Tables 2.14 and 2.15, respectively, address only symmetric distributions, additional analyses associated with asymmetric distributions may yield unanticipated results.

TABLE 2.14. Simulated power $(1 - \hat{\beta})$ comparisons for specified values of v, given $\alpha = 0.05$ and the LS values in Table 2.13.

Distribution	v							
	0.25	0.5	1.0	1.5	2.0	3.0	4.0	6.0
Laplace	.6835	.7044	.7084	.6733	.6154	.5159	.4562	.3802
logistic	.5094	.5507	.5930	.5971	.5835	.5338	.4884	.4226
$t(1)$, Cauchy	.8859	.8612	.6936	.3902	.2861	.2356	.2187	.1938
$t(2)$, $SK(2)$	.8332	.8456	.8180	.7069	.5875	.4744	.4255	.3639
$t(3)$	.7271	.7537	.7642	.7184	.6482	.5457	.4941	.4237
$t(5)$	.5769	.6153	.6496	.6423	.6117	.5423	.4922	.4217
$t(10)$	.5697	.6096	.6582	.6717	.6646	.6195	.5731	.5082
$t(20)$	.5376	.5825	.6363	.6584	.6591	.6292	.5945	.5313
$t(50)$	.4956	.5437	.5975	.6220	.6294	.6110	.5803	.5262
$t(\infty)$, normal	.5031	.5541	.6083	.6361	.6461	.6312	.6053	.5543
$SK(0.25)$	.7814	.2779	.0874	.0532	.0462	.0393	.0368	.0339
$SK(0.5)$	.7763	.4394	.1176	.0538	.0461	.0405	.0379	.0314
$SK(1)$	.7510	.6715	.4074	.1958	.1490	.1319	.1227	.1091
$SK(2.5)$	.6062	.6398	.6529	.6023	.5365	.4535	.4059	.3503
$SK(5)$	.4715	.5213	.5833	.6152	.6271	.6223	.6069	.5729
$SK(10)$	.4908	.5358	.5982	.6439	.6814	.7382	.7649	.7969
$SK(25)$	.4645	.4990	.5560	.6021	.6423	.7150	.7703	.8410
$SK(50)$	.4304	.4555	.5102	.5601	.6005	.6768	.7359	.8147
$SK(100)$	.3688	.3966	.4419	.4860	.5316	.6040	.6674	.7583

2.9   Permutation Version of One-Way ANOVA

Let the usual one-way analysis-of-variance (ANOVA) statistic be denoted by

$$F = \frac{MS_{Treatment}}{MS_{Error}},$$

where n_i is the number of objects in the ith of g groups, $N = \sum_{i=1}^{g} n_i$ is the total number of objects, x_{ki} is the response measurement on the kth object in the ith group,

$$MS_{Treatment} = \frac{1}{g-1} \sum_{i=1}^{g} n_i \left(\bar{x}_i - \bar{x} \right)^2,$$

$$MS_{Error} = \frac{1}{N-g} \sum_{i=1}^{g} \sum_{k=1}^{n_i} \left(x_{ki} - \bar{x}_i \right)^2,$$

and

$$SS_{Total} = (g-1)MS_{Treatment} + (N-g)MS_{Error},$$

TABLE 2.15. Simulated significance ($\hat{\alpha}$) comparisons for specified values of v, given $\alpha = 0.05$ and LS $= 0$.

Distribution	0.25	0.5	1.0	1.5	2.0	3.0	4.0	6.0
				v				
Laplace	.0449	.0467	.0482	.0525	.0545	.0523	.0523	.0515
logistic	.0455	.0473	.0500	.0523	.0537	.0546	.0524	.0521
$t(1)$, Cauchy	.0460	.0474	.0489	.0515	.0524	.0504	.0470	.0389
$t(2)$, $SK(2)$	.0449	.0467	.0480	.0526	.0545	.0534	.0516	.0484
$t(3)$	.0421	.0436	.0458	.0497	.0514	.0506	.0496	.0479
$t(5)$	.0454	.0472	.0497	.0529	.0545	.0538	.0523	.0516
$t(10)$	.0452	.0470	.0502	.0525	.0540	.0546	.0523	.0517
$t(20)$	.0453	.0468	.0497	.0522	.0539	.0538	.0519	.0514
$t(50)$	.0455	.0470	.0499	.0525	.0540	.0540	.0522	.0509
$t(\infty)$, normal	.0457	.0469	.0502	.0526	.0540	.0537	.0523	.0506
$SK(0.25)$	.0534	.0485	.0615	.0518	.0448	.0417	.0360	.0330
$SK(0.5)$	.0494	.0540	.0454	.0421	.0384	.0327	.0294	.0249
$SK(1)$	.0470	.0482	.0492	.0523	.0532	.0506	.0462	.0391
$SK(2.5)$	.0448	.0468	.0487	.0528	.0544	.0540	.0525	.0498
$SK(5)$	.0459	.0472	.0503	.0527	.0530	.0523	.0517	.0495
$SK(10)$	.0464	.0482	.0498	.0516	.0528	.0527	.0522	.0494
$SK(25)$	.0468	.0483	.0501	.0523	.0530	.0530	.0505	.0488
$SK(50)$	.0472	.0486	.0503	.0521	.0531	.0524	.0510	.0481
$SK(100)$	.0467	.0488	.0503	.0519	.0528	.0522	.0512	.0480

with

$$\bar{x}_i = \frac{1}{n_i} \sum_{k=1}^{n_i} x_{ki},$$

where $i = 1, ..., g$, and

$$\bar{x} = \frac{1}{N} \sum_{i=1}^{g} \sum_{k=1}^{n_i} x_{ki}.$$

When $r = 1$, $v = 2$, $K = N$, and $C_i = (n_i - 1)/(N - g)$ for $i = 1, ..., g$, it is easily shown that δ is a permutation version of the F statistic. The relationship between δ and F in this case (Berry and Mielke, 1983b; Mielke and Berry, 1994)[2] is given by

$$N\delta = \frac{2(NA_2 - A_1^2)}{N - g + (g-1)F},$$

[2]Adapted and reprinted with permission of the American Educational Research Association from P.W. Mielke, Jr. and K.J. Berry. Permutation tests for common locations among samples with unequal variances. *Journal of Educational and Behavioral Statistics*, 1994, 19, 217–236. Copyright © 1994 by the American Educational Research Association.

where $A_1 = \sum_{I=1}^{N} x_I$, $A_2 = \sum_{I=1}^{N} x_I^2$, and x_I is the response measurement on the Ith of N objects. If $g = 2$, then $F = t^2$ where t is the two-sample t test statistic. The permutation version of the F test given here is commonly called the Fisher–Pitman permutation test (Fisher, 1935; Pitman, 1938). Also, $\mu = 2SS_{Total}/(N-1)$ and $\delta = 2MS_{Error}$ yield the relation given by

$$\delta = \frac{1}{N-g}\left[(N-1)\mu - 2(g-1)MS_{Treatment}\right].$$

Because μ is fixed for a given univariate sample and $MS_{Treatment}$ depends only on differences among group means, δ depends solely on the differences among the group means. Thus, the statistical inference is completely un-affected by differences in scale (i.e., variance) among the g groups (Berry and Mielke, 2002; Johnston et al., 2004).

Consider the statistic F under the usual normality assumption where one value of the ith of g groups is designated as w and is allowed to vary while the remaining $N-1$ values are fixed. When w becomes either very large or very small, relative to the $N-1$ fixed values, the value of F approaches

$$\frac{(N-g)(N-n_i)}{(g-1)N(n_i-1)}. \tag{2.1}$$

If $n_i = N/g$, then the value of F approaches unity. This result explains the overwhelming influence of a single value relative to a fixed set of values for the F test. On the other hand, with $v = 1$, the P-value is relatively unaffected by the presence of a single extreme value.

To demonstrate that permutation tests with $v = 1$ are robust, consider the data given in Table 2.16 for comparing two groups of sizes $n_1 = n_2 = 13$. While 25 of the $N = 26$ univariate values are fixed, one value of group 1, designated by y, is allowed to vary in order to determine its effect on the exact two-sided P-values. Extreme examples of y and their associated P-values are given in Table 2.17. The three P-values of Table 2.17 associated with each value of y correspond to the permutation tests with $v = 1$ and $v = 2$, and with the two-sample t test, respectively. The permutation test P-values with $v = 1$ for low and high values of y, relative to the 25 fixed values, are 4.04×10^{-6} and 9.81×10^{-5}, respectively. The P-values are stable, consistent, and are not affected by the extreme magnitudes of y in either direction. In contrast, the permutation test P-values with $v = 2$ are 4.04×10^{-6} for small values of y and 1.000 for large values of y, relative to the fixed values. Finally, the two-sample (nonpermutation) t test P-values approach a common P-value (i.e., 0.327) as y becomes either very small or very large, relative to the fixed values. Due to the extreme values of y, the two-sample t test is unable to detect the obvious difference in location between groups 1 and 2, as shown in Expression (2.1). Effect size is used by Endler and Mielke (2005) to indicate other alternative data set patterns that are detectable with MRPP based on $v = 1$ (see Section 2.3.5). The results of Table 2.17

TABLE 2.16. Frequencies of observed values for groups 1 and 2 with $N = 26$ subjects assigned to $g = 2$ groups with $n = 13$ subjects in each group.

Value	Group 1	Group 2
445.6	1	0
445.7	2	0
445.8	4	0
445.9	4	1
446.0	1	3
446.1	0	4
446.2	0	3
446.3	0	2
y	1	0

TABLE 2.17. Exact two-sided P-value comparisons of δ-based permutation tests with $v = 1$ and $v = 2$ and the two-sample t test for the data set in Table 2.16.

	Permutation test		Two-sample
y	$v = 1$	$v = 2$	t test
107.7	4.04×10^{-6}	4.04×10^{-6}	0.322
437.7	4.04×10^{-6}	4.04×10^{-6}	0.153
443.7	4.04×10^{-6}	4.04×10^{-6}	1.16×10^{-2}
444.7	4.04×10^{-6}	4.04×10^{-6}	5.69×10^{-4}
445.7	4.04×10^{-6}	4.04×10^{-6}	5.84×10^{-7}
446.7	9.81×10^{-5}	9.82×10^{-3}	9.16×10^{-3}
447.7	9.81×10^{-5}	0.430	0.320
449.7	9.81×10^{-5}	1.000	1.000
453.7	9.81×10^{-5}	1.000	0.617
783.7	9.81×10^{-5}	1.000	0.333

imply that Euclidean distance based permutation methods are so robust to extreme values that they seldom need the data manipulation techniques devised for squared Euclidean distance based permutation methods such as truncations and rank order statistic transformations.

2.10   Euclidean and Hotelling Commensuration

Whenever there are two or more responses for each subject, the response measurements may be expressed in different units, which must be made commensurate (i.e., standardized) before analysis. Let $y'_I = (y_{1I}, ..., y_{rI})$ for $I = 1, ..., N$ denote N noncommensurate r-dimensional values ($r \geq 2$).

The corresponding N commensurate r-dimensional values denoted by $x'_I = (x_{1I}, ..., x_{rI})$ for $I = 1, ..., N$ are given by $x_{jI} = y_{jI}/\phi_j$, where

$$\phi_j = \left[\sum_{I<J} | y_{jI} - y_{jJ} |^v \right]^{1/v}$$

for $j = 1, ..., r$. The commensurated data have the desired property that

$$\sum_{I<J} | x_{jI} - x_{jJ} |^v = 1$$

for $j = 1, ..., r$ and any $v > 0$. This commensuration procedure is based on the distance between the r response measurements of subjects ω_I and ω_J and is given by the distance function

$$\Delta_{I,J} = \left[\sum_{j=1}^r (x_{jI} - x_{jJ})^2 \right]^{v/2},$$

where $v > 0$. The commensuration is termed Euclidean commensuration when $v = 1$ (Berry and Mielke, 1992). An alternative commensuration, termed Hotelling commensuration, is based on the distance function

$$\Delta_{I,J} = \left[(y_I - y_J)' S^{-1} (y_I - y_J) \right]^{v/2},$$

where S is the $r \times r$ variance-covariance matrix given by

$$S = \begin{bmatrix} \dfrac{1}{N} \sum_{I=1}^N (y_{1I} - \bar{y}_1)^2 & \cdots & \dfrac{1}{N} \sum_{I=1}^N (y_{1I} - \bar{y}_1)(y_{rI} - \bar{y}_r) \\ \vdots & & \vdots \\ \dfrac{1}{N} \sum_{I=1}^N (y_{rI} - \bar{y}_r)(y_{1I} - \bar{y}_1) & \cdots & \dfrac{1}{N} \sum_{I=1}^N (y_{rI} - \bar{y}_r)^2 \end{bmatrix},$$

$v > 0$, and

$$\bar{y}_j = \frac{1}{N} \sum_{I=1}^N y_{jI}$$

for $j = 1, ..., r$ (Mielke and Berry, 1994).

Multivariate permutation methods based on Euclidean commensuration involve $g \geq 2$, $C_k = n_k/K$, and $v = 1$. In contrast, multivariate permutation methods based on Hotelling commensuration involve $g \geq 2$, $C_k = (n_k - 1)/(K - g)$, and either $v = 1$ or $v = 2$. If $v = 2$, $N = K$, and Hotelling commensuration is invoked, then the identity relating δ and the multivariate analysis-of-variance Bartlett–Nanda–Pillai (BNP) trace test statistic $V^{(s)}$, where $s = \min(g - 1, r)$, is

$$\delta = \frac{2\left(r - V^{(s)}\right)}{N - g}$$

(Anderson, 1984, pp. 326–328; Bartlett, 1939; Mielke, 1991; Mielke and Berry, 1994; Nanda, 1950; Pillai, 1955).

To establish the relationship between δ and $V^{(s)}$, an alternative notation is used. Let

$$H = \sum_{k=1}^{g} n_k \left(\bar{w}_k - \bar{w}\right)\left(\bar{w}_k - \bar{w}\right)'$$

and

$$E = \sum_{k=1}^{g} \sum_{j=1}^{n_k} \left(w_{jk} - \bar{w}_k\right)\left(w_{jk} - \bar{w}_k\right)',$$

where $w'_{jk} = (w_{1jk}, ..., w_{rjk})$ and w_{ijk} denotes the ith response measurement of subject j in group k,

$$\bar{w}_k = \frac{1}{n_k} \sum_{j=1}^{n_k} w_{jk},$$

and

$$\bar{w} = \frac{1}{N} \sum_{k=1}^{g} \sum_{j=1}^{n_k} w_{jk},$$

since

$$N = \sum_{k=1}^{g} n_k.$$

Then, the BNP statistic is given by

$$V^{(s)} = \text{trace}\left[H\left(E + H\right)^{-1}\right] = \sum_{i=1}^{s} \theta_i,$$

where $\theta_1 \geq \cdots \geq \theta_s$ are the s ordered eigenvalues of $H\left(E + H\right)^{-1}$ and $s = \min\left(g - 1, r\right)$. With respect to this alternative notation, consider the statistic

$$\delta = \sum_{k=1}^{g} C_k \xi_k$$

characterized by a Hotelling commensuration distance function with $v = 2$, $C_k = \left(n_k - 1\right) / \left(N - g\right)$, and the average between-subject difference, which may be expressed as

$$\xi_k = \binom{n_k}{2}^{-1} \sum_{h<j} (w_{hk} - w_{jk})' (E + H)^{-1} (w_{hk} - w_{jk})$$

$$= 2 \text{ trace} \left[(E + H)^{-1} S_k \right],$$

where

$$S_k = (n_k - 1)^{-1} \sum_{j=1}^{n_k} (w_{jk} - \bar{w}_k)(w_{jk} - \bar{w}_k)'$$

for $k = 1, ..., g$. The identity $E = (E + H) - H$ then establishes

$$\delta = \frac{2 \left(r - V^{(s)} \right)}{N - g}$$

since

$$\delta = \frac{2}{N - g} \text{ trace} \left[(E + H)^{-1} E \right]$$

$$= \frac{2}{N - g} \left(r - \sum_{i=1}^{s} \theta_i \right)$$

$$= \frac{2}{N - g} \left(r - V^{(s)} \right).$$

The identity relating the two-sample Hotelling T^2 statistic (Hotelling, 1931) to $V^{(s)}$ when $g = 2$ is

$$V^{(1)} = \frac{T^2}{N - 2 + T^2}.$$

When $g = 2$, then the Hotelling T^2 test is an exact test under the multivariate normality assumptions. In addition to the BNP trace test statistic, three classical multivariate test statistics (Anderson, 1984, pp. 321–330) can also be expressed in terms of the s ordered eigenvalues $\theta_1 \geq \cdots \geq \theta_s$ and are equivalent to the two-sample Hotelling T^2 test statistic when $g = 2$. The Lawley–Hotelling trace test statistic is

$$\sum_{i=1}^{s} \frac{\theta_i}{1 - \theta_i},$$

Roy's maximum root test statistic is $\theta_1 / (1 - \theta_1)$, and Wilks' likelihood-ratio test statistic is

$$\prod_{i=1}^{s} (1 - \theta_i).$$

If $g > 2$, exact procedures for the BNP trace test are generally unknown when the multivariate normality assumptions are true. However, an excellent saddle-point approximation by Butler et al. (1992) is available for the general case of the BNP trace test. It must be emphasized that the Butler et al. (1992) saddle-point approximation requires that the multivariate normality assumptions be satisfied.

2.11 Power Comparisons

Simulated power comparisons for location shifts of five uncorrelated bivariate distributions (Mielke and Berry, 1994) indicate that (1) MRPP with Euclidean commensuration, Hotelling commensuration and $v = 1$, and Hotelling commensuration and $v = 2$, perform almost equally well for the bivariate normal distribution; (2) MRPP with Hotelling commensuration and $v = 2$ performs better than either MRPP with Euclidean commensuration or MRPP with Hotelling commensuration and $v = 1$, for the bivariate uniform distribution; and (3) both MRPP with Euclidean commensuration and MRPP with Hotelling commensuration and $v = 1$ performs much better than MRPP with Hotelling commensuration and $v = 2$, for the bivariate exponential, lognormal, and Cauchy distributions. A related study involved simulated power comparisons for location shifts of five correlated bivariate distributions (Mielke and Berry, 1999).[3]

If the location shift is parallel to the major axis of a correlated bivariate distribution, as shown in Figure 2.11, then MRPP with Euclidean commensuration performs better than either MRPP with Hotelling commensuration and $v = 1$ or MRPP with Hotelling commensuration and $v = 2$ for all five correlated bivariate distributions. If the location shift is parallel to the minor axis of a correlated bivariate distribution, as shown in Figure 2.12, then MRPP with Hotelling commensuration and $v = 2$ performs better than the two other versions of MRPP for the correlated bivariate normal and uniform distributions. Finally, if the location shift is parallel to the minor axis of a correlated bivariate distribution, then MRPP with Hotelling commensuration and $v = 1$ performs better than the two other versions of MRPP for the correlated bivariate exponential, lognormal, and Cauchy distributions. Although the influence of extreme values for $v = 1$ and $v = 2$ has been discussed for the univariate case, the following detailed examination demonstrates the effects of distance functions based on $v = 1$ and $v = 2$ in power comparisons involving the bivariate normal and bivariate Cauchy probability distributions.

---

[3] Adapted and reprinted with permission of the American Educational Research Association from P.W. Mielke, Jr. and K.J. Berry. Multivariate tests for correlated data in completely randomized designs. *Journal of Educational and Behavioral Statistics*, 1999, 24, 109–131. Copyright © 1999 by the American Educational Research Association.

Monte Carlo simulations are used to obtain power comparisons for permutation tests. The power comparisons in the present analysis are based on bivariate data from two selected probability distributions consisting of the bivariate normal and the bivariate Cauchy probability distributions. Each of the bivariate probability distributions is based on two independent univariate probability distributions. The density function of the univariate normal probability distribution is

$$f(x) = \frac{1}{\sqrt{2\pi}} e^{-x^2/2}$$

with mean, variance, skewness, and kurtosis of 0, 1, 0, and 0, respectively. The density function of the univariate Cauchy probability distribution is

$$f(x) = \left[\pi \left(1 + x^2\right)\right]^{-1}$$

with infinite variance and with mean, skewness, and kurtosis undefined. Interestingly, the Cauchy and normal distributions are extreme cases of the t probability distribution associated with 1 and ∞ degrees-of-freedom, respectively. Two specific test sizes ($\alpha = 0.01$ and $\alpha = 0.05$) are considered. Each estimate of α ($\hat{\alpha}$) and each estimate of power ($1 - \hat{\beta}$) involves a set of 100,000 simulations based on transformed real uniform random numbers on $[0,1)$ generated from a common seed using REAL FUNCTION UNI. If U is a value generated by REAL FUNCTION UNI, then the associated normal and Cauchy distribution values are $\Psi(U)$ and $\tan[\pi(U - 0.5)]$, respectively, where $\Psi(U)$ is a standard normal quantile approximation given in Kennedy and Gentle (1980, pp. 90–95). Each comparison involves two groups, where the first group is a control group and the location of the second group is shifted by a specified amount for each dimension (ϵ_1, ϵ_2), which depends on the probability distribution in question, the group sizes, and the specified correlation. Of course, no location shifts are used to evaluate $\hat{\alpha}$, and the prescribed location shifts are applied to both dimensions in the second group to obtain $1 - \hat{\beta}$. Both equal ($n_1 = n_2 = 20$) and unequal ($n_1 = 30$, $n_2 = 15$) sample sizes are considered, and ϵ_1 and ϵ_2 are applied in the same direction for each dimension to the subjects in the second group. Finally, five specified correlations are considered: $R = -0.8$, $R = -0.6$, $R = 0.0$, $R = +0.6$, and $R = +0.8$, where R is the Pearson product-moment correlation coefficient. Mielke and Berry (1994, 1999) consider three additional bivariate probability distributions in addition to the normal and Cauchy: the bivariate uniform, bivariate exponential, and bivariate lognormal.

The P-values for the permutation tests are based on the Pearson type III approximation. Computation of P-values by resampling where each P-value is based on $L = 100,000$ is impractical for the present purpose since $100,000^2$ simulations are computationally overwhelming. The three permutation tests consist of (1) Euclidean commensuration, (2) Hotelling commensuration with $v = 1$, and (3) Hotelling commensuration with $v = 2$,

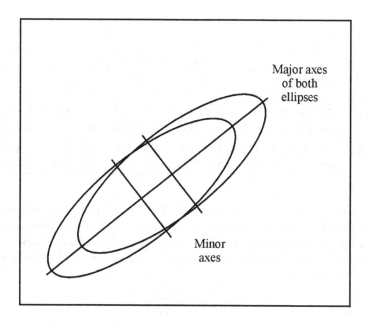

FIGURE 2.11. Bivariate location shifts where Euclidean commensuration is superior to Hotelling commensuration.

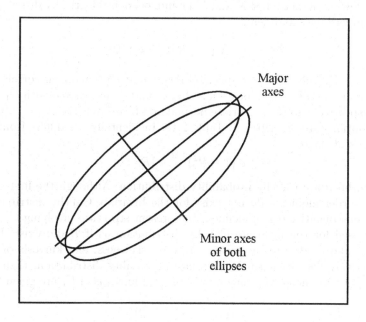

FIGURE 2.12. Bivariate location shifts where Hotelling commensuration is superior to Euclidean commensuration.

TABLE 2.18. Bivariate location shifts (ϵ_1, ϵ_2) for sample configurations, five specified correlations, and two probability distributions.

		Specified correlations (R)									
Distri-	Sample	−0.8		−0.6		0.0		+0.6		+0.8	
bution	sizes	U_1	U_2	U_1	U_2	U_1	U_2	U_1	U_2	U_1	U_2
Normal	20, 20	0.4	0.4	0.5	0.5	0.6	0.6	0.7	0.7	0.8	0.8
	30, 15	0.3	0.5	0.4	0.6	0.5	0.7	0.6	0.8	0.7	0.9
Cauchy	20, 20	1.2	1.2	1.5	1.5	1.8	1.8	2.1	2.1	2.4	2.4
	30, 15	0.9	1.5	1.2	1.8	1.5	2.1	1.8	2.4	2.1	2.7

which is the permutation version of the BNP trace test. Also included is the BNP trace test under the usual normality assumptions. Because only two groups are considered, the BNP trace test reduces to the two-sample Hotelling T^2 test. Thus, the probability values of the modified observed BNP trace statistic,

$$\frac{(n_1 + n_2 - r - 1)\, T^2}{(n_1 + n_2 - 2)\, r},$$

are obtained from Snedecor's F distribution with r *df* in the numerator and $n_1 + n_2 - r - 1$ *df* in the denominator.

The bivariate ($r = 2$) correlated response data sets were constructed in the following manner. Let X and Y be independent identically distributed random variables and define

$$U_1 = X\left(1 - R^2\right)^{1/2} + YR$$

and $U_2 = Y$, where R is the specified Pearson product-moment correlation between U_1 and U_2. The location shifts, ϵ_1 and ϵ_2, associated with U_1 and U_2, respectively, for the bivariate normal and bivariate Cauchy probability distributions are described in Table 2.18. Incidentally, U_1 differs from U_2 by the scale factor

$$\left(1 - R^2\right)^{1/2} + |R|$$

for the bivariate Cauchy probability distribution. Although the first- and second-order moments do not exist for the bivariate Cauchy distribution and, consequently, R is undefined, the present structure involving U_1 and U_2 is used for the bivariate Cauchy distribution as if R did exist. If μ, σ^2, γ_1, and γ_2 denote the mean, variance, skewness, and kurtosis of U_2, respectively, for the normal univariate probability distribution, then the corresponding mean, variance, skewness, and kurtosis of U_1 are given by

$$\mu\left[\left(1 - R^2\right)^{1/2} + R\right],$$

$$\sigma^2,$$

$$\gamma_1 \left[\left(1 - R^2\right)^{3/2} + R^3 \right],$$

and

$$\gamma_2 \left[\left(1 - R^2\right)^{2} + R^4 \right],$$

respectively.

The verification of the linear transformation was tested in the following manner. A total of 10,000,000 independent (X, Y) pairs of pseudorandom numbers was generated for both of the bivariate probability distributions. The linear transformation of the paired X and Y values yielded U_1 and U_2, where R was specified to be -0.8, -0.6, 0.0, $+0.6$, and $+0.8$ for both of the bivariate probability distributions. Pearson product-moment correlations were obtained between the 10,000,000 paired values of U_1 and U_2 for both of the bivariate probability distributions and each of the five specified values of R. The results listed here indicate that the linear transformation works very well for the bivariate normal probability distribution. However, the bivariate Cauchy probability distribution yields results that deviate from the specified correlation values. Since even the first two moments do not exist for the bivariate Cauchy probability distribution, convergence cannot be expected and the Cauchy distribution remains an informative but pathological example.

R	Normal	Cauchy
-0.8	-0.80012	-0.88261
-0.6	-0.60007	-0.72612
0.0	$+0.00043$	-0.00000
$+0.6$	$+0.60050$	$+0.72612$
$+0.8$	$+0.80031$	$+0.88261$

An unanticipated result of the power analysis involves the orientation of the location shifts and the direction (negative or positive) of the bivariate correlation. Location shifts parallel to the major axis of the bivariate data scatterplot yield different results from location shifts of the same magnitude that are parallel to the minor axis of the bivariate data scatterplot. Experimental designs that yield combinations of negative or positive correlation and same- or opposite-signed location shifts are quite common. The following two bivariate examples illustrate the interaction between correlation and joint location shifts.

First, consider two negatively correlated variables such as weight and self-esteem of high-school students. Measurements on both variables are taken before and after the introduction of a three-month regimen of diet and fitness conditioning supervised by nutrition and exercise science personnel. The location shifts are opposite signed $(-, +)$ for weight and self-esteem, respectively, and the joint location shift is parallel to the major axis. A similar example would be two positively correlated variables and same-signed location shifts $(-, -$ or $+, +)$ where the joint location shift also is parallel to the major axis.

TABLE 2.19. Estimated test size $\hat{\alpha}$ and power $1 - \hat{\beta}$ for the bivariate normal distribution based on 100,000 simulations for five specified correlation values, $n_1 = n_2 = 20$, and the equal location shifts listed in Table 2.18.

		Permutation tests							Bartlett–
Corre-lation	Test size	Euclidean commensuration		Hotelling commensuration				Nanda–Pillai test	
				$v = 1$		$v = 2$			
R	α	$\hat{\alpha}$	$1 - \hat{\beta}$	$\hat{\alpha}$	$1 - \hat{\beta}$	$\hat{\alpha}$	$1 - \hat{\beta}$	$\hat{\alpha}$	$1 - \hat{\beta}$
−0.8	.01	.00971	.09375	.01011	.78848	.01012	.80911	.00996	.80696
	.05	.04838	.38817	.04969	.93034	.05134	.94308	.04913	.94021
−0.6	.01	.00962	.25004	.01011	.64997	.01012	.67393	.00996	.67081
	.05	.04804	.57848	.04969	.85307	.05134	.87407	.04913	.86972
0.0	.01	.01011	.38047	.01011	.35430	.01012	.37174	.00996	.36896
	.05	.04949	.62366	.04969	.60833	.05134	.63675	.04913	.62926
+0.6	.01	.01052	.39710	.01011	.28946	.01012	.30385	.00996	.30097
	.05	.04786	.63516	.04969	.53542	.05134	.56345	.04913	.55529
+0.8	.01	.01070	.47075	.01011	.34963	.01012	.36736	.00996	.36428
	.05	.04857	.70821	.04969	.60223	.05134	.63033	.04913	.62284

Second, consider two positively correlated variables such as the number of hours spent studying for an examination and scores on the examination for college sophomores. Measurements on both variables are taken before and after a two-week concentrated workshop designed to develop improved and efficient study skills. The location shifts are opposite-signed $(-, +)$ for hours spent studying and scores on the examination, respectively, and the joint location shift is parallel to the minor axis. A similar example would be two negatively correlated variables and same-signed $(-, -$ or $+, +)$ location shifts where the joint location shift also is parallel to the minor axis.

The results of the power analyses for the normal and Cauchy probability distributions are contained in Tables 2.19 through 2.22. Five specified correlation values $(R = -0.8, R = -0.6, R = 0.0, R = +0.6,$ and $R = +0.8)$ are evaluated, two alpha levels $(\alpha = 0.01$ and $\alpha = 0.05)$ are considered, equal $(n_1 = n_2 = 20)$ and unequal $(n_1 = 30, n_2 = 15)$ sample sizes are tested, and same-signed $(+, +)$ equal and unequal location shifts are examined. Because positive and negative correlations having the same absolute values are included, same-signed $(-, -$ or $+, +)$ and opposite-signed $(-, +$ or $+, -)$ location shifts yield essentially the same results. In Tables 2.19 through 2.22, each $\hat{\alpha}$ value and each $1 - \hat{\beta}$ value is based on 100,000 Monte Carlo simulations using a common seed of 29 for the pseudorandom number generator REAL FUNCTION UNI. Specific location shifts for each analysis are given in Table 2.18.

TABLE 2.20. Estimated test size $\hat{\alpha}$ and power $1 - \hat{\beta}$ for the bivariate normal distribution based on 100,000 simulations for five specified correlation values, $n_1 = 30$, $n_2 = 15$, and the unequal location shifts listed in Table 2.18.

		Permutation tests						Bartlett–	
		Euclidean		Hotelling commensuration				Nanda–	
Corre- lation	Test size	commensuration		$v = 1$		$v = 2$		Pillai test	
R	α	$\hat{\alpha}$	$1 - \hat{\beta}$	$\hat{\alpha}$	$1 - \hat{\beta}$	$\hat{\alpha}$	$1 - \hat{\beta}$	$\hat{\alpha}$	$1 - \hat{\beta}$
−0.8	.01	.01037	.10344	.01041	.79614	.01005	.81886	.00989	.81762
	.05	.04763	.40183	.04958	.93200	.05227	.94525	.05041	.94398
−0.6	.01	.01026	.26216	.01041	.65974	.01005	.68789	.00989	.68563
	.05	.04770	.58797	.04958	.85705	.05227	.87775	.05041	.87470
0.0	.01	.01045	.39234	.01041	.37066	.01005	.39257	.00989	.38915
	.05	.04958	.63589	.04958	.62279	.05227	.65297	.05041	.64855
+0.6	.01	.01037	.40885	.01041	.32461	.01005	.34372	.00989	.34095
	.05	.04818	.64735	.04958	.57173	.05227	.60064	.05041	.59521
+0.8	.01	.01031	.48506	.01041	.41634	.01005	.43832	.00989	.43560
	.05	.04879	.72092	.04958	.66536	.05227	.69426	.05041	.68979

2.11.1 The Normal Probability Distribution

The power analyses for the bivariate normal probability distribution are contained in Tables 2.19 and 2.20. Table 2.19 summarizes the power analyses based on the equal sample sizes and equal location shifts listed in Table 2.18. In Table 2.19, all $\hat{\alpha}$ values are very close to the specified α values. Inspection of Table 2.19 reveals that for $R = -0.8$ the Euclidean commensuration permutation test (EC) has low power relative to the three other tests, the Hotelling commensuration permutation test with $v = 1$ (HC1) has better power, the Hotelling commensuration permutation test with $v = 2$ (HC2) is the most powerful of the four tests, and the Bartlett–Nanda–Pillai trace test (BNP) has approximately the same power as HC2. These results hold for both $\alpha = 0.01$ and $\alpha = 0.05$. In general, the same pattern is observed for $R = -0.6$. For $R = 0.0$, a change is apparent. Here, for $\alpha = 0.01$, EC is the most powerful test, HC1 is the least powerful, and HC2 and BNP are intermediate in power and approximately equal. For $\alpha = 0.05$, HC2 is the most powerful test, BNP is next, EC is slightly less powerful than BNP, and HC1 is the least powerful test. These results are consistent with the findings in Mielke and Berry (1994), where only $R = 0.0$ was considered. It should be noted that, overall, there is very little difference in power among the four tests when $R = 0.0$. For $R = +0.6$ and $R = +0.8$, EC is the most powerful test, HC1 is the least powerful test, HC2 is slightly better than HC1, and BNP has about the same power as HC2. The results are consistent for both $\alpha = 0.01$ and $\alpha = 0.05$. While BNP

TABLE 2.21. Estimated test size $\hat{\alpha}$ and power $1 - \hat{\beta}$ for the bivariate Cauchy distribution based on 100,000 simulations for five specified correlation values, $n_1 = n_2 = 20$, and the equal location shifts listed in Table 2.18.

		Permutation tests						Bartlett–
		Euclidean		Hotelling commensuration				Nanda–
Corre-lation	Test size	commensuration		$v = 1$		$v = 2$		Pillai test
R	α	$\hat{\alpha}$	$1 - \hat{\beta}$	$\hat{\alpha}$	$1 - \hat{\beta}$	$\hat{\alpha}$	$1 - \hat{\beta}$	$\hat{\alpha}$	$1 - \hat{\beta}$
−0.8	.01	.00917	.21274	.00950	.70344	.00872	.35644	.00128	.24429
	.05	.04847	.46463	.04989	.82958	.05211	.49017	.01734	.39025
−0.6	.01	.00921	.35289	.00950	.66283	.00872	.31098	.00128	.19646
	.05	.04937	.60019	.04989	.81704	.05211	.45204	.01734	.34866
0.0	.01	.00939	.48505	.00950	.46964	.00872	.19990	.00128	.10471
	.05	.04989	.68774	.04989	.68014	.05211	.34354	.01734	.23931
+0.6	.01	.00954	.48485	.00950	.38577	.00872	.16894	.00128	.08703
	.05	.04953	.68873	.04989	.58348	.05211	.30091	.01734	.20629
+0.8	.01	.00947	.58832	.00950	.42648	.00872	.19141	.00128	.10650
	.05	.04942	.77449	.04989	.60909	.05211	.32107	.01734	.22759

is uniformly most powerful for detecting location shifts among a specified class of tests, neither EC nor HC1 belongs to this class of tests.

Table 2.20 summarizes the power analyses based on the unequal sample sizes and unequal location shifts listed in Table 2.18. For $R = -0.8$, EC has less power and the three other tests are similar and relatively more powerful, for both $\alpha = 0.01$ and $\alpha = 0.05$, as with equal sample sizes. For $R = -0.6$ the same pattern holds, but the differences are less extreme, and for $R = 0.0$ there are no appreciable differences among the four tests. For $R = +0.6$ and $R = +0.8$, EC is more powerful than the three other tests, HC2 and BNP are nearly identical, and HC1 is slightly more powerful than HC2 and BNP. This relationship is the same for $\alpha = 0.01$ and $\alpha = 0.05$.

For the bivariate normal probability distribution, when the joint location shift of U_1 and U_2 is parallel to the major axis (i.e., same-signed location shifts and positive R or opposite-signed location shifts and negative R), EC provides the most power. On the other hand, when the joint location shift of U_1 and U_2 is parallel to the minor axis (i.e., same-signed location shifts and negative R or opposite-signed location shifts and positive R), then HC2 and BNP provide the most power for the bivariate normal probability distribution. These results hold for equal and unequal sample sizes, equal and unequal location shifts, and $\alpha = 0.01$ and $\alpha = 0.05$.

TABLE 2.22. Estimated test size $\hat{\alpha}$ and power $1 - \hat{\beta}$ for the bivariate Cauchy distribution based on 100,000 simulations for five specified correlation values, $n_1 = 30$, $n_2 = 15$, and the unequal location shifts listed in Table 2.18.

Corre-lation	Test size	Permutation tests						Bartlett–Nanda–Pillai test	
		Euclidean commensuration		Hotelling commensuration					
				$v = 1$		$v = 2$			
R	α	$\hat{\alpha}$	$1 - \hat{\beta}$	$\hat{\alpha}$	$1 - \hat{\beta}$	$\hat{\alpha}$	$1 - \hat{\beta}$	$\hat{\alpha}$	$1 - \hat{\beta}$
−0.8	.01	.00991	.23353	.01008	.72430	.01079	.33957	.00243	.22628
	.05	.04641	.49575	.04757	.85421	.05121	.47794	.02478	.37736
−0.6	.01	.00996	.36613	.01008	.67803	.01079	.29223	.00243	.17987
	.05	.04664	.61871	.04757	.83798	.05121	.43727	.02478	.33489
0.0	.01	.01001	.46799	.01008	.45489	.01079	.18093	.00243	.09685
	.05	.04722	.67646	.04757	.66708	.05121	.31761	.02478	.22494
+0.6	.01	.00995	.50368	.01008	.38009	.01079	.16097	.00243	.08982
	.05	.04827	.70434	.04757	.55420	.05121	.27840	.02478	.19967
+0.8	.01	.01012	.60706	.01008	.44073	.01079	.19115	.00243	.11498
	.05	.04797	.79073	.04757	.59869	.05121	.31120	.02478	.22909

2.11.2   The Cauchy Probability Distribution

The power analyses for the bivariate Cauchy probability distribution are contained in Tables 2.21 and 2.22. Table 2.21 summarizes the power analyses based on the equal sample sizes and equal location shifts listed in Table 2.18. In Table 2.21, all $\hat{\alpha}$ values approximate the specified α values, except for the BNP $\hat{\alpha}$ values, which are substantially lower, due to the fact that the bivariate normality assumption is not met. Inspection of Table 2.21 indicates that for $R = -0.8$ and $\alpha = 0.01$, EC has low power relative to the three other tests, HC1 has the highest power, HC2 is third on power, and BNP has a little more power than EC. For $R = -0.6$, HC1 has the greatest power, EC is second, HC2 is third, and BNP is a distant fourth. For $R = 0.0$, $R = +0.6$, and $R = +0.8$, EC possesses the greatest power, HC1 is next in power, HC2 is a distant third, and BNP has, relatively speaking, exceedingly low power.

Table 2.22 summarizes the power analyses based on the unequal sample sizes and unequal location shifts listed in Table 2.18. In general, for $R = -0.8$ and $R = -0.6$, EC has low power, HC1 has the highest power, and HC2 and BNP are second and third in power, respectively, but are closer to EC than to HC1. An exception occurs for $R = -0.6$ and $\alpha = 0.05$ where, although HC1 still has the greatest power, EC has more power than either HC2 or BNP. For $R = 0.0$, $R = +0.6$, and $R = +0.8$, EC has the greatest power, HC1 is next, and HC2 and BNP are third and fourth in power, respectively.

For the bivariate Cauchy probability distribution, when the joint location shift of U_1 and U_2 is parallel to the major axis (i.e., same-signed location shifts and positive R or opposite-signed location shifts and negative R), EC provides the most power. However, when the joint location shift of U_1 and U_2 is parallel to the minor axis, i.e., same-signed location shifts and negative R or opposite-signed location shifts and positive R, then HC1 provides the most power. HC1 performs much better than HC2 for all cases of the bivariate Cauchy distribution due to the Euclidean nature of the HC1 distance function (i.e., $v = 1$). It is notable that the $\hat{\alpha}$ values closely approximate the specified α values for the three permutation tests, i.e., EC, HC1, and HC2, since the moment structure of the bivariate Cauchy distribution is undefined. These results hold for equal and unequal sample sizes, equal and unequal location shifts, and $\alpha = 0.01$ and $\alpha = 0.05$.

2.11.3   Noncentrality and Power

The present results provide data for examining linearity between the BNP test's noncentrality parameter (τ^2) and the estimated power $(1 - \hat{\beta})$ of the four multivariate tests. Since the BNP trace test in these simulations is the two-sample Hotelling T^2 test with $r = 2$, the noncentrality parameter for the BNP trace test (Anderson, 1984, p. 113) is given by

$$\tau^2 = \frac{n_1 \, n_2}{n_1 + n_2} \begin{pmatrix} \epsilon_1 \\ \epsilon_2 \end{pmatrix}' \begin{pmatrix} 1 & R \\ R & 1 \end{pmatrix}^{-1} \begin{pmatrix} \epsilon_1 \\ \epsilon_2 \end{pmatrix} = \frac{n_1 \, n_2 \left(\epsilon_1^2 - 2R\epsilon_1\epsilon_2 + \epsilon_2^2 \right)}{(n_1 + n_2)\left(1 - R^2\right)},$$

where ϵ_1 and ϵ_2 are the corresponding location shifts for U_1 and U_2 listed in Table 2.18. The 16 correlation values between τ^2 and $1 - \hat{\beta}$ given in Table 2.23 involve two values of α, two bivariate distributions, and four multivariate tests. Each of the correlation values in Table 2.23 is based on the ten paired τ^2 and $1 - \hat{\beta}$ values associated with the five values of R and the two distinct location shift and sample size combinations. High positive correlations occur for both the BNP and HC2 tests. Although high positive correlations also occur for HC1, the obviously reduced correlation value for the bivariate Cauchy probability distribution is attributed to the modified behavior of HC1 relative to BNP and HC2. In contrast to the three other tests, the negative correlation values obtained for EC indicate the entirely different nature of this test.

2.11.4   Synopsis

Considered in this section are completely randomized multivariate experimental designs in which a sample of subjects is randomly partitioned into g mutually exclusive groups that are randomly assigned to distinct treatments and in which the r response variables are correlated to some degree.

TABLE 2.23. Correlations between the noncentrality parameter τ^2 and estimated power $1 - \hat{\beta}$.

Distribution	Test size α	Euclidean commensuration	Hotelling commensuration		Bartlett–Nanda–Pillai test
			$v = 1$	$v = 2$	
Normal	0.01	−0.94335	0.99713	0.99606	0.99615
	0.05	−0.88708	0.98745	0.98503	0.98499
Cauchy	0.01	−0.91087	0.97128	0.98523	0.99191
	0.05	−0.89378	0.92641	0.97132	0.98537

Power comparisons are provided for four tests (a Euclidean commensuration permutation test, a Hotelling commensuration permutation test with $v = 1$, a Hotelling commensuration permutation test with $v = 2$, and the Bartlett–Nanda–Pillai trace test), two bivariate probability distributions (normal and Cauchy), five levels of correlation ($R = -0.8$, $R = -0.6$, $R = 0.0$, $R = +0.6$, and $R = +0.8$), two specified α values ($\alpha = 0.01$ and $\alpha = 0.05$), equal ($n_1 = n_2 = 20$) and unequal ($n_1 = 30$ and $n_2 = 15$) sample sizes, and equal and unequal location shifts.

For both bivariate probability distributions, EC has more power than HC1, HC2, or BNP when the location shifts are parallel to the major axis of the bivariate scatterplots of the correlated responses. This conclusion holds for equal and unequal sample sizes and for equal and unequal location shifts. For the bivariate normal probability distribution, HC2 and BNP have the highest power, HC1 has less power, and EC has the least power when the location shifts are parallel to the minor axis of the bivariate scatterplots of the correlated responses. These results hold for equal or unequal sample sizes and for equal or unequal location shifts. For the Cauchy probability distribution, HC1 has more power than HC2, BNP, and EC when the location shifts are parallel to the minor axis of the bivariate scatterplots of the correlated responses. For the uncorrelated ($R = 0.0$) bivariate probability distributions, EC has the highest power for the bivariate Cauchy distribution, and HC2 and BNP have the highest power for the bivariate normal probability distribution. The poor power characteristics attributed to the BNP trace test for the bivariate Cauchy distribution also pertain to the Lawley–Hotelling trace, Roy's maximum root, and Wilks' likelihood-ratio statistics since these four tests are equivalent when $g = 2$.

For reasons of utility and practicality, the power comparisons presented here are limited to bivariate distributions. It is clear, however, that the documented problems will be compounded for designs with three or more response variables. In these cases, there may exist complex correlation structures and/or directions of correlation among the r response variables, the distributions associated with the r response variables may be substantially different, the location shift may be a complex composite of major and minor axes in the r-dimensional scatterplot of data points, or combinations of these possibilities may exist.

In practice, even for the simple bivariate case, an investigator must be familiar enough with the data to know whether the underlying correlations are positive or negative. In addition, a correct anticipation of the directional changes of the location shifts is essential for choosing the appropriate statistic. In those cases where the directions of the underlying correlations or the location shifts cannot be anticipated in advance, it is recommended that all three permutation tests (i.e., EC, HC1, and HC2) be employed. For the true multivariate case with three or more response variables, the approach of employing all three permutation tests is seemingly unavoidable.

2.12 Summary

The motivation and description of multiresponse permutation procedures (MRPP) are presented in this chapter. The principal attractions of MRPP as an analysis procedure are a reliance on randomization and a choice of various distance functions. Both exact and approximate methods for obtaining P-values are described. The relationship of MRPP to classical univariate and multivariate statistical methods, based on $v = 2$, is described. The advantage of $v = 1$ over $v = 2$ is demonstrated for data involving extreme values, i.e., methods based on $v = 1$ are far more robust to violations of basic assumptions than methods based on $v = 2$. Analyses of multivariate correlated data may be vastly improved with new techniques based on normal and Cauchy distributions. Chapter 3 describes additional applications of MRPP.

3

Additional MRPP Applications

MRPP is an effective procedure for analyzing data in a wide variety of contexts. The ability to vary weighting and commensuration, utilize a variety of distance functions, include an excess group, measure agreement, accommodate extreme values, and incorporate both univariate and multivariate data make MRPP a powerful and versatile analysis technique. In this chapter, further applications of MRPP are described. Included are applications of MRPP to autoregressive patterns, two-way contingency tables, agreement measures, cyclic data, generalized runs tests, rank-order data, and environmental influence on educational achievement.

3.1   Autoregressive Pattern Detection Methods

Consider a variation of MRPP where $r \geq 1$, $g = N$, B is ∞, $n_i = 1$ ($i = 1, ..., g$), a meaningful ordering exists for the objects $\omega_1, ..., \omega_N$ (e.g., occurrences in time), $x'_I = [x_{1I}, ..., x_{rI}]$ denotes a vector of r response measurements for each of N objects ω_I ($I = 1, ..., N$), $M = N!$, and

$$\Delta_{I,J} = \left[\sum_{k=1}^{r} (x_{kI} - x_{kJ})^2 \right]^{v/2} .$$

Then, the variation of the MRPP statistic given by

$$\delta = \frac{1}{N-1} \sum_{I=2}^{N} \Delta_{I-1,I}$$

suggests first-order autoregressive occurrences when δ is small (Mielke, 1991; Walker et al., 1997). Thus, the P-value $= P(\delta \leq \delta_o \,|\, H_0)$ and the mean, variance, and skewness of δ under H_0 are given by

$$\mu = D(1),$$

$$\sigma^2 = \frac{N-2}{N(N-1)^2} \left[(N-1) D(2) - 2 (N-2) D(2') + (N-3) D(2'') \right],$$

and

$$\gamma = \frac{(N-4)W}{N^2(N-1)^3 \sigma^3},$$

respectively, where

$$
\begin{aligned}
W = {} & (N-1)(N-2)D(3') - 6(N-2)^2 D(3) \\
& + 4(N-3)(N-5)D(3''''') \\
& + (N-2)(N-3) \left[3D(3'') + 4D(3^{***}) \right] \\
& + 4(N-2)D(3^*) + 6(N-3)(N-4) \left[D(3^{**}) - 2D(3''') \right]
\end{aligned}
$$

yields an approximate Pearson type III distribution P-value. The 12 definitional equations for $D(\cdot)$ are given in Section 2.3. If $r = 1$ and $v = 2$, this approach yields a permutation version of the Durbin and Watson (1950) test for serial correlation. For the special case when $r = v = 2$, the permutation test based on statistic δ is the randomization test due to Solow (1989) based on the Schoener (1981) t^2 statistic.

Suppose $N = ij + k$, where i, j, and k are integers such that $i \geq 1$, $j \geq 1$, and $0 \leq k < i$. Then, the jth order autoregressive pattern of this finite sequence is defined as

$$\omega_1, \ \omega_{j+1}, \ \omega_{2j+1}, \ ..., \ \omega_2, \ \omega_{j+2}, \ \omega_{2j+2}, \ ..., \ \omega_j, \ \omega_{2j}, \ ..., \ \omega_{ij}$$

and each partial sequence of objects (e.g., $\omega_2, \omega_{j+2}, \omega_{2j+2}, ...$) is completed before returning to the beginning of the sequence. Thus, $j - 1$ returns will occur for the jth order autoregressive pattern (N is fairly large and j is quite small in most applications). In the present context, the analysis of the jth order autoregressive pattern involves replacement of the first-order autoregressive pattern with the jth-order autoregressive pattern. Although the $j - 1$ returns may reduce the sensitivity of the test for detecting an alternative hypothesis, the permutation test is perfectly valid under H_0.

To illustrate an MRPP autoregressive analysis, consider two analyses of the first-order autoregressive patterns in the two sequential data sets listed in Table 3.1. Both these data sets consist of $N = 10$ sequential univariate values, i.e., $r = 1$. An exact permutation analysis with $v = 1$ of the first-order autoregressive pattern of data set 1 yields an observed δ (δ_o) given by $\delta_o = 1.8889$. The exact P-value of a δ as extreme or more extreme than δ_o is $1038/3{,}628{,}800 = 0.2860 \times 10^{-3}$. A resampling approximation

TABLE 3.1. Example data set for first-order autoregressive association.

Order	Data set 1	Data set 2
1	12	7
2	13	9
3	11	6
4	8	12
5	6	5
6	4	3
7	3	11
8	2	8
9	5	2
10	7	4

with $L = 1,000,000$ yields $\delta_o = 1.8889$ and a P-value of 0.2940×10^{-3}. The Pearson type III approximation yields $\delta_o = 1.8889$, $\mu = 4.6000$, $\sigma^2 = 0.6872$, $\gamma = -0.1628$, and $T_o = -3.2705$, with a P-value of 0.1163×10^{-2}. An exact permutation analysis with $v = 1$ of the first-order autoregressive pattern of data set 2 yields $\delta_o = 4.3333$ and the exact P-value of a δ as extreme or more extreme than δ_o is $2,515,248/3,628,800 = 0.6931$. A resampling approximation with $L = 1,000,000$ yields $\delta_o = 4.3333$ and a P-value of 0.6936. The Pearson type III approximation yields $\delta_o = 4.3333$, $\mu = 4.0222$, $\sigma^2 = 0.4607$, $\gamma = -0.1588$, and $T_o = 0.4584$, with a P-value of 0.6691. A first-order autoregressive pattern clearly exists for data set 1, but is not distinguishable for data set 2.

A typical autoregressive pattern investigation might involve the El Niño–La Niña association with sea-surface temperatures over time at a number of Pacific Ocean locations. Such an investigation could conceptually involve sea-surface temperature measurements at specific times of the annual cycle from, say, $r = 75$ locations during the past $N = 55$ years. The purpose of such an investigation is to establish the existence of, identify, and isolate an autoregressive pattern from purely chance phenomena. Other applications have involved determining the significance of spatial dependence in a geological setting (Walker et al., 1997).

As a specific example of the detection technique for identifying autoregressive patterns, consider an attempt to examine possible first- and second-order autoregressive patterns in the sequential data listed in Table 3.2 and displayed in Figure 3.1. These data consist of $N = 29$ sequential bivariate (x and y) values, i.e., $r = 2$. Since $29! = 0.8842 \times 10^{31}$, an exact permutation analysis is not feasible for these data. A resampling approximation analysis with $v = 1$ of the first-order autoregressive pattern with $L = 1,000,000$ yields $\delta_o = 1.5364$ and a P-value of 0.2500×10^{-3}. The Pearson type III approximation analysis yields $\delta_o = 1.5364$, $\mu = 2.1123$, $\sigma^2 = 0.0263$,

TABLE 3.2. Example data set for first- and
second-order autoregressive association.

Order	x	y
1	1.6	3.0
2	3.2	2.8
3	3.0	3.4
4	1.4	4.0
5	0.0	3.2
6	2.0	2.0
7	3.2	1.8
8	3.6	1.0
9	3.2	0.6
10	2.2	0.0
11	2.2	3.4
12	4.0	3.0
13	2.6	4.0
14	1.2	3.4
15	0.4	2.6
16	2.2	2.6
17	3.8	2.2
18	3.0	1.4
19	3.6	0.0
20	2.0	0.6
21	2.6	3.0
22	3.6	3.6
23	2.0	3.8
24	0.6	3.6
25	1.4	1.8
26	2.8	2.4
27	4.0	1.6
28	2.6	0.8
29	2.8	0.2

$\gamma = -0.1000$, $T_o = -3.5488$, and a P-value of 0.3694×10^{-3}. Also, a resampling approximation analysis with $v = 1$ of the second-order autoregressive pattern with $L = 1,000,000$ yields $\delta_o = 2.2546$ and a P-value of 0.8072. The Pearson type III approximation analysis yields $\delta_o = 2.2546$, $\mu = 2.1123$, $\sigma^2 = 0.0263$, $\gamma = -0.1000$, $T_o = 0.8775$, and a P-value of 0.8089. Although a first-order autoregressive pattern appears to exist, a second-order autoregressive pattern is not distinguishable from noise within these data.

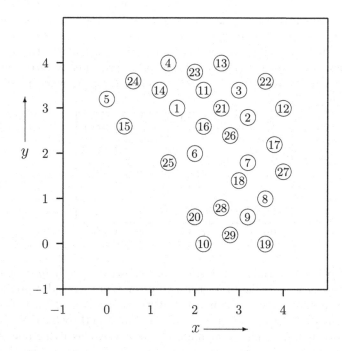

FIGURE 3.1. Plot of the autoregressive data in Table 3.2.

3.2   Asymmetric Two-Way Contingency Table Analyses

A common problem confronting researchers is the analysis of a cross-classification table where both variables are nominal, i.e., categorical; see Berry and Mielke, 1985a, 1986.[1] Goodman and Kruskal (1954) present an asymmetrical proportional-reduction-in-error prediction measure, t_a, for the analysis of a random sample of two cross-classified categorical variables. Consider a random sample of two cross-classified unordered polytomies, A and B, with A the dependent variable and B the independent variable. The Goodman and Kruskal (1954) statistic t_a is a measure of the relative reduction in prediction error where two types of errors are defined. The first type of error is the error in prediction based solely on knowledge of the distribution of the independent variable. This error is termed error of the

---

[1]Adapted and reprinted with permission of Sage Publications, Inc. from K.J. Berry and P.W. Mielke, Jr. Goodman and Kruskal's tau-b statistic: a nonasymptotic test of significance. *Sociological Methods & Research*, 1985, 13, 543–550. Copyright © 1985 by Sage Publications, Inc.

first kind (E_1) and consists of the expected number of errors when predicting the r independent variable categories from the observed distribution of the marginals of the independent variable. The second type of error is the error in prediction based on knowledge of the distribution of both the independent and dependent variables. This error is termed error of the second kind (E_2) and consists of the expected number of errors when predicting

B	A				Sum
	a_1	a_2	$\cdots$	a_g	
b_1	n_{11}	n_{12}	$\cdots$	n_{1g}	N_1
b_2	n_{21}	n_{22}	$\cdots$	n_{2g}	N_2
$\vdots$	$\vdots$	$\vdots$	$\ddots$	$\vdots$	$\vdots$
b_r	n_{r1}	n_{r2}	$\cdots$	n_{rg}	N_r
Sum	n_1	n_2	$\cdots$	n_g	N

the r independent variable categories from knowledge of the g dependent variable categories. To illustrate the two error types, consider predicting b_1 only from knowledge of its marginal distribution, $N_1, ..., N_r$. It is clear that N_1 out of N cases are in category b_1, but exactly which N_1 of the N cases are unknown. The probability of incorrectly classifying one of the N cases in category b_1 by chance is $(N - N_1)/N$. Since there are N_1 such classifications required, the number of expected erroneous classifications is $N_1(N - N_1)/N$ and, for all r categories of B, the independent variable, the number of expected errors of the first kind is given by

$$E_1 = \sum_{i=1}^{r} \frac{N_i (N - N_i)}{N}.$$

To predict $n_{11}, ..., n_{r1}$ from the dependent category a_1, the probability of incorrectly classifying one of the n_1 cases in cell n_{11} by chance is $(n_1 - n_{11})/n_1$. Since there are n_{11} such classifications required, the number of incorrect classifications is $n_{11}(n_1 - n_{11})/n_1$ and, for all gr cells, the number of expected errors of the second kind is given by

$$E_2 = \sum_{j=1}^{g} \sum_{i=1}^{r} \frac{n_{ij} (n_j - n_{ij})}{n_j}.$$

Goodman and Kruskal's t_a statistic is then defined as

$$t_a = \frac{E_1 - E_2}{E_1}.$$

A computed value of t_a indicates the proportional reduction in prediction error given knowledge of the distribution of the dependent variable A over

and above knowledge of only the distribution of the independent variable
B. Goodman and Kruskal's statistic t_a is an asymmetrical measure of association when polytomy B is the independent variable and polytomy A
is the dependent variable. As defined, t_a is a point estimator of Goodman
and Kruskal's population parameter τ_a for the population from which the
sample of N cases is obtained. If polytomy B is considered the dependent variable and polytomy A is considered the independent variable, then
Goodman and Kruskal's statistic t_b and parameter τ_b are analogously defined. For a 2×2 cross-classification table, t_a and t_b yield identical values
and are both equal to the squared Pearson fourfold point correlation, ϕ^2,
defined as

$$\phi^2 = \frac{\chi^2}{N},$$

where χ^2 is the Pearson chi-squared test statistic for a 2×2 cross-classification table. Note that ϕ^2 is a special case of the squared Pearson product-
moment correlation coefficient, r^2, for two dichotomous variables.

3.2.1 Development of the Problem

While parameter τ_a norms properly from 0 to 1, possesses a clear and
meaningful proportional-reduction-in-error interpretation (Costner, 1965),
and is characterized by high intuitive and factorial validity (Hunter, 1973),
statistic t_a presents difficulties whenever the null hypothesis (H_0) posits
that H_0: $\tau_a = 0$ (Margolin and Light, 1974). The problem is due to the fact
that t_a is not asymptotically normal when $\tau_a = 0$. Because, in practice, the
vast majority of null hypotheses test H_0: $\tau_a = 0$, the problem is pervasive
and the applicability of statistic t_a is severely circumscribed.

Although t_a and τ_a were developed by Goodman and Kruskal in 1954, it
was not until 1963 that the asymptotic normality was established and an
asymptotic variance was given for t_a, but only for $0 < \tau_a < 1$ (Goodman
and Kruskal, 1963). Unfortunately, the asymptotic variance for t_a given in
1963 was found to be incorrect, and it was not until 1972 that the correct
asymptotic variance for t_a when $0 < \tau_a < 1$ was obtained (Goodman
and Kruskal, 1972). In 1971, Light and Margolin (1971) developed R^2, an
analysis-of-variance technique for categorical response variables, sometimes
called CATANOVA. They apparently were unaware that R^2 was identical
to t_a and that they had asymptotically solved the longstanding problem of
testing H_0: $\tau_a = 0$. The identity between R^2 and t_a was first recognized by
Särndal (1974) and later discussed by Margolin and Light (1974), where
they showed that $t_a(N-1)(r-1)$ is asymptotically distributed as the
χ^2 distribution with $(r-1)(g-1)$ degrees-of-freedom under H_0: $\tau_a = 0$ as N becomes infinite. Haberman (1982) presented a general measure
of concentration for multinomial responses, which includes Goodman and
Kruskal's t_a for the special case involving a single independent variable.
An asymptotic test including both categorical and continuous independent

variables is provided by Haberman (1982) and, with a single independent variable, it is equivalent to the χ^2 test of Margolin and Light (1974).

3.2.2 A Nonasymptotic Solution

The Goodman and Kruskal (1963, 1972) test when $0 < \tau_a < 1$, the Margolin and Light (1974) test for $\tau_a = 0$, and the encompassing procedures of Haberman (1982) are all asymptotic solutions. To develop a nonasymptotic solution (Berry and Mielke, 1985a, 1986), consider two cross-classified un-ordered polytomies, A and B, with A the dependent variable where $r \geq 2$ and $g \geq 2$. If each of the N cases is represented by a binary column vector v of dimension r, with a single row entry set to 1 to indicate the classification of the case and the remaining $r - 1$ row entries set to 0, then an r by N matrix may be defined by $\mathbf{V} = [v_1, v_2, ..., v_N]$.

If $\Delta_{I,J} = 1 - v_I' v_J$, then $\Delta_{I,J}$ is 0 if $v_I = v_J$ and 1 otherwise. Thus, $\Delta_{I,J}$, the difference between cases I and J, is 1 if I and J occur in different rows (i.e., are different on the independent variable, B) of the observed cross-classification. The variation for categorical responses in the jth category of A $(j = 1, ..., g)$ is given by

$$\xi_j = \binom{n_j}{2}^{-1} \sum_{I<J} \Delta_{I,J} \Psi_j (v_I) \, \Psi_j (v_J),$$

where $\sum_{I<J}$ is the sum over all I and J such that $1 \leq I < J \leq N$ and $\Psi_j (v_1)$ is an indicator function that is 1 if v_1 belongs to the jth category of A and 0 otherwise for $j = 1, ..., g$. Thus defined, the value of ξ_j represents the average between-case difference for all $\binom{n_j}{2}$ differences within the jth category of the dependent variable A and is zero when all cases in the jth category are concentrated in a single category of the independent variable B.

The MRPP test statistic of interest is the weighted average of the ξ_j values $(j = 1, ..., g)$ and is given by

$$\delta_a = \sum_{j=1}^{g} C_j \xi_j,$$

where $K = N$ (i.e., no excess group), $\sum_{j=1}^{g} C_j = 1$, and $C_j = (n_j - 1)/(K-g)$ for $j = 1, ..., g$. Thus, in an analysis-of-variance context, C_j is the proportion of the within degrees-of-freedom contributed by the jth category of the dependent variable, A. The present choice of $C_j = (n_j - 1)/(K - g)$ dictates the relationship between t_a and δ_a, but a corresponding test based on $C_j = n_j/K$ would be a natural alternative since degrees-of-freedom are meaningless in the permutation context.

An efficient computational form for δ_a is

$$\delta_a = \frac{N - \sum\limits_{i=1}^{r}\sum\limits_{j=1}^{g} \frac{n_{ij}^2}{n_j}}{N - g},$$

and t_a, defined in terms of δ_a, may be obtained by

$$t_a = 1 - \frac{N\,(N-g)\,\delta_a}{N^2 - \sum\limits_{i=1}^{r} N_i^2} = \frac{N\sum\limits_{i=1}^{r}\sum\limits_{j=1}^{g}\frac{n_{ij}^2}{n_j} - \sum\limits_{i=1}^{r} N_i^2}{N^2 - \sum\limits_{i=1}^{r} N_i^2}.$$

Under H_0: $\tau_a = 0$, each of the

$$M_a = \frac{N!}{\prod\limits_{j=1}^{g} n_j!}$$

possible permutations of the N cases over the g categories of the dependent variable A is equally probable with n_j fixed ($j = 1, ..., g$). The exact probability of the observed t_a value is the proportion of the M_a possible values of t_a equal to or greater than the observed t_a value or, equivalently, the proportion of δ_a values equal to or less than the observed δ_a value. Alternatively, a resampling approximation or a moment approximation based on the Pearson type III probability distribution may be used. Because the Pearson type III distribution is a standardized gamma distribution, it includes the χ^2 distribution as a special case. This variation of MRPP yields a major computational simplification since the symmetric function model parameters analytically simplify from their definitional sum forms to the easily computed polynomial forms given by

$$D\,(1) = D(2) = D(3) = R_1/N^{(2)},$$

$$D\,(2') = D(3') = (R_2 - R_1)\,/N^{(3)},$$

$$D\,(3^*) = (2R_2 - NR_1)\,/N^{(3)},$$

$$D\,(2'') = D\,(3'') = \left[R_1\,(R_1 + 2) - 4R_2\right]\Big/N^{(4)},$$

$$D\,(3^{**}) = \left[R_3 - (N + 4)\,R_2 + R_1\,(R_1 + N + 1)\right]\Big/N^{(4)},$$

$$D\,(3^{***}) = (R_3 - 3R_2 + 2R_1)\,/N^{(4)},$$

$$D\,(3''') = \left[R_2\,(R_1 + 4N + 14) - 6R_3 - R_1\,(5R_1 + 2N + 4)\right]\Big/N^{(5)},$$

TABLE 3.3. Cross-classification of political party affiliation (A) and candidate preference (B).

Preference	Affiliation (A)			
(B)	a_1	a_2	a_3	Sum
b_1	5	1	3	9
b_2	47	6	2	55
Sum	52	7	5	64

and

$$D\left(3''''\right) = \left[R_1\left(R_1^2 + 30R_1 + 8N + 16\right) + 40R_3\right.$$
$$\left. - R_2\left(12R_1 + 24N + 64\right)\right] \Big/ N^{(6)},$$

where

$$N^{(m)} = \frac{N!}{(N-m)!}$$

for $m = 1, ..., 6$;

$$R_k = \sum_{i=1}^{r} N_i(N - N_i)^k$$

for $k = 1, 2,$ and 3; and

$$N_i = \sum_{I=1}^{g} n_{iI}$$

for $i = 1, ..., r$. A necessary condition for the asymptotic normality of the MRPP statistic is that $D\left(2'\right) - D\left(2''\right) \to \epsilon$ as $N \to \infty$, where $\epsilon > 0$ (O'Reilly and Mielke, 1980). An interesting feature in the present context is that

$$D\left(2'\right) - D\left(2''\right) = -\frac{(r-1)\,N^2\,(N-r)}{r^2 N^{(4)}}$$

if $N_i = N/r$ for $i = 1, ..., r$. Thus, asymptotic normality of the MRPP statistic can never occur in this instance since $D(2') - D(2'')$ converges to 0 as $N \to \infty$.

3.2.3 Examples

Suppose $N = 64$ individuals are asked about their political party affiliation (variable A) and preference for one of two political candidates (variable B). The results are given in Table 3.3. Variable A consists of three categories: Republican (a_1), Democrat (a_2), and Independent (a_3). Variable B consists of two categories: candidates I (b_1) and II (b_2). If the null hypothesis posits that political party affiliation (A) does not depend on candidate preference (B), then H_0: $\tau_a = 0$,

$$v_1 = \begin{bmatrix} 1 \\ 0 \end{bmatrix}, \quad v_2 = \begin{bmatrix} 1 \\ 0 \end{bmatrix}, \quad v_3 = \begin{bmatrix} 1 \\ 0 \end{bmatrix}, ..., \quad v_{64} = \begin{bmatrix} 0 \\ 1 \end{bmatrix},$$

and

$$V = \begin{bmatrix} 1 & 1 & 1 & 0 & 0 & 1 & 0 & 0 & \cdots & 0 \\ 0 & 0 & 0 & 1 & 1 & 0 & 1 & 1 & \cdots & 1 \end{bmatrix}.$$

For these data, $N = 64$, $r = 2$, $v = 1$, $g = 3$, $K = N$, $n_1 = 52$, $n_2 = 7$, $n_3 = 5$, $C_j = (n_j - 1)/(K - g)$, and the specified truncation constant (also termed B) is ∞. The $\binom{64}{2}$ $\Delta_{I,J}$ values are $\Delta_{1,2} = 0$, $\Delta_{1,3} = 0$, $\Delta_{1,4} = 2^{1/2}, \Delta_{1,5} = 2^{1/2}, ..., \Delta_{63,64} = 0$, $\xi_1 = \binom{5}{2}^{-1}(6 \times 2^{1/2}) = 0.8485$, $\xi_2 = \binom{7}{2}^{-1}(6 \times 2^{1/2}) = 0.4041$, $\xi_3 = \binom{52}{2}^{-1}(235 \times 2^{1/2}) = 0.2506$, and $\delta_a = [(5-1)/(64-3)](0.8485) + [(7-1)/(64-3)](0.4041) + [(52-1)/(64-3)](0.2506) = 0.3049$. Thus, the MRPP analysis yields $\delta_a = 0.3049$, $\mu_a = 0.3472$, $\sigma_a^2 = 0.1352 \times 10^{-3}$, $\gamma_a = -3.1423$, $T_a = -3.6392$, and $t_a = 0.1497$. A computed value of $t_a = 0.1497$ indicates a 15 percent reduction in the number of prediction errors given knowledge of the distribution of candidate preference (B) over knowledge of only the distribution of political party affiliation (A). The adjusted t_a value of Margolin and Light (1974) is $t_a(N - 1)(r - 1) = (0.1497)(64 - 1)(2 - 1) = 9.4324$ and, with $(r - 1)(g - 1) = (2 - 1)(3 - 1) = 2$ degrees-of-freedom (df), the asymptotic χ^2 P-value is 0.8949×10^{-2}. In comparison, a resampling approximation with $L = 1,000,000$ yields a P-value of 0.2281×10^{-1}, the Pearson type III P-value is 0.1412×10^{-1}, and the exact P-value is 0.2290×10^{-1}.

It should be noted that the skewness of t_a under the asymptotic model is 2.0 because the asymptotic distribution is χ^2 with 2 df, thus causing the asymptotic skewness of t_a to be $(8/df)^{1/2} = 2.0$. In contrast, the nonasymptotic skewness of t_a is 3.1423 (the sign is reversed due to the relationship between t_a and δ_a). The use of the asymptotic skewness value instead of the nonasymptotic skewness value often yields questionable probability values since the asymptotic assumption is not satisfied.

If, for illustrative purposes, the null hypothesis posits that candidate preference (B) does not depend on political party affiliation (A) in this particular election, then Table 3.3 can be transposed, H_0: $\tau_b = 0$,

$$v_1 = \begin{bmatrix} 1 \\ 0 \\ 0 \end{bmatrix}, \quad v_2 = \begin{bmatrix} 1 \\ 0 \\ 0 \end{bmatrix}, \quad v_3 = \begin{bmatrix} 1 \\ 0 \\ 0 \end{bmatrix}, ..., \quad v_{64} = \begin{bmatrix} 0 \\ 0 \\ 1 \end{bmatrix},$$

and

$$V = \begin{bmatrix} 1 & 1 & 1 & 0 & 0 & 0 & 0 & 0 & \cdots & 0 \\ 0 & 0 & 0 & 1 & 0 & 0 & 0 & 0 & \cdots & 0 \\ 0 & 0 & 0 & 0 & 1 & 1 & 1 & 1 & \cdots & 1 \end{bmatrix}.$$

For these data, $N = 64$, $r = 3$, $v = 1$, $g = 2$, $K = N$, $n_1 = 9$, $n_2 = 55$, $C_j = (n_j - 1)/(K - g)$, and the specified truncation constant is ∞. The $\binom{64}{2}$ $\Delta_{I,J}$ values are $\Delta_{1,2} = 0$, $\Delta_{1,3} = 0$, $\Delta_{1,4} = 2^{1/2}$, $\Delta_{1,5} = 2^{1/2}$, ..., $\Delta_{63,64} = 0$, $\xi_1 = \binom{9}{2}^{-1}(23 \times 2^{1/2}) = 0.9035$, $\xi_2 = \binom{55}{2}^{-1}(388 \times 2^{1/2}) = 0.3695$, and $\delta_b = [(9-1)/(64-2)](0.9035) + (55-1)/(64-2)](0.3695) = 0.4384$. Thus, the MRPP analysis yields $\delta_b = 0.4384$, $\mu_b = 0.4623$, $\sigma_b^2 = 0.6691 \times 10^{-4}$, $\gamma_b = -3.3112$, $T_b = -2.9186$, and $t_b = 0.6670 \times 10^{-1}$. A value of $t_b = 0.6670 \times 10^{-1}$ indicates a seven percent reduction in the number of prediction errors given knowledge of the distribution of political party affiliation (A) over knowledge of only the distribution of candidate preference (B). The adjusted t_b value of Margolin and Light (1974) is $t_b(N - 1)(r - 1) = (0.6670 \times 10^{-1})(64 - 1)(3 - 1) = 8.4039$ and, with $(r - 1)(g - 1) = (3 - 1)(2 - 1) = 2$ df, the asymptotic χ^2 P-value is 0.1497×10^{-1}. In comparison, a resampling approximation with $L = 1,000,000$ yields a P-value of 0.1891×10^{-1}, the Pearson type III P-value is 0.2464×10^{-1}, and the exact P-value is 0.1895×10^{-1}. For this example, the skewness of t_b under the asymptotic model is 2.0, whereas the nonasymptotic skewness is 3.3112.

The previous examples illustrate that the asymptotic approach yields probability values that may be questionable. The skewness specified by the asymptotic model may differ considerably from the nonasymptotic skewness value whenever cross-classification tables possess unbalanced marginals, a condition commonly encountered in survey research. Although the asymptotic and nonasymptotic tests routinely yield similar results when large samples and balanced marginals are encountered, the nonasymptotic test is superior for small samples and/or unbalanced marginals.

A further example shows that the P-values associated with t_a and t_b may be exceedingly different for a given contingency table. The data of this example consist of $N = 77$ responses involving a 3×5 contingency table.

4	7	2	9	0	22
1	5	2	7	5	20
4	5	9	17	0	35
9	17	13	33	5	77

For the t_a analysis, $N = 77$, $r = 3$, $v = 1$, $g = 5$, $K = N$, $n_1 = 9$, $n_2 = 17$, $n_3 = 13$, $n_4 = 33$, $n_5 = 5$, $C_j = (n_j - 1)/(K - g)$, and the specified truncation constant is ∞. The MRPP analysis for t_a yields $\delta_a = 0.8439$, $\mu_a = 0.9232$, $\sigma_a^2 = 0.6053 \times 10^{-3}$, $\gamma_a = -0.9264$, $T_a = -3.2195$, and $t_a = 0.1339$. The exact P-value is 0.6859×10^{-2}, a resampling P-value with $L = 1,000,000$ is 0.6992×10^{-2}, and the Pearson type III P-value is

0.6874×10^{-2}. The adjusted t_a value is $t_a(N-1)(r-1) = (0.1339)(77 - 1)(3-1) = 20.3528$ and, with $(r-1)(g-1) = (3-1)(5-1) = 8$ df, the asymptotic χ^2 P-value is 0.9072×10^{-2}. For the t_b analysis, $N = 77, r = 5$, $v = 1, g = 3, K = N, n_1 = 22, n_2 = 20, n_3 = 35, C_j = (n_j - 1)/(K - g)$, and the specified truncation constant is ∞. The MRPP analysis for t_b yields $\delta_b = 1.0174, \mu_b = 1.0334, \sigma_b^2 = 0.2308 \times 10^{-3}, \gamma_b = -1.2436, T_b = -1.0468$, and $t_b = 0.4130 \times 10^{-1}$. The exact P-value is 0.1380, a resampling P-value with $L = 1,000,000$ is 0.1380, and the Pearson type III P-value is 0.1402. The adjusted t_b value is $t_b(N-1)(r-1) = (0.4130 \times 10^{-1})(77-1)(5-1) = 12.5552$ and, with $(r-1)(g-1) = (5-1)(3-1) = 8$ df, the asymptotic χ^2 P-value is 0.1281.

3.2.4 Null Hypotheses

If the population models associated with τ_a and τ_b involve p_{ij} being the limit of n_{ij}/N as $N \to \infty$, $p_{i.} = \sum_{j=1}^{g} p_{ij}$, $p_{.j} = \sum_{i=1}^{r} p_{ij}$, and $p_{..} = 1$, then τ_a and τ_b can be defined as

$$\tau_a = \frac{\displaystyle\sum_{j=1}^{g}\sum_{i=1}^{r} \frac{p_{ij}^2}{p_{.j}} - \sum_{i=1}^{r} p_{i.}^2}{1 - \displaystyle\sum_{i=1}^{r} p_{i.}^2}$$

and

$$\tau_b = \frac{\displaystyle\sum_{i=1}^{r}\sum_{j=1}^{g} \frac{p_{ij}^2}{p_{i.}} - \sum_{j=1}^{g} p_{.j}^2}{1 - \displaystyle\sum_{j=1}^{g} p_{.j}^2},$$

respectively. Consequently, H_0: $\tau_a = 0$ or H_0: $\tau_b = 0$ implies that

$$\sum_{i=1}^{r}\left(\sum_{j=1}^{g} \frac{p_{ij}^2}{p_{.j}} - p_{i.}^2\right) = \sum_{i=1}^{r}\sum_{j=1}^{g} \frac{(p_{ij} - p_{i.}p_{.j})^2}{p_{.j}} = 0$$

or

$$\sum_{j=1}^{g}\left(\sum_{i=1}^{r} \frac{p_{ij}^2}{p_{i.}} - p_{.j}^2\right) = \sum_{j=1}^{g}\sum_{i=1}^{r} \frac{(p_{ij} - p_{i.}p_{.j})^2}{p_{i.}} = 0,$$

respectively. Thus, the null hypotheses $\tau_a = 0$, $\tau_b = 0$, and independence ($p_{ij} = p_{i.}p_{.j}$ for $i = 1, ..., r$ and $j = 1, ..., g$) are equivalent. Power comparisons between the asymptotic and nonasymptotic tests based on statistics t_a and t_b were conducted on four different table configurations ($r \times g = 2 \times 4$, 3×4, 4×4, and 5×4) with two sample sizes ($N = 20$ and $N = 50$) (Berry and Mielke, 1988a). Each of the eight combinations of r by g and N was analyzed under both the null hypothesis, where each cell proportion, p_{ij}, was set equal to $1/(rg)$, and a selected alternative hypothesis designed to produce probability values within the range of the significance levels of interest, i.e., $\alpha = 0.10$, 0.05, and 0.01.

3.2.5   Extension to Multiple Binary Choices

Instead of the Goodman and Kruskal test's restriction to one value of $x_{I1}, ..., x_{Ir}$ being 1 and the remaining $r-1$ values being 0, consider the case where each of the r x_{Ij} values can be 1 or 0 (Berry and Mielke, 2003a).[2] Even though analyses of these multivariate data are a direct application of MRPP, the following paragraph shows that this approach was not considered.

Surveys and other studies often include questions for which respondents may select any number of categories, i.e., cafeteria or multiple-response questions. Coombs (1964, pp. 295–297, 305–317) and Levine (1979) refer to this type of question as a "pick any/r" type question, where "pick any/r" instructs the subject to choose any or all of r categories. For example, subjects may be requested to list every magazine to which they subscribe, queried as to which attributes they like about a service or product, or asked to choose names of friends from a list of classmates. Frequently, it is of interest to determine whether the multiple responses differ among specified groups. However, multiple-response questions are often difficult to analyze as the answers are not independent (Agresti and Liu, 1999; Babbie, 2001, p. 240; Stark and Roberts, 1996, p. 159). Current methods that are used to analyze multiple-response data are limited to assessments of contingency, independence, and the magnitude of predictive association among the responses (Agresti and Liu, 1999, 2001; Bilder and Loughin, 2001; Bilder et al., 2000; Decady and Thomas, 2000; Loughin and Scherer, 1998; Umesh, 1995). These methods are not designed to test for differences among groups within the multiple-response structure.

The MRPP analysis of multiple binary category choices may be conceptualized as a binary argument problem in which N subjects choose any or all of r presented categories and the responses for each subject are coded as binary, i.e., 1 if the category is selected and 0 if the category is not selected. The subjects are a priori classified into g distinct groups and the groups are compared on the multiple responses. Specifically, let $\Omega = \{\omega_1, ..., \omega_N\}$ be a finite sample of subjects that is representative of a target population, let $x_{I1}, ..., x_{Ir}$ denote r binary response measurements for subject ω_I for

---

[2]Adapted and reprinted with permission of Psychological Reports from K.J. Berry and P.W. Mielke, Jr. Permutation analysis of data with multiple binary category choices. *Psychological Reports*, 2003, 92, 91–98. Copyright © 2003 by Psychological Reports.

$I = 1, ..., N$, and let $S_1, ..., S_g$ designate an exhaustive partitioning of the N subjects into g disjoint treatment groups of sizes $n_1, ..., n_g$ where $n_i \geq 2$ for $i = 1, ..., g$, $K = N$, and

$$\sum_{i=1}^{g} n_i = N.$$

The response of each of the N subjects is a single r-dimensional column vector of size $r \times 1$ in which each argument of the response vector is either a 0 or 1. The total number of distinct responses for a subject in this context is 2^r. Clearly, a simple 1-dimensional sum, or arithmetic mean, of the r 0 and 1 values for a single subject does not describe the data in question for the binary argument problem. The analysis of the multiple responses depends on the statistic given by

$$\delta = \sum_{i=1}^{g} C_i \xi_i,$$

where $C_i = n_i/N$.

The null hypothesis (H_0) of no differences in the response structures among the g groups specifies that each of the

$$M = \frac{N!}{\displaystyle\prod_{i=1}^{g} n_i!}$$

possible allocations of the N r-dimensional response measurements to the g treatment groups is equally likely. If $n_0 = 0$ and

$$N_i = N - \sum_{j=0}^{i-1} n_j,$$

then

$$M = \prod_{i=1}^{g-1} \binom{N_i}{n_i}.$$

Under H_0, the permutation distribution of δ assigns equal probabilities to the resulting M values of δ. Because small values of δ imply a concentration of similar scores within the g treatment groups, H_0 is rejected when the observed value of δ, δ_o, is small.

It is important to distinguish between the r-dimensional binary argument problem and an r-dimensional contingency table problem. The r-dimensional contingency problem has received considerable attention in the literature (Agresti and Liu, 1999, 2001; Bilder and Loughin, 2001; Bilder et al., 2000; Decady and Thomas, 2000; Loughin and Scherer, 1998; Umesh,

TABLE 3.4. Elementary school children: Reading example 1.

Girls			Boys		
A	B	C	A	B	C
1	0	0	0	0	1
1	0	1	1	0	1
1	1	0	0	1	1
1	1	0	1	0	1
1	1	0	0	0	0
0	1	1	0	0	1
1	1	1	0	1	1
1	1	0	0	0	1
			0	0	1
			0	0	1
			1	1	0

1995), whereas the binary argument problem has suffered from a lack of interest. To illustrate the permutation tests, consider three examples of applications in which g groups are compared on r responses and each respondent is allowed to select any one of the 2^r possible arrangements of categorical responses.

Example 1

Suppose that a class of elementary school children is assigned three books to read over the summer. Upon their return to school, the children are surveyed as to which of the three books they read. The $r = 3$ response categories are books A, B, and C, each of $N = 19$ students is allowed to choose any of the $2^3 = 8$ possible response arrangements, and the $g = 2$ groups consist of $n_1 = 8$ girls and $n_2 = 11$ boys. Table 3.4 lists the row vectors of observed binary responses from the eight possible response arrangements for each child, where a 1 indicates that a book was read and a 0 indicates that a book was not read.

The exact permutation analysis based on $M = 75,582$ possible allocations yields $\delta_o = 0.9520$ with an exact P-value of $685/75,582 = 0.009063$, the resampling permutation procedure based on $L = 1,000,000$ resamplings yields an approximate P value of 0.009086, and the Pearson type III moment approximation permutation analysis yields an approximate P-value of 0.007429. Because the exact analysis is obviously preferred for this example, the resampling and moment approximation P-values are included to demonstrate that they provide reasonable approximations to the exact P-value. In all three cases, there is a low probability that the differences in books read between girls and boys can be attributed to chance under H_0.

TABLE 3.5. Elementary school children: Reading example 2.

Girls		Boys	
A	B	A	B
1	0	1	1
1	0	1	1
1	0	1	1
1	0	1	1
1	0	1	1
1	0	1	1
0	1	0	0
0	1	0	0
0	1	0	0
0	1	0	0
0	1	0	0
0	1	0	0

Example 2

Some statistics are specifically designed to test for differences among responses and other statistics are designed to measure similarities among responses. In various studies it is commonplace to design experiments for which a test of differences is requisite, e.g., an F test in a one-way analysis of variance design. To clarify the function of the δ test statistic as a test for differences, consider a modification of the data in Example 1.

Suppose that a class of elementary school students is assigned two books to read over the summer, then the students are surveyed as to which of the two books they read. The $r = 2$ response categories are books A and B, each of $N = 24$ students may choose any of the $2^2 = 4$ possible response arrangements, and the $g = 2$ groups consist of $n_1 = 12$ girls and $n_2 = 12$ boys. In addition, assume that half of the girls read book A only and the other half of the girls read book B only, while half of the boys read both books and the other half of the boys read neither book. Table 3.5 lists the row vectors of observed binary responses from the four possible response arrangements for each child, where a 1 indicates that a book was read and a 0 indicates that a book was not read. In one sense, the data are the same for the girls and the boys, as there are 12 books read by both the girls and boys. In another sense, the data are different for the girls and the boys, as the selection of books read by the girls differs from the boys.

The exact permutation analysis based on $M = 2{,}704{,}156$ possible allocations yields $\delta_o = 0.7714$ with an exact P-value of $19{,}606/2{,}704{,}156 = 0.007250$, the resampling permutation procedure based on $L = 1{,}000{,}000$ resamplings yields an approximate P-value of 0.007172, and the Pearson type III moment approximation permutation analysis yields an approximate P-value of 0.007235. Thus, the δ test statistic detects the selection differences in reading choices between girls and boys.

Example 3

Consider a third example in which $N = 262$ Kansas pig farmers were asked, "What are your primary sources of veterinary information?" The farmers chose as many sources as applied from $r = 5$ response categories: (A) professional consultant, (B) veterinarian, (C) state or local extension service, (D) magazines, and (E) feed companies and representatives. The farmers were also asked their highest attained level of education, providing $g = 5$ educational groups with $n_1 = 88$ high school graduates, $n_2 = 16$ vocational school graduates, $n_3 = 31$ 2-year college graduates, $n_4 = 113$ 4-year college graduates, and $n_5 = 14$ other graduates. The data are from Bilder et al. (2000, p. 1287) and have been analyzed and discussed in an r-dimensional contingency table context by Loughin and Scherer (1998), Agresti and Liu (1999), Bilder et al. (2000), Decady and Thomas (2000), and Bilder and Loughin (2001). In this example, the veterinary information data are analyzed in an r-dimensional binary argument context.

Table 3.6 lists the frequencies and row vectors of the observed binary vectors from the $2^5 = 32$ possible response arrangements for each farmer, where a 1 indicates that the source of information was used and a 0 indicates that the information source was not used. An exact analysis of the veterinary information data is not feasible since $M \doteq 4.2196 \times 10^{144}$ is the number of possible permutations. The resampling permutation procedure based on $L = 1,000,000$ resamplings yields $\delta_o = 1.3601$ with an approximate P-value of 0.127263, and the Pearson type III moment approximation procedure yields an approximate P-value of 0.127958. Here, the δ test statistic detects no definitive differences in sources of veterinary information among the five educational groups.

3.3   Measurement of Agreement

A common problem in data analysis is the measurement of the degree of relationship between a nominal independent variable and a dependent variable, which may be nominal, ordinal, or interval. Some representative examples are the measured relationships between religious affiliation (Catholic, Jewish, Protestant) and voting behavior (Democrat, Independent, Republican), between gender (female, male) and any attitudinal question that is Likert-scaled (strongly agree, agree, disagree, strongly disagree), and between marital status (single, married, widowed, divorced) and number of work days missed each year (0, 1, 2, ...), respectively. Additionally, there may be interest in the degree of relationship between a nominal independent variable and a multivariate dependent variable such as an object's position

TABLE 3.6. Frequencies of responses for the veterinary information data from five information sources and level of education scored as high school (HS), vocational school (VS), 2–year college (2C), 4–year college (4C), and other (O).

Source of information					Level of education				
A	B	C	D	E	HS	VS	2C	4C	O
0	0	0	0	0	0	0	0	0	0
0	0	0	0	1	8	1	6	16	1
0	0	0	1	0	17	3	6	30	1
0	0	0	1	1	4	1	2	2	1
0	0	1	0	0	5	4	2	17	2
0	0	1	0	1	1	0	0	1	1
0	0	1	1	0	3	0	1	6	1
0	0	1	1	1	3	0	0	0	1
0	1	0	0	0	9	3	4	11	1
0	1	0	0	1	7	0	1	2	0
0	1	0	1	0	1	0	0	1	0
0	1	0	1	1	2	0	2	0	0
0	1	1	0	0	0	0	0	1	1
0	1	1	0	1	0	0	0	0	1
0	1	1	1	0	1	0	3	3	0
0	1	1	1	1	8	2	3	4	0
1	0	0	0	0	9	0	0	11	1
1	0	0	0	1	0	0	0	0	0
1	0	0	1	0	0	0	0	0	1
1	0	0	1	1	0	0	0	0	0
1	0	1	0	0	0	0	1	0	0
1	0	1	0	1	0	0	0	0	0
1	0	1	1	0	0	1	0	1	0
1	0	1	1	1	0	0	0	0	0
1	1	0	0	0	2	0	0	0	0
1	1	0	0	1	0	0	0	0	0
1	1	0	1	0	0	0	0	0	0
1	1	0	1	1	0	0	0	0	0
1	1	1	0	0	0	0	0	1	0
1	1	1	0	1	0	0	0	0	0
1	1	1	1	0	1	1	0	2	0
1	1	1	1	1	7	0	0	4	1

in a three-dimensional matrix defined by occupational prestige, income in dollars, and years of education, where a researcher may not want to suffer the loss of information engendered by compositing the three measurements into a univariate index of socioeconomic status. The generalized measure of agreement, $\Re$, provides for the analysis of a nominal independent variable with any number or combination of nominal, ordinal, or interval dependent variables (Berry and Mielke, 1992). As stated in Section 2.3.5, $\Re$ may be considered a measure of effect size.

3.3.1   Interval Dependent Variables

As in Chapter 2, let $\Omega = \{\omega_1, ..., \omega_N\}$ indicate a finite collection of N objects, let $x'_I = [x_{1I}, ..., x_{rI}]$ denote a vector of r commensurate interval-level response measurements for object ω_I $(I = 1, ..., N)$, and let $S_1, ..., S_g$ represent an exhaustive a priori partitioning of the N objects comprising Ω into g disjoint categories, where $n_i \geq 2$ is the number of objects in category S_i $(i = 1, ..., g)$. In addition, let

$$\Delta_{I,J} = \left[\sum_{k=1}^{r} (x_{kI} - x_{kJ})^2 \right]^{v/2}$$

be the symmetric distance function value of the r response measurements associated with objects ω_I and ω_J, where $v > 0$. If $v = 1$, then $\Delta_{I,J}$ is the ordinary Euclidean distance between response measurements. Let

$$\xi_i = \binom{n_i}{2}^{-1} \sum_{I<J} \Delta_{I,J} \Psi_i(\omega_I) \Psi_i(\omega_J)$$

represent the average between-object difference for all objects within category S_i $(i = 1, ..., g)$, where $\sum_{I<J}$ is the sum over all I and J such that $1 \leq I < J \leq N$, and $\Psi_i(\cdot)$ is an indicator function given by

$$\Psi_i(\omega_I) = \begin{cases} 1 & \text{if } \omega_I \in S_i, \\ 0 & \text{otherwise.} \end{cases}$$

Then, the average within-category difference, weighted by the number of objects n_i in category S_i $(i = 1, ..., g)$, is defined as

$$\delta = \sum_{i=1}^{g} C_i \xi_i,$$

where $C_i > 0$, $\sum_{i=1}^{g} C_i = 1$, and $C_i = n_i/N$ $(i = 1, ..., g)$.

Whenever there are multiple response measurements for each object (i.e., $r \geq 2$), the response variables may possess different units of measurement and must be made commensurate, i.e., rescaled to attain a standardization among the multivariate measurements. As in Chapter 2, let

$y'_I = [y_{1I}, ..., y_{rI}]$, where $I = 1, ..., N$, denote N noncommensurate r-dimensional values $(r \geq 2)$. The corresponding N Euclidean commensurate r-dimensional values $x'_I = [x_{1I}, ..., x_{rI}]$ for $I = 1, ..., N$ are given by $x_{jI} = y_{jI}/\phi_j$, where

$$\phi_j = \sum_{I < J} |y_{jI} - y_{jJ}|.$$

As defined, the Euclidean commensurated data have the desired property that

$$\sum_{I < J} |x_{jI} - x_{jJ}| = 1$$

for $j = 1, ..., r$. Euclidean commensuration ensures that the resulting inferences are independent of the units of the individual response measurements and invariant to linear transformations of the response measurements.

If δ_j denotes the jth value among the M possible values of δ, then the expected value of δ under H_0 is defined by

$$E[\delta \mid H_0] = \mu = \frac{1}{M} \sum_{j=1}^{M} \delta_j$$

and, since δ reflects differences within categories, the within-category measure of agreement is given by

$$\Re = 1 - \frac{\delta}{\mu}.$$

$\Re$ is a chance-corrected measure of both agreement and/or effect size, reflecting the amount of agreement in excess of what would be expected by chance. $\Re$ attains a maximum value of unity when the agreement between the nominal independent variable and the interval dependent variable(s) is perfect, i.e., dependent variable scores are identical within each of the g categories of the nominal independent variable. $\Re$ attains a value of zero when the agreement is equal to what is expected by chance (i.e., $E[\Re \mid H_0] = 0$). Like all chance-corrected measures, $\Re$ occasionally will be slightly negative when agreement is less than what is expected by chance.

Because $\Re$ is a simple linear transformation of δ, a test of significance for δ is also a test of significance for $\Re$. Thus, the probability value for an observed δ (δ_o) is the probability, under the null hypothesis, given by P-value $= P(\delta \leq \delta_o \mid H_0)$. The exact probability of the observed $\Re$ $(\Re_o)$ is the proportion of the M possible values of $\Re$ equal to or greater than $\Re_o$ or, equivalently, the proportion of δ values equal to or less than δ_o. Since $\Re$ is based on a permutation structure, it requires no simplifying assumptions about the underlying population distribution. Finally, $\Re$ is completely data dependent, i.e., all the information on which $\Re$ is based comes from the available sample.

TABLE 3.7. Semantic differential data with $N = 15$ subjects.

Subject	Gender	Semantic differential		
		Evaluation	Potency	Activity
1	F	4.5	5.5	3.9
2	F	2.4	6.0	2.7
3	F	2.7	5.8	3.8
4	F	3.6	6.5	4.5
5	F	4.3	5.6	4.0
6	F	2.5	5.9	2.8
7	F	2.8	5.7	4.0
8	F	3.5	6.4	4.4
9	M	6.4	3.5	6.1
10	M	5.6	4.2	5.5
11	M	5.2	3.1	5.6
12	M	6.2	3.6	6.0
13	M	5.7	4.3	5.7
14	M	5.2	3.0	5.8
15	M	6.1	3.6	6.2

Interval Example

Consider an example application where it is desired to measure the degree of agreement between gender, i.e., a nominal independent variable, and scores on three dimensions of the semantic differential, i.e., interval dependent variables. The semantic differential is based on ratings by subjects of a number of concepts (e.g., mother, fate, success) on a set of bipolar adjective scales (e.g., severe–lenient, active–passive, rational–intuitive). Osgood et al., (1957) factor analyzed the scales into the three well-known dimensions of evaluation, potency, and activity. These three dimensions are the ones usually employed in semantic differential research and have been replicated and corroborated in many different studies and populations. Let eight female subjects and seven male subjects be scored on the three dimensions of the semantic differential: evaluation, potency, and activity. The data are listed in Table 3.7. For these data, $N = 15$, $r = 3$, $v = 1$, $g = 2$, $K = N$, $n_1 = 8$, $n_2 = 7$, $C_i = n_i/N$, and B is ∞. The MRPP analysis with Euclidean commensuration yields $\delta_o = 0.7529 \times 10^{-2}$, $\mu = 0.1726 \times 10^{-1}$, $\sigma^2 = 0.1192 \times 10^{-5}$, $\gamma = -2.3142$, $T_o = -8.9137$, and $\Re_o = 0.5638$. In this example, the exact P-value of a δ equal to or less than $\delta_o = 0.7529 \times 10^{-2}$ is the probability of an $\Re$ value equal to or greater than $\Re_o = 0.5638$ is $1/6435 = 0.1554 \times 10^{-3}$. For comparison, a resampling approximation P-value with $L = 1{,}000{,}000$ is 0.1680×10^{-3}, and the Pearson type III P-value is 0.9864×10^{-4}.

3.3.2   Ordinal Dependent Variables

Researchers are often faced with the problem of measuring the degree of relationship between a nominal independent variable and one or more ordinal dependent variables. A number of measures of association have been advanced specifically for a nominal independent variable and a single ordinal dependent variable: Cureton's (1956, 1968) rank-biserial correlation coefficient, Freeman's (1965) theta (θ_{ON}), Crittenden and Montgomery's (1980) ν, which is a modification of Freeman's (1965) θ_{ON} to ensure a proportional-reduction-in-error interpretation, Agresti's (1981) $\bar{\alpha}$ and $\bar{\delta}$ measures, and Piccarreta's (2001) $\hat{\tau}_o$ coefficient. None of these measures has gained much popularity in the research literature. The rank-biserial correlation coefficient is defined only for a dichotomous nominal variable; consequently, its use is limited. Because the sampling distributions of both θ_{ON} and ν are unknown, the development of corresponding tests of significance has not been possible. In addition, because Cureton's (1956, 1968), Freeman's (1965), and Crittenden and Montgomery's (1980) measures are Kendall-type coefficients, they are based on unweighted agreements and inversions of paired-score differences. Because the scoring system codes any pairwise difference simply as the sign of the difference and ignores the magnitude of the difference, a substantial amount of information is lost in the process of measuring the relationship (Reynolds, 1977). Piccarreta's (2001) $\hat{\tau}_o$ coefficient is a generalization of Goodman and Kruskal's (1954) τ coefficient for a nominal independent variable and a nominal dependent variable.

Although the focus here is on measuring the relationship between a nominal independent variable and ordinal dependent variables, it should be noted that Hubert (1974) has defined θ_{NO}, a modification of Freeman's θ_{ON} for an ordinal independent variable and a nominal dependent variable. Again, the sampling distribution remains unknown. In addition, a symmetric version of Freeman's θ_{ON} has been independently proposed by Särndal (1974), Hubert (1974), Crittenden and Montgomery (1980), and Agresti (1981), which they term κ, θ_{SYM}, I (i.e., IOTA), and $\bar{\delta}$, respectively. Agresti (1981) has developed the asymptotic sampling distribution of $\bar{\delta}$. Finally, models for describing patterns of nominal/ordinal association (e.g., logit and log-linear) have been developed. For deficiencies of the model approach in this application, see Agresti (1981, pp. 527–528).

$\Re$ is directly applicable, without modification, to a nominal independent variable and dependent variables that are ordinal. Ordinal variables, in this context, include the range of dependent variables from fully ranked data, where each subject is assigned a unique rank from 1 to N based on the conversion of original scores to ranks, to having N subjects associated with a limited number of ordinal categories. This second case differs from the first in that an investigator does not have original data to convert to ranks but encounters only a crude ordering of the subjects into categories, such as low, medium, and high, in the data collection process. In such a case, a simple assignment of ordered values (such as 1, 2, and 3, to low, medium, and high, respectively) to the categories may be used rather than the assigned values associated with tied ranks. This attribute is especially important in the social sciences where categorical variables such as marital status (single, married, widowed, divorced) may be cross-classified with ordinal variables such as Likert scales where, a question is scored as strongly agree, agree, neutral, disagree, and strongly disagree.

Ordinal Example

Consider a second example, where it is desired to measure the degree of relationship between political affiliation (a nominal independent variable) and scores on two dimensions of socioeconomic status (ordinal dependent variables). Let 8 Democrats and 12 Republicans be scored on two ordinal dependent variables: years of education and occupational prestige, both measured in quintiles. The data are listed in Table 3.8. For these data, $N = 20$, $r = 2$, $v = 1$, $g = 2$, $K = N$, $n_1 = 8$, $n_2 = 12$, $C_i = n_i/N$, and B is ∞. The MRPP analysis with Euclidean commensuration yields $\delta_o = 0.6043 \times 10^{-2}$, $\mu = 0.8342 \times 10^{-2}$, $\sigma^2 = 0.7716 \times 10^{-7}$, $\gamma = -1.6169$, $T_o = -8.2767$, and $\Re_o = 0.2756$. The exact probability of an $\Re$ value equal to or greater than $\Re_o = 0.2756$ is $2/125{,}970 = 0.1588 \times 10^{-4}$. For comparison, a resampling approximation P-value with $L = 1{,}000{,}000$ is 0.1800×10^{-4}, and the Pearson type III P-value is 0.3366×10^{-4}.

3.3.3 Nominal Dependent Variables

$\Re$ is easily adapted to measure the degree of relationship between a nominal independent variable and a nominal dependent variable. If the categories of the dependent variable are considered as r dimensions of the variable, then each subject can be assigned a binary vector of length r with $r - 1$ values of 0 and a single value of 1 corresponding to the category of the dependent variable in which the subject is classified, e.g., for four categories labeled 'A,' 'B,' 'C,' and 'D' and a subject who has checked 'C,' $x' = [0\ 0\ 1\ 0]$.

Nominal Example

Consider a third example, where it is desired to measure the degree of relationship between rural–urban residence (a nominal independent variable) and marital status (a nominal dependent variable). Let 10 rural residents and 14 urban residents be classified on four dimensions of marital status: single, married, widowed, and divorced. The data are listed in Table 3.9. For these data, $N = 24$, $r = 4$, $v = 1$, $g = 2$, $K = N$, $n_1 = 10$, $n_2 = 14$, $C_i = n_i/N$, and B is ∞. The MRPP analysis with Euclidean commensuration yields $\delta_o = 0.4949 \times 10^{-2}$, $\mu = 0.6223 \times 10^{-2}$, $\sigma^2 = 0.7696 \times 10^{-7}$, $\gamma = -1.8283$, $T_o = -4.5916$, and $\Re_o = 0.2047$. The

TABLE 3.8. Socioeconomic status data with $N = 20$ subjects.

Subject	Political affiliation	Socioeconomic status	
		Education	Prestige
1	D	5	3
2	D	4	5
3	D	5	4
4	D	2	3
5	D	2	5
6	D	3	4
7	D	4	2
8	D	2	4
9	R	2	1
10	R	2	1
11	R	1	2
12	R	3	1
13	R	1	2
14	R	2	1
15	R	1	2
16	R	1	1
17	R	3	1
18	R	1	2
19	R	2	3
20	R	3	2

exact probability of an $\Re$ value equal to or greater than $\Re_o = 0.2047$ is $7657/1{,}961{,}256 = 0.3904 \times 10^{-2}$. For comparison, a resampling approximation P-value with $L = 1{,}000{,}000$ is 0.3963×10^{-2}, and the Pearson type III P-value is 0.3190×10^{-2}.

3.3.4 Mixed Dependent Variables

A distinctive advantage of the MRPP approach to measuring agreement is the ability to analyze sets of dependent variables that are mixed: nominal, ordinal, and/or interval. Each interval or ordinal dependent variable contributes one dimension to the analysis, and each nominal dependent variable contributes one dimension for each category of the nominal variable.

Mixed Example

Consider a fourth example where it is desired to measure the degree of relationship between religious affiliation (a nominal independent variable) and birth experience, measured as a mixture of three dependent variables: one

TABLE 3.9. Marital status data with $N = 24$ subjects.

Subject	Residence	Single	Married	Widowed	Divorced
			Marital status		
1	R	0	0	0	1
2	R	0	1	0	0
3	R	0	1	0	0
4	R	0	1	0	0
5	R	0	1	0	0
6	R	0	1	0	0
7	R	0	1	0	0
8	R	0	1	0	0
9	R	0	1	0	0
10	R	1	0	0	0
11	U	0	0	0	1
12	U	0	0	0	1
13	U	0	0	0	1
14	U	0	1	0	0
15	U	0	1	0	0
16	U	1	0	0	0
17	U	1	0	0	0
18	U	1	0	0	0
19	U	1	0	0	0
20	U	1	0	0	0
21	U	0	0	1	0
22	U	0	0	1	0
23	U	0	0	1	0
24	U	0	0	1	0

interval, one ordinal, and one nominal. Let four Protestant mothers, five Catholic mothers, and six Jewish mothers be scored on five dimensions of the birth experience, with hours in labor constituting the interval-level variable, birth weight (measured as above normal, normal, and below normal) constituting the ordinal dependent variable, and type of anesthesia (local, general, and none) constituting the nominal dependent variable. One of the five dimensions represents the interval variable, one dimension represents the ordinal variable, and three dimensions (one for each category) represent the nominal variable. The data are listed in Table 3.10. For these data, $N = 15$, $r = 5$, $v = 1$, $g = 3$, $K = N$, $n_1 = 4$, $n_2 = 5$, $n_3 = 6$, $C_i = n_i/N$, and B is ∞. The MRPP analysis with Euclidean commensuration yields $\delta_o = 0.2229 \times 10^{-1}$, $\mu = 0.2803 \times 10^{-1}$, $\sigma^2 = 0.2440 \times 10^{-5}$, $\gamma = -0.8296$, $T_o = -3.6713$, and $\Re_o = 0.2046$. The exact probability of an $\Re$ value equal to or greater than $\Re_o = 0.2046$ is $1792/630{,}630 = 0.2842 \times 10^{-2}$.

TABLE 3.10. Birth experience data with $N = 15$ subjects.

Subject	Religion	Hours in labor	Birth weight	Anesthesia Local	Anesthesia General	Anesthesia None
1	P	20	3	0	0	1
2	P	15	3	0	1	0
3	P	10	2	0	0	1
4	P	8	3	0	1	0
5	C	10	3	0	1	0
6	C	8	2	0	1	0
7	C	8	2	0	1	0
8	C	6	1	0	1	0
9	C	5	1	0	0	1
10	J	12	3	1	0	0
11	J	10	2	1	0	0
12	J	5	1	0	1	0
13	J	5	1	1	0	0
14	J	5	1	1	0	0
15	J	4	1	1	0	0

For comparison, a resampling approximation P-value with $L = 1,000,000$ is 0.2796×10^{-2}, and the Pearson type III P-value is 0.2874×10^{-2}.

3.3.5 Relationships with Existing Statistics

As is the case with any new statistical procedure, there are certain relationships with existing methods. It should be noted that the choice of $C_i = n_i/N$ is simply the number of subjects in the ith category of the nominal independent variable divided by the total number of subjects. In the subsequent comparisons with existing methods, the maximum likelihood argument based on the normal probability distribution dictates that $C_i = (n_i - 1)/(N - g)$. This alternative C_i is the number of degrees-of-freedom associated with the ith category of the nominal independent variable divided by the total degrees-of-freedom over all g nominal categories. In a permutation context, degrees-of-freedom are not relevant because they are a consequence of fitting parameters in a maximum likelihood context. In addition, $v = 1$, which is associated with ordinary Euclidean distances, is now replaced by $v = 2$, which also results from the maximum likelihood argument based on the normal distribution. Finally, it should be noted that $\Re$ is a median-based measure of agreement if $v = 1$, whereas $\Re$ is a mean-based measure of agreement if $v = 2$. For clarification, and as noted in Chapter 2, consider the pairwise sum of univariate ($r = 1$) symmetric distance functions given by

$$\sum_{I<J} \Delta_{I,J} = \sum_{I<J} |x_I - x_J|^v,$$

where $x_1, ..., x_N$ are univariate response variables and $\sum_{I<J}$ is the sum over all I and J such that $1 \le I < J \le N$. Let $x_{1,N} \le \cdots \le x_{N,N}$ be the order statistics associated with $x_1, ..., x_N$. If $v = 1$, then the inequality given by

$$\sum_{I=1}^{N} |N - 2I + 1||x_{I,N} - \theta| \ge \sum_{I<J} |x_I - x_J|$$

holds for all θ, and equality holds if θ is the median of $x_1, ..., x_N$. If $v = 2$, then the inequality given by

$$N \sum_{I=1}^{N} (x_I - \theta)^2 \ge \sum_{I<J} (x_I - x_J)^2$$

holds for all θ, and equality holds if and only if θ is the mean of $x_1, ..., x_N$.

Interval Dependent Variable

The permutation version of one-way analysis of variance (ANOVA) is a special case of the permutation method with a single dependent variable. Specifically,

$$\Re = \frac{F - 1}{F + (N - g)/(g - 1)},$$

where $r = 1$, $v = 2$, and $C_i = (n_i - 1)/(N - g)$. In addition, the unbiased correlation ratio ε^2 (Kelley, 1935) is identical to $\Re$ when $r = 1$, $v = 2$, and $C_i = (n_i - 1)/(N - g)$. Since ε^2, in an analysis-of-variance context, is identical to the shrunken squared correlation coefficient $\hat{R}^2$ (Cohen and Cohen, 1975, p. 188) in a regression context, then $\hat{R}^2$ (i.e., the unbiased estimator of the squared population Pearson correlation coefficient) is also identical to $\Re$. Finally, the permutation version of one-way multivariate analysis of variance (MANOVA) is a special case of the permutation method when $r \ge 2$, $v = 2$, $C_i = (n_i - 1)/(N - g)$, and

$$\Delta_{I,J} = \left[(x_I - x_J)' \hat{\Sigma}^{-1} (x_I - x_J) \right]^{v/2},$$

where $\hat{\Sigma}$ is the $r \times r$ variance-covariance matrix described in Section 2.9.

Ordinal Dependent Variable

In the previous discussion pertaining to an interval-level dependent variable, ε^2 can be associated with an unbiased squared correlation coefficient involving the Kruskal–Wallis (1952) test, where the rank-order statistics replace the interval-level observations in the one-way analysis of variance. However, the requirement of a complete ordering of all subjects from 1 to N precludes its use in many applications. Consequently, the more general statistic, $\Re$, which is applicable to either fully ranked or partially ranked observations, is potentially more useful. In addition, since the Kruskal–Wallis (1952) test is the rank-order analog of one-way ANOVA, then the rank-order analog of one-way MANOVA is attained by substitution.

Nominal Dependent Variable

If $C_i = (n_i - 1)/(N - g)$ and r represents the number of categories in a nominal dependent variable, then

$$\Re = \frac{N-1}{N-g}\left(t - \frac{g-1}{N-1}\right),$$

where t is Goodman and Kruskal's (1954) statistic associated with g categories of a nominal independent variable and r categories of a nominal dependent variable (Berry and Mielke, 1985a). Finally, it should be observed that the previously noted degrees-of-freedom, from the maximum likelihood approach based on the normal distribution, is an integral component of Goodman and Kruskal's (1954) statistic t for cross-classified categorical data.

3.4   Analyses Involving Cyclic Data

Suppose a study is concerned with comparing groups of points on the surface of an m-dimensional hypersphere. If x_I and x_J denote two of N points on the surface of a unit m-dimensional hypersphere centered at the origin, then $\sum_{k=1}^{m} x_{kI}^2 = 1$ for $I = 1, ..., N$ and the symmetric distance measure is the arc length in radians given by

$$\Delta_{I,J} = \cos^{-1}\left(\sum_{k=1}^{m} x_{kI} x_{kJ}\right).$$

If $m = 2$, let θ_I and θ_J denote the positions in radians of the Ith and Jth points on the edge of a unit circle where $0 \le \theta_I < 2\pi$ for $I = 1, ..., N$. Then, the symmetric distance measure is alternatively given by

$$\Delta_{I,J} = \min\left(|\theta_I - \theta_J|, 2\pi - |\theta_I - \theta_J|\right).$$

This representation is especially convenient for group comparisons involving cyclic data such as wind directions or temporal occurrence patterns during either days or years. For example, if the Ith event occurs h_I days after the first day of a year, then $0 \le h_I < 365$ and $\theta_I = 2\pi h_I/365$. Furthermore, suppose $\theta_{1I}, ..., \theta_{cI}$ denote c multiresponse cyclic measurements in radians of the Ith of N objects. Then, the transformation given by

$$x_{1I} = \cos(\theta_{1I}),$$

$$x_{2I} = \sin(\theta_{1I})\cos(\theta_{2I}),$$

$$\vdots \qquad \vdots$$

$$x_{cI} = \sin(\theta_{1I})\sin(\theta_{2I}) \cdots \sin(\theta_{c-1,I})\cos(\theta_{cI}),$$

$$x_{c+1,I} = \sin(\theta_{1I})\sin(\theta_{2I}) \cdots \sin(\theta_{c-1,I})\sin(\theta_{cI}),$$

yields the basis for MRPP analyses of c-dimensional cyclic data since, in the present context, $m = c+1$ and $x_{1I}, ..., x_{c+1,I}$ denote the coordinates of a point on a unit hypersphere having $c+1$ dimensions (Mielke, 1986).

Similarly, suppose groups involving both wind direction and velocity are compared. Let θ_I and v_I be the polar coordinates denoting direction in radians and velocity for the Ith of N measurements, respectively. Then, $x_{1I} = v_I \cos(\theta_I)$ and $x_{2I} = v_I \sin(\theta_I)$ are the corresponding Cartesian coordinates. Here, the symmetric distance measure ($\Delta_{I,J}$) of MRPP analyses is again the Euclidean distance based on the Ith and Jth Cartesian coordinates. The following examples illustrate applications to circular data with $m = 2$ and spherical data with $m = 3$. Further discussion of circular and spherical data is given by Jammalamadaka and Sengupta (2001) and Mardia and Jupp (2000).

3.4.1 Analysis of Circular Data

Of interest is the possibility that the occurrence of a specific type of crime is influenced by annual temperature cycles. The hypothetical data of Table 3.11 consist of specific dates when 9 of these crime events occurred in Melbourne, Australia and 14 of these same crime events occurred in Seattle, U.S.A. If, for example, crime events occurred on 18 February and 23 October, then the recorded values h_I in Table 3.11 are the Julian calendar dates 48 and 295, respectively (a nonleap year is assumed), $\theta_I = 2\pi h_I/365$, and

$$\Delta_{I,J} = \min\left(|\theta_I - \theta_J|,\ 2\pi - |\theta_I - \theta_J|\right).$$

Under H_0, the temporal distributions of occurrences are the same for both locations. Since the temperature cycles are reversed at these two locations, there might be a possibility of detecting such an alternative. The MRPP analysis for these data involves $N = 23$, $m = 2$, $g = 2$, $n_1 = 9$, $n_2 = 14$, $K = N$, $C_i = n_i/K$, and B is ∞. Then, $\delta_0 = 1.3094$, $\mu = 1.6160$, $\sigma^2 = 0.3590 \times 10^{-2}$, $\gamma = -1.6814$, $T_0 = -5.1176$, and the Pearson type III

TABLE 3.11. Julian dates of 9 crime events in Melbourne, Australia and 14 crime events in Seattle, U.S.A.

Melbourne	Seattle
354	291
1	189
54	312
127	217
39	142
340	278
47	212
151	361
84	133
	244
	319
	201
	303
	255

P-value is 0.1510×10^{-2}. Since there are $M = 817{,}190$ possible permutations and 1044 δ values as extreme or more extreme than $\delta_0 = 1.3094$, the exact P-value is 0.1278×10^{-2}.

3.4.2   Analysis of Spherical Data

Geophysicists and archaeologists have long known that the direction and intensity of Earth's magnetic field have varied throughout prehistoric times. Many soils contain magnetic materials that, when heated, assume the direction and intensity of Earth's magnetic field at the time of heating. When soils containing ferromagnetic materials are cooled after heating, the magnetic particles align themselves with the direction of Earth's magnetic field and retain this direction permanently unless reheated. Thus, if the changes in direction of Earth's magnetic field are known, it is possible to date collected fired material by comparing the magnetic direction of the collected sample with a record of the changes in the direction of Earth's magnetic field. MRPP is an ideal procedure for the purpose of detecting sample differences among archaeomagnetic polar directions based on collected samples from, for example, fired hearths, or among palaeomagnetic polar directions based on collected materials from, for example, lava flows. The application of MRPP is demonstrated here with archaeomagnetic data.

In archaeomagnetic research, it is often necessary to draw two or more samples of specimens from their respective archaeological features (such as in situ walls, floors, kilns, ovens, and hearths) and to test whether the magnetic directions of the features are identical. For example, archaeomagnetists often need to know whether similar archaeomagnetic dates (i.e., polar directions) were produced by the same thermal event. In addition, it is important to know whether directional differences obtained from instruments made by different laboratories and/or instruments of different types are comparable. The problem in all its manifestations arises because archaeological materials imperfectly record and preserve magnetic directions, magnetometers are unable to measure remanent magnetism perfectly, and it is usually not possible to measure the entire archaeological feature of interest. Repeated measurements on large sample sets reduce the uncertainty in estimating ancient directions, but when two or more samples produce different magnetic directions, the question remains as to whether the sample differences in estimated magnetic directions are merely due to sampling and measurement error or instead reflect actual differences among the archaeological features from which the samples were drawn.

A Parametric Approach

The F test, first proposed by Watson (1956), is widely used in archaeomagnetic research to address the problem by testing the hypothesis that two or more archaeological features possess identical magnetic directions. Unfortunately, the F test is limited in its applicability by a number of requirements that are often difficult to satisfy (Engebretson and Beck, 1978; Larochelle, 1967a, 1967b; Onstott, 1980; Watson, 1956; Watson and Irving, 1957; Watson and Williams, 1956). In particular, the F test requires that both populations possess equal precision parameters (i.e., homogeneity of variance) and that the directions of magnetism follow a normal probability density function on a sphere (Fisher, 1953). In addition, the F test utilizes a squared-distance measure that may give disproportionate importance to outliers. Because of these requirements, use of the F test should be limited to situations in which the requisite conditions can be satisfied. Note that, for example, such uncontrollable variables as variation in grain size, variation in magnetic mineralogy, and instrument noise, all of which are common in archaeomagnetic research, may cause unequal variances in samples.

A Permutation Approach

The usual approach when comparing magnetic directions is to statistically compare the sample mean directions. If the assumptions of equal variances and normality are satisfied, then large mean sample differences imply directional differences among two or more features (Watson, 1956). In contrast, MRPP is based on the within-sample average of the arc distances between surface points on a sphere, where a surface point is merely the location at which a direction of magnetism intersects Earth's surface and is calculated from the remanent magnetism of a single specimen from an archaeological feature. In addition, MRPP requires that each of the $N!$ possible specimen assignments to the N surface points is equally probable under H_0, avoids the wrapping problem associated with a normal distribution on a sphere, and permits analyses of two or more samples that may be of equal or unequal sizes. In archaeomagnetic applications, the surface points are described by the latitude and longitude of virtual geomagnetic polar locations. Although MRPP can compare sample directions (i.e., declination and inclination) as easily and accurately as surface points (Mielke, 1984, 1986; Mielke and Berry, 2000a), in this application sample directions are converted to virtual geomagnetic polar locations because this is the most common method used by archaeologists to compare archaeomagnetic samples.

Let $\Omega = (\omega_1, ..., \omega_N)$ designate a finite population of N specimens. In the case of archaeomagnetic research, surface points are determined for each specimen from the directions of magnetism (Irving, 1964, pp. 43–44). Let the latitude (λ_s) and longitude (ϕ_s) of the collection site be known, and let the declination (D_i) relative to the meridian of the site (ϕ_s) and the inclination (I_i) of a specimen (ω_i) be determined ($i = 1, ..., N$). Then, the latitude (λ_i) and longitude (ϕ_i) for the surface point associated with specimen ω_i ($i = 1, ..., N$) are given by

$$\lambda_i = \sin^{-1}\left[\sin\left(\lambda_s\right)\cos\left(\psi_i\right) + \cos\left(\lambda_s\right)\sin\left(\psi_i\right)\cos\left(D_i\right)\right],$$

where $-90° \leq \lambda_i \leq +90°$ and

$$\phi_i = \phi_s + \sin^{-1}\left[\cos\left(\psi_i\right)\sin\left(D_i\right)/\cos\left(\lambda_i\right)\right],$$

where $0° \leq \phi_i \leq 360°$ when $\cos\left(\psi_i\right) \geq \sin\left(\lambda_s\right)\sin\left(\lambda_i\right)$, or

$$\phi_i = \phi_s + 180° - \sin^{-1}\left[\cos\left(\psi_i\right)\sin\left(D_i\right)/\cos\left(\lambda_i\right)\right],$$

where $0° \leq \phi_i \leq 360°$ when $\cos\left(\psi_i\right) < \sin\left(\lambda_s\right)\sin\left(\lambda_i\right)$, and the colatitude, ψ_i, is given by

$$\psi_i = \cot^{-1}\left[0.5\tan\left(I_i\right)\right],$$

where $0° \leq \psi_i \leq 180°$. The Cartesian coordinates (x_i, y_i, z_i) for the surface point on a unit sphere associated with specimen ω_i ($i = 1, ..., N$) are obtained from

$$x_i = \cos\left(\lambda_i\right)\cos\left(\phi_i\right),$$

$$y_i = \cos\left(\lambda_i\right)\sin\left(\phi_i\right),$$

and

$$z_i = \sin\left(\lambda_i\right).$$

Let $S_1, ..., S_g$ represent an exhaustive partitioning of the N specimens comprising Ω into g disjoint samples, let n_i be the number of specimens in the ith sample, and let $\Delta_{j,k}$ be the arc distance among the surface points associated with specimens ω_j and ω_k, namely,

$$\Delta_{j,k} = \cos^{-1}\left(x_j x_k + y_j y_k + z_j z_k\right).$$

The MRPP test statistic, δ, is then defined as

$$\delta = \sum_{i=1}^{g} \frac{n_i}{N}\, \xi_i,$$

where

$$\xi_i = \binom{n_i}{2}^{-1} \sum_{j<k} \Delta_{j,k} \Psi_i\left(\omega_j\right) \Psi_i\left(\omega_k\right)$$

is the average arc distance among the surface points associated with the ith sample $(i = 1, ..., g)$, $\sum_{j<k}$ is the sum over all j and k such that $1 \leq j < k \leq N$, and $\Psi_i(\cdot)$ is an indicator function given by

$$\Psi_i\left(\omega_j\right) = \begin{cases} 1 & \text{if } \omega_j \in S_i, \\ 0 & \text{otherwise.} \end{cases}$$

Thus defined, δ is the weighted within-sample average of the arc distances among corresponding surface points on a unit sphere, where the weight (n_i/N) is the proportional contribution of the number of specimens in the ith sample. Utilizing δ, consider H_0: the a priori samples $S_1, ..., S_g$ correspond to a random distribution of the surface points $\omega_1, ..., \omega_N$ to the g samples, with fixed size structure $n_1, ..., n_g$, versus H_1: the distribution is not random. If H_0 is rejected, there is evidence of a meaningful difference in surface-point locations on the unit sphere among the g samples. If δ_o is the observed value of δ, then the P-value is given by

$$P\text{-value} = P\left(\delta \leq \delta_o \mid H_0\right).$$

Application of the Permutation Approach

In archaeomagnetic (palaeomagnetic) research, it is often necessary to draw two or more samples of specimens from their respective archaeological (geological) features and test whether the magnetic directions of the samples are from a common population of directions. To demonstrate MRPP for evaluating directional differences on a unit sphere, consider the following application drawn from archaeomagnetic research (Mielke et al., 1991).

Archaeomagnetic collection involves removing 0.5-inch cubes of burned archaeological features (encased in one-cubic-inch plaster molds) to a laboratory for measurement of remanent magnetization. The orientation of each specimen is determined in situ before removal. Archaeomagnetists are interested in knowing whether or not the standard orienting technique using a magnetic compass is accurate. It is possible that local magnetic anomalies may influence the accuracy and/or precision with which a magnetic compass will record a specimen's orientation.

A sun compass orients a specimen independently of local magnetic fields, but a sun compass is useless on cloudy days or in shady locations, and the definition of the shadow cast by a sun compass prohibits the determination of directions finer than $0.5°$ of arc. Therefore, a test was devised to determine whether the two collecting instruments produce identical results for independent samples drawn from a small isolated hearth. In this application, the entire rim of an experimentally fired hearth yielded a total of 20 specimens. The latitude and longitude of the hearth were $\lambda_s = 40.03°$ N latitude and $\phi_s = 251.24°$ E longitude. Unrestricted randomization by a coin toss determined whether each specimen's orientation was measured by the sun compass or the magnetic compass. Eight (n_1) specimens were measured with the magnetic compass (S_1) and 12 (n_2) specimens were measured with the sun compass (S_2). The directions of all $N = 20$ specimens were measured on a spinner magnetometer after magnetic cleaning. Values for I, D, x, y, and z for each specimen from the sun compass and magnetic compass samples are presented in Table 3.12. For the data in Table 3.12, $N = 20$, $m = 3$, $g = 2$, $K = N$, $n_1 = 8$, $n_2 = 12$, $C_i = n_i/N$, and B is ∞. The MRPP analysis of the data in Table 3.12 yields $\delta_o = 0.1961$, $\mu = 0.2066$, $\sigma^2 = 0.3488 \times 10^{-4}$, $\gamma = -1.6941$, $T_o = -1.7863$, and the Pearson type III P-value is 0.0611. Because there are $M = 125{,}970$ possible permutations and 7731 δ values as extreme or more extreme than $\delta_o = 0.1961$, the exact P-value is 0.0614. These values suggest the possibility that the magnetic compass and the sun compass are not providing the same results and indicate that additional tests of the accuracy and precision of the two types of collecting instruments should be considered.

3.5 Analyses Based on Generalized Runs

Suppose that each of N objects is associated with a position in an arbitrary space (termed a node) and that each pair of objects is either linked or not linked. If ω_I and ω_J are linked, then $\Delta_{I,J} = 1$; otherwise, $\Delta_{I,J} = 0$. Furthermore, zero or more links may emanate from each node. Either an isolated node with no links or a collection of sequentially linked objects is termed a tree, provided there are no closed circuits (cycles) of links. A cycle of three or more links occurs when it is possible to return to an object by a sequence of linked objects where no link is repeated. As with other MRPP analyses, the number of objects in classified group S_i is $n_i \geq 2$ and the number of unclassified objects is $n_{g+1} \geq 0$. If objects ω_I and ω_J are both linked and belong to the same classified group, then ω_I and ω_J are connected objects; otherwise, ω_I and ω_J are nonconnected objects.

TABLE 3.12. Spinner results and coordinates for magnetic and sun compass samples from an experimental hearth after demagnetization.

I	D	x	y	z
Magnetic compass				
63.8925	353.8238	−0.1032	−0.0698	0.9922
68.5391	358.3221	−0.0829	−0.1879	0.9787
65.8246	6.6206	0.0270	−0.1601	0.9867
39.3117	358.5600	0.0760	0.2962	0.9521
64.4793	351.0394	−0.1388	−0.0743	0.9875
59.2503	344.5506	−0.1989	0.0485	0.9788
68.9326	343.5224	−0.2379	−0.1622	0.9576
63.9768	356.1613	−0.0763	−0.0792	0.9939
Sun compass				
59.8150	4.4251	0.0513	−0.0310	0.9982
58.6753	3.7364	0.0508	−0.0069	0.9987
59.2786	349.7595	−0.1316	0.0356	0.9907
63.6060	2.7799	0.0031	−0.0971	0.9953
67.7262	353.3333	−0.1300	−0.1539	0.9796
66.5547	343.9890	−0.2269	−0.1060	0.9681
57.5229	12.4841	0.1677	−0.0349	0.9852
66.2503	7.7520	0.0349	−0.1743	0.9841
60.5099	6.6361	0.0728	−0.0549	0.9958
56.1073	5.1267	0.0861	0.0307	0.9958
64.8497	7.7744	0.0485	−0.1453	0.9882
62.8736	13.1101	0.1259	−0.1341	0.9829

A run consists of either a nonconnected object, any unclassified object, or a collection of sequentially connected objects. If L is the number of links, t is the number of trees, R is the number of runs, and the MRPP analysis is based on

$$C_i = \frac{\binom{n_i}{2}}{\sum_{j=1}^{g} \binom{n_j}{2}}$$

for $i = 1, ..., g$, then the defining equation that relates L, t, R, and the MRPP statistic δ is given by

$$R = L + t - \delta \sum_{i=1}^{g} \binom{n_i}{2}. \tag{3.1}$$

Since small values of R suggest that H_0 may be suspect, Expression (3.1) relating δ and R implies that the exact MRPP P-value is

$$P\left(\delta \geq \delta_o \mid H_0\right) = \frac{\text{number of } \delta \text{ values} \geq \delta_o}{M},$$

where δ_o is the observed value of δ and

$$M = \frac{N!}{\displaystyle\prod_{i=1}^{g+1} n_i!}.$$

In particular, the classical two-sample runs test due to Wald and Wolfowitz (1940) involves $K = N$, $L = N - 1$, $t = 1$, and $g = 2$.

3.5.1 Wald–Wolfowitz Runs Test

Consider a single tree ($t = 1$) where each inner node has two links and the two outer nodes have only one link. In this case, each node is occupied by either the symbol O or the symbol X, where the total sequence consists of m Os and n Xs and $m \leq n$. A run is a sequence of like symbols that are bounded by either the other symbol or no symbol. Then, R is the number of runs of Os and Xs. Under the null hypothesis, the ordered sequence of Os and Xs is purely random. The exact probability distribution of R is given by

$$P(R = r) = 2 \binom{m-1}{s-1} \binom{n-1}{s-1} \binom{m+n}{m}^{-1}$$

when $r = 2s$, and

$$P(R = r) = \left(\frac{m+n}{s} - 2\right) \binom{m-1}{s-1} \binom{n-1}{s-1} \binom{m+n}{m}^{-1}$$

when $r = 2s + 1$ ($1 \leq s \leq m \leq n$). The exact P-value of the runs test is the probability under the null hypothesis of obtaining a value of R less than or equal to the observed value of R, say x, and is given by

$$P\text{-value} = \sum_{r=2}^{x} P(R = r).$$

If both m and n are large, the approximate distribution of R under the null hypothesis is given by

$$\frac{R - \mu_R}{\sigma_R} \left(\overset{\text{d}}{=}\right) N(0, 1),$$

where

$$\mu_R = \frac{2mn}{m+n} + 1$$

and

$$\sigma_R^2 = \frac{2mn\,(2mn - m - n)}{(m+n)^2(m+n-1)}.$$

To illustrate the Wald–Wolfowitz runs test, consider the following sequence:

$$\underbrace{\text{X X}}\ \underbrace{\text{O O O O}}\ \underbrace{\text{X X}}\ \underbrace{\text{O}}\ \underbrace{\text{X X}}\ \underbrace{\text{O O O}}\ \underbrace{\text{X}},$$

where $L = 14$ links, $t = 1$ tree, $g = 2$ groups, $m = 7$ Xs, $n = 8$ Os, $R = 7$ runs, and $2 \leq r \leq 7$. When $r = 2$, then r is even, $s = 1$, and $P(R = 2)$ is

$$2\binom{7-1}{1-1}\binom{8-1}{1-1}\binom{7+8}{7}^{-1} = \frac{1}{6435}.$$

When $r = 3$, then r is odd, $s = 1$, and $P(R = 3)$ is

$$\left(\frac{7+8}{1} - 2\right)\binom{7-1}{1-1}\binom{8-1}{1-1}\binom{7+8}{7}^{-1} = \frac{13}{6435}.$$

When $r = 4$, $s = 2$ and $P(R = 4)$ is $42/6435$. When $r = 5$, $s = 2$ and $P(R = 5)$ is $231/6435$. When $r = 6$, $s = 3$ and $P(R = 6)$ is $315/6435$. When $r = 7$, $s = 3$ and $P(R = 7)$ is $945/6435$. The P-value is the sum of the probabilities for $r = 2, ..., 7$, which is $1547/6435 = 0.2404$. A runs test involving three or more distinct symbols is much more complicated.

3.5.2   Generalized Runs Test

The generalization of the Wald–Wolfowitz runs test was initially suggested by Whaley (1983) and immediately extends the Wald–Wolfowitz runs test to $g \geq 2$, $t \geq 1$, nodes with zero and more links, and the inclusion of unclassified objects. Applications include almost any variety of transect analysis. Finally, if one or more cycles do exist, then the MRPP analysis remains valid; however, Expression (3.1) relating δ and R no longer holds.

To illustrate the generalized runs test, consider the example data set given in Table 3.13 with $L = 14$ links, $t = 3$ trees, and $g = 2$ groups with an excess (unclassified) group. Group S_1 contains $n_1 = 8$ similar objects indicated by $\triangle$s, group S_2 contains $n_2 = 5$ similar objects indicated by $\diamond$s, and the excess group S_{g+1} contains $n_{g+1} = 4$ objects indicated by $\square$s. Since $N = 17$ and $N - K = n_{g+1}$, $K = 13$. Table 3.13 contains the $\binom{17}{2} = 136$ $\Delta_{I,J}$ values, where the four $\triangle$s in tree number 1 are labeled 1 through 4 from left to right and from top to bottom, the two $\triangle$s in tree number 2 are labeled 5 and 6 from left to right, and the two $\triangle$s in tree number 3 are labeled 7 and 8 from left to right. The five $\diamond$s are labeled from 9 to 13 in an analogous manner starting with tree number 1 and ending with tree number 3. Finally, the four $\square$s are labeled from 14 to 17 in the same manner starting with tree number 1 and ending with tree number 3.

TABLE 3.13. Values of $\Delta_{I,J}$, where $I < J$, for the $t = 3$ trees.

I	2	3	4	5	6	7	8	9	10	11	12	13	14	15	16	17
1	1	0	0	0	0	0	0	0	0	0	0	0	0	0	0	0
2		1	0	0	0	0	0	1	0	0	0	0	0	1	0	0
3			1	0	0	0	0	0	0	0	0	0	0	0	0	0
4				0	0	0	0	0	0	0	0	0	0	0	0	0
5					1	0	0	0	0	0	0	0	0	0	0	0
6						0	0	0	0	0	0	0	0	0	1	0
7							1	0	0	0	0	0	0	0	0	0
8								0	0	0	0	1	0	0	0	1
9									0	0	0	0	0	0	0	0
10										1	0	0	0	0	0	0
11											1	0	0	0	1	0
12												0	0	0	0	0
13													0	0	0	0
14														1	0	0
15															0	0
16																0

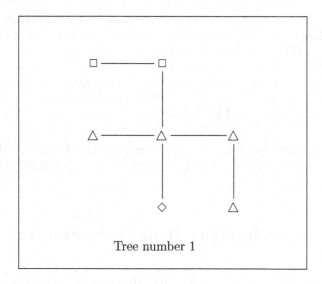

Tree number 1

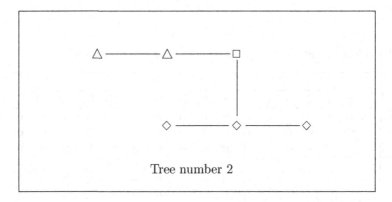

Tree number 2

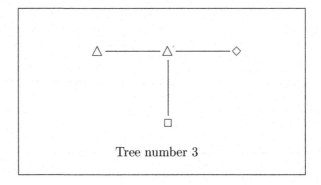

Tree number 3

The MRPP analysis yields $\delta_o = 0.1842$, $\mu = 0.1029$, $\sigma^2 = 0.1610 \times 10^{-2}$, $\gamma = 0.1181$, $T_o = 2.0253$, and a Pearson type III P-value of 0.2446×10^{-1}. A resampling approximation with $L = 1,000,000$ yields $\delta_o = 0.1842$, and a P-value of 0.4549×10^{-1}. Because there are

$$M = \frac{N!}{\prod_{i=1}^{g+1} n_i!} = \frac{17!}{8!\,5!\,4!} = 3{,}063{,}060$$

possible permutations of the $N = 17$ objects, of which 139,407 δ values are equal to or greater than $\delta_o = 0.1842$, the exact P-value is $139{,}407/3{,}063{,}060 = 0.4551 \times 10^{-1}$.

3.6 Analyses Involving Rank-Order Statistics

In a completely randomized design, the substitution of rank-type score functions for observed data values in MRPP results in univariate and multivariate g-sample rank tests adjusted for tied values. Since the initial motivation for replacing observed data with rank-order statistics in the two-sample t test and one-way analysis-of-variance statistics was to diminish the influence of extreme values, this approach involved an effort to compensate for the nonmetric geometry problem associated with $v = 2$. Since all but the ordering structure of raw data is lost when rank-order transformations are employed, the use of $v = 1$ may accomplish this same purpose without a monumental loss of data-related information. When $r > 1$, the range of each response is from 1 to N, and consequently this provides another way to create the commensurated data.

3.6.1 An Extended Class of Rank Tests

For each of the r responses, suppose an untied univariate value x_I ($I = 1, ..., N$) is replaced with the rank-order statistic function given by

$$h\left(R_I\right) = \begin{cases} |R_I - (N+1)/2|^w & \text{if } R_I > (N+1)/2, \\ 0 & \text{if } R_I = (N+1)/2, \\ -|R_I - (N+1)/2|^w & \text{if } R_I < (N+1)/2, \end{cases}$$

where $w > -1$ and R_I is the rank-order statistic of x_I, an integer from 1 to N. If tied values are present, replace tied x_I values with the average of the corresponding R_I values as if there had been no tied values.

Let statistic $\delta_{w,v}$ designate the univariate ($r = 1$) MRPP rank test specified by w and v. If $N = K$ and $C_i = (n_i - 1)/(K - g)$ for $i = 1, ..., g$, then $\delta_{1,2}$ is equivalent to the Kruskal–Wallis test (Kruskal and Wallis, 1952; Mielke, 1986). In addition, if $g = 2$, then $\delta_{1,2}$ is equivalent to the two-sided Wilcoxon–Mann–Whitney test (Mann and Whitney, 1947; Wilcoxon, 1945). If there are no ties, then the simplified symmetric function model parameters of $\delta_{1,2}$ (Mielke et al., 1981b) are given by

$$D(1) = \frac{N(N+1)}{6},$$

$$D(2) = \frac{2N^2 - 3}{5} D(1),$$

$$D(2') = \frac{1}{2} D(2),$$

$$D(2'') = \frac{(N-1)(5N+6)}{30} D(1),$$

$$D(3) = \frac{(N^2 - 2)(3N^2 - 5)}{14} D(1),$$

$$D(3') = \frac{19N^4 - 7N^3 - 79N^2 + 7N + 75}{210} D(1),$$

$$D(3^*) = \frac{N(N^2 - 1)(N + 2)}{60} D(1),$$

$$D(3'') = \frac{14N^4 - 6N^3 - 59N^2 + N + 50}{210} D(1),$$

$$D(3''') = \frac{1}{2} D(3''),$$

$$D(3'''') = \frac{35N^4 - 14N^3 - 143N^2 + 2N + 120}{1260} D(1),$$

$$D(3^{**}) = \frac{49N^4 - 4N^3 - 184N^2 - 11N + 150}{1260} D(1),$$

and

$$D(3^{***}) = \frac{58N^4 - 52N^3 - 283N^2 + 67N + 300}{1260} D(1).$$

The corresponding simplified symmetric function model parameters of $\delta_{1,1}$ (Mielke et al., 1981b) are given by

$$D(1) = \frac{N + 1}{3},$$

$$D(2) = \frac{N}{2} D(1),$$

$$D(2') = \frac{7N + 4}{20} D(1),$$

$$D(2'') = \frac{5N + 4}{15} D(1),$$

$$D(3) = \frac{3N^2 - 2}{10} D(1),$$

$$D(3') = \frac{11N^2 + 4N - 6}{60} D(1),$$

$$D(3'') = \frac{5N^2 + 3N - 2}{30} D(1),$$

$$D(3''') = \frac{49N^2 + 59N + 6}{420} D(1),$$

$$D(3'''') = \frac{35N^2 + 49N + 12}{315} D(1),$$

$$D(3^*) = \frac{N(N+2)}{10} D(1),$$

$$D(3^{**}) = \frac{51N^2 + 59N - 2}{420} D(1),$$

and

$$D(3^{***}) = \frac{18N^2 + 13N - 4}{140} D(1).$$

Estimated significance levels and location-shift power comparisons of the MRPP rank tests associated with $\delta_{1,1}$, $\delta_{1,2}$, $\delta_{2,1}$, and $\delta_{2,2}$ are given in Tables 3.14 and 3.15. These tables specifically involve $N = 80$, $r = 1$, $g = 2$, $n_1 = n_2 = 40$, $K = N$, $C_1 = C_2 = 0.5$, and B is ∞. The power comparisons in Table 3.15 are based on two location shifts (0.5σ and 0.7σ, where σ is the standard deviation of the distribution in question) for each of five distributions: Laplace (i.e., double exponential), logistic, normal, uniform, and a U-shaped distribution with density function $3x^2/2$ for $-1 < x < 1$. Each estimated significance value of $\alpha = 0.001$ and $\alpha = 0.01$ is based on 10,000,000 simulations, and each power comparison is based on 1,000,000 simulations. The estimated significance values of Table 3.14 indicate that the Pearson type III critical values are satisfactory. The power comparisons among $\delta_{1,1}$, $\delta_{1,2}$, $\delta_{2,1}$, and $\delta_{2,2}$ indicate that (1) $\delta_{1,1}$ is best for the Laplace distribution when α is 0.001 and 0.01 and the logistic distribution when α is 0.001, (2) $\delta_{1,2}$ is best for the logistic distribution when α is 0.01, (3) $\delta_{2,1}$ is best for the normal distribution when α is 0.001 and the U-shaped distribution when α is 0.001 and 0.01, and (4) $\delta_{2,2}$ is best for the normal distribution when α is 0.01 and the uniform distribution when α is 0.001 and 0.01. Because $\delta_{1,2}$ corresponds to the Wilcoxon–Mann–Whitney test, which is asymptotically most powerful for detecting logistic distribution location shifts among the class of linear rank tests, this asymptotic result is not contradicted by the power values of $\delta_{1,1}$, since $\delta_{1,1}$ does not correspond to any linear rank test. Because no basis exists for asymptotic comparisons between $\delta_{1,1}$ and $\delta_{1,2}$, a multitude of questions arise about asymptotically most powerful rank tests, distributions, values of v, and sample sizes.

3.6.2 Asymptotically Most Powerful Rank Tests and v

Consider a two-sample linear rank test statistic given by

$$H = \sum_{I=1}^{N} h(R_I) U_I,$$

where $h(R_I)$ is the rank function of x_I and $U_I = 1$ if $\omega_I \in S_1$, and 0 otherwise. Also consider the MRPP statistic δ with $r = 1$, $v = 2$, $g = 2$,

TABLE 3.14. Estimated significance levels for 10,000,000 simulated samples of size $n_1 = n_2 = 40$ based on the Pearson type III distribution critical values.

α	$\delta_{1,1}$	$\delta_{1,2}$	$\delta_{2,1}$	$\delta_{2,2}$
0.001	0.00102	0.00094	0.00105	0.00092
0.01	0.01002	0.01003	0.00995	0.01010

TABLE 3.15. Estimated powers for 1,000,000 simulated samples for size $n_1 = n_2 = 40$ against location shifts of 0.5σ and 0.7σ.

Distri-bution	α	0.5σ				0.7σ			
		$\delta_{1,1}$	$\delta_{1,2}$	$\delta_{2,1}$	$\delta_{2,2}$	$\delta_{1,1}$	$\delta_{1,2}$	$\delta_{2,1}$	$\delta_{2,2}$
Laplace	0.001	0.272	0.236	0.203	0.152	0.641	0.587	0.533	0.426
	0.01	0.546	0.510	0.449	0.389	0.862	0.834	0.787	0.716
Logistic	0.001	0.152	0.150	0.148	0.131	0.443	0.442	0.433	0.393
	0.01	0.379	0.387	0.367	0.358	0.721	0.730	0.707	0.691
Normal	0.001	0.112	0.119	0.122	0.118	0.350	0.369	0.375	0.369
	0.01	0.311	0.332	0.324	0.338	0.635	0.664	0.653	0.671
Uniform	0.001	0.075	0.103	0.144	0.195	0.252	0.319	0.435	0.525
	0.01	0.245	0.309	0.379	0.476	0.537	0.617	0.728	0.805
U-shaped	0.001	0.538	0.504	0.932	0.914	0.785	0.689	0.992	0.978
	0.01	0.861	0.774	0.993	0.984	0.977	0.889	1.000	0.997

$n_1 = n$, $n_2 = N - n$, $K = N$, $C_i = (n_i - 1)/(K - g)$, and B is ∞. Then, the identity relating H and δ (Mielke, 1984) is given by

$$N(N - 2)\delta = 2 \left[NA_2 - A_1^2 - \frac{(NH - nA_1)^2}{n(N - n)} \right],$$

where

$$A_1 = \sum_{I=1}^{N} h(R_I)$$

and

$$A_2 = \sum_{I=1}^{N} \left[h(R_I) \right]^2.$$

Consequently, all two-sample linear rank tests may be analyzed utilizing MRPP. To indicate the scope of two-sample linear rank tests that have been studied, consider the following three infinite classes of linear rank tests (Mielke, 1972) designated by Class I, Class II, and Class III and given by Class I:

$$h(R_I) = R_I^w, \text{ for } w > 0,$$

Class II:
$$h(R_I) = |R_I - (N + 1)/2|^w, \text{ for } w > 0,$$

and Class III:

$$h(R_I) = \begin{cases} |R_I - (N + 1)/2|^w & \text{if } R_I > (N + 1)/2, \\ 0 & \text{if } R_I = (N + 1)/2, \\ -|R_I - (N + 1)/2|^w & \text{if } R_I < (N + 1)/2, \end{cases}$$

for $w > -1$. Given that $v = 2$, the asymptotic properties of each test within these three classes is well known (Mielke 1972, 1974; Mielke and Sen, 1981), including the specific distribution for which each test is asymptotically most powerful for detecting a location or scale shift. Some specific tests with $v = 2$ follow: Class I includes the Wilcoxon–Mann–Whitney test when $w = 1$ (Mann and Whitney, 1947; Wilcoxon, 1945) and the Taha test when $w = 2$ (Duran and Mielke, 1968; Grant and Mielke, 1967; Taha, 1964); Class II includes the Ansari–Bradley test when $w = 1$ (Ansari and Bradley, 1960) and the Mood test when $w = 2$ (Mood, 1954); Class III includes the Brown–Mood median test when $w = 0$ (Brown and Mood, 1951; Mood, 1954), the Wilcoxon–Mann–Whitney test when $w = 1$, and a modified squared-rank test when $w = 2$ (Mielke, 1974).

If $v = 2$, then Class I with parameter $w > 0$ is asymptotically optimum in detecting scale shifts for the kappa distribution (Mielke, 1973; Mielke and Johnson, 1973) with cumulative distribution function (*cdf*) and probability density function (*pdf*) given by

$$F(x) = \begin{cases} \left[(x^w/w) / (1 + x^w/w) \right]^{1/w} & \text{if } 0 \le x, \\ 0 & \text{if } x \le 0, \end{cases}$$

and

$$f(x) = \begin{cases} w^{-1/w} (1 + x^w/w)^{-(w+1)/w} & \text{if } 0 \le x, \\ 0 & \text{if } x < 0, \end{cases}$$

respectively. A related point is that the generalized beta distribution of the second kind (Mielke and Johnson, 1974) and other distributions (Mielke, 1975, 1976) were motivated by the kappa distribution. If $v = 2$, then Class I with parameter $w > 0$ is asymptotically optimum in detecting location shifts for the generalized logistic distribution with *cdf* and *pdf* given by

$$F(x) = \left[(e^{wx}/w) / (1 + e^{wx}/w) \right]^{1/w}$$

and

$$f(x) = (e^{wx}/w)^{1/w} (1 + e^{wx}/w)^{-(w+1)/w},$$

respectively. The generalized logistic distribution is the logistic distribution when $w = 1$. If $v = 2$, then Class II with parameter $w > 0$ is asymptotically optimum in detecting scale shifts for the symmetric kappa distribution with cdf and pdf given by

$$F(x) = \begin{cases} 0.5 \left\{ 1 + \left[(x^w/w)/(1 + x^w/w) \right]^{1/w} \right\} & \text{if } 0 \leq x, \\ 0.5 \left\{ 1 - \left[(|x|^w/w)/(1 + |x|^w/w) \right]^{1/w} \right\} & \text{if } x \leq 0, \end{cases}$$

and

$$f(x) = 0.5 w^{-1/w} \left(1 + |x|^w/w \right)^{-(w+1)/w},$$

respectively. The symmetric kappa distribution is the Student t distribution with two degrees-of-freedom when $w = 2$. If $v = 2$, then Class III with parameter $w > -1$ is asymptotically optimum in detecting location shifts for the omega distribution (Copenhaver and Mielke, 1977) with cdf and pdf implicitly given by

$$F(x(p)) = p,$$

$$f(x(p)) = \left[2 (w + 1) \right]^{-1} \left(1 - |2p - 1|^{w+1} \right),$$

and

$$x(p) = \int_{0.5}^{p} \left[f(x(z)) \right]^{-1} dz,$$

where $0 < p < 1$. The omega distribution is the Laplace (double exponential) distribution when $w = 0$ and is the logistic distribution when $w = 1$. An incidental comment is that the quantal response assay method termed quantit analysis (Copenhaver and Mielke, 1977; Magnus et al., 1977) is based on the omega distribution.

Since the asymptotic null distribution of statistic H in most cases is $N(\mu_H, \sigma_H^2)$, where

$$\mu_H = \frac{nA_1}{N}$$

and

$$\sigma_H^2 = \frac{n(N - n)(NA_2 - A_1^2)}{N^2(N - 1)},$$

the use of this asymptotic distribution as an approximation for the null distribution of H when N is of small or moderate size is suspect. In contrast, the approximate nonasymptotic null distribution provided by MRPP, which depends on the three exact moments of δ, accounts for small and moderate sample sizes. Of course, the extension of the rank tests to $v \neq 2$ requires the MRPP approximation.

The class of rank tests investigated by Mielke (1972, 1974) and Mielke and Sen (1981) is confined to linear rank test statistics based on $v = 2$ such as statistic H with asymptotic conditions, i.e., very large sample sizes. An

TABLE 3.16. Value of location shift (LS) for the generalized logistic distribution with parameter w.

w	LS
0.1	7.5
0.25	2.75
0.5	1.75
1.0	1.25
2.0	0.75
5.0	0.5
10.0	0.4

TABLE 3.17. Simulated power $(1 - \hat{\beta})$ comparisons for the generalized logistic distribution with parameter w given specified values of v, $\alpha = 0.05$, and the LS values listed in Table 3.16.

w	v							
	0.25	0.5	1.0	1.5	2.0	3.0	4.0	6.0
0.1	0.4305	0.4649	0.5098	0.5356	0.5425	0.5354	0.5181	0.4815
0.25	0.3326	0.3547	0.3867	0.4046	0.4099	0.3995	0.3835	0.3556
0.5	0.4093	0.4336	0.4615	0.4753	0.4800	0.4712	0.4448	0.4023
1.0	0.5492	0.5650	0.5875	0.5989	0.6068	0.5904	0.5652	0.5129
2.0	0.4826	0.4986	0.5195	0.5308	0.5353	0.5288	0.5133	0.4737
5.0	0.5133	0.5589	0.5939	0.6026	0.6074	0.6011	0.5938	0.5753
10.0	0.5521	0.6273	0.6729	0.6819	0.6894	0.6928	0.6864	0.6626

open question is the small sample performance of linear rank tests compared to corresponding rank tests based on alternative distance functions, i.e., $v \neq 2$. To shed light on this question, two-sample simulated location-shift power comparisons involving seven cases of Class I ($w = 0.1$, 0.25, 0.5, 1.0, 2.0, 5.0, and 10.0) were made for eight choices of v (0.25, 0.5, 1.0, 1.5, 2.0, 3.0, 4.0, and 6.0). The same value of w corresponds to both the rank-order statistic and the generalized logistic distribution parameter for each case. The location shifts of the second sample values associated with each value of w are given in Table 3.16. The simulated powers in Table 3.17 are based on 10,000 randomly simulated Pearson type III P-values for each two-sample test, where the sample sizes of each simulated test are $n_1 = n_2 = 20$ and the level of significance is $\alpha = 0.05$. Attainment of P-values by resampling where each P-value is based on $L = 100,000$ is impractical for the present purpose since $10,000 \times 100,000$ simulations is a computational burden. An immediate feature of Table 3.17 is that the largest simulated power occurs when $v = 2.0$ for six of the seven cases (for $w = 10.0$, the largest simulated power occurs when $v = 3.0$). The power analyses of Mielke (1972) were purely asymptotic, but the simulated power comparisons in Table 3.17 suggest that analogous results carry over reasonably well for small sample sizes in many situations.

Specific applications involving these classes of rank tests include analyses of weather modification experiments (Grant and Mielke, 1967; Mielke, 1974, 1995; Mielke et al., 1970, 1971, 1981c, 1982). Finally, the motivation for using rank transformations to avoid problems with extreme values when $v = 2$ is moot when $v = 1$; thus, the loss of information regarding the original data when a rank transformation is used may be irrelevant.

3.7   Analyses of Metal Contamination and Learning Achievement

Determining causes of learning difficulties in children and the subsequent poor ratings of elementary schools is elusive due to the complexity of the situation.[3] Learning involves a panoply of activities and interactions including parental support, student preparedness, teacher skills, and institutional infrastructures. Children are particularly vulnerable to environmental toxins in their early developmental years (ages 12–24 months) and are especially susceptible to neurotoxic effects from metals such as lead (Bearer, 2000; Cohen Hubal et al., 2000).

Environmental contamination as a cause of neurotoxicity in children is suspected to be one factor affecting abilities and behaviors connected with learning. A potential source of learning and behavior problems is the quality of the community environment where preschool children live prior to attending their local school. In New Orleans, a pre-Katrina study compared soil lead on elementary school properties with soil lead on neighboring residential properties (Mielke et al., 2005a). The New Orleans study focused on the qualities of the environments of elementary school communities of New Orleans and their potential impact on children's learning achievement. Two databases were used to evaluate the conditions of the environment and human health response. The measure of environmental quality is the metal content of elementary school community soils of New Orleans. The city had previously been systematically surveyed and a database consisting of analysis of soil samples for nine metals: lead (Pb), zinc (Zn), cadmium (Cd), nickel (Ni), manganese (Mn), copper (Cu), chromium (Cr), cobalt (Co), and vanadium (V) stratified by census tracts had been assembled (Mielke et al., 2000). The Multiple Metal Accumulation (MMA) value is simply the sum of the nine individual metal values.

---

[3]Adapted and reprinted with permission of Elsevier Inc. from H.W. Mielke, K.J. Berry, P.W. Mielke, Jr., E.T. Powell, and C.R. Gonzales. Multiple metal accumulation as a factor in learning achievement with various New Orleans elementary school communities. *Environmental Research*, 2005, 97, 67–75. Copyright © 2004 by Elsevier Inc.

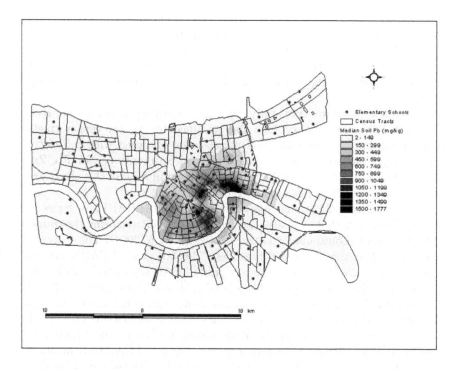

FIGURE 3.2. Locations of metropolitan New Orleans elementary district schools ($n = 111$) overlaid on a map of the multiple metal accumulation in urban soils.

Learning achievement is a potentially sensitive measure of the human health response to environmental stressors (May, 2000). The measures used for learning achievement were the standardized test scores of the Louisiana Educational Assessment Program (LEAP) 4th grade public elementary school students (Louisiana Department of Education, 2001). The null hypothesis tested here is that there is no association between metal contaminated soils of elementary school attendance districts and learning achievement of students attending New Orleans elementary schools.

3.7.1 Methods

Geographic Information Science was used to assemble the data for this study. The components include: attendance district schools and their assignment to census tracts, soil metal data by census tracts, and LEAP score data by census tracts. The analysis of the data sets are based on MRPP.

Paired community metal data and student achievement scores were available for 128 elementary schools in metropolitan New Orleans. In New Orleans, 17 magnet schools that drew students from beyond the local neighborhood had also been established. The remaining 111 schools were attendance district schools that drew students directly from the local community. Each of 94 among a total of 286 census tracts contained at least 1 of these remaining 111 elementary schools: 79 census tracts contained 1 school, 14 census tracts contained 2 schools, and 1 census tract contained 4 schools.

The soil samples for this study were systematically collected between February 1998 and January 2000 and stratified by the 286 census tracts of metropolitan New Orleans. Soil metals were analyzed with a Spectro Inductively Coupled Plasma Atomic Emission Spectroscope, for Pb, Zn, Cd, Ni, Mn, Cu, Cr, Co, and V. The environmental data of this study are medians of nine soil metals analyzed for each census tract.

The Louisiana Educational Assessment Program (LEAP) is a series of standardized tests that evaluates the progress of students during the course of their studies (Louisiana Department of Education, 2001). The tests are administered to the 4th and 8th grades. The 4th grade LEAP scores of students are more likely than the 8th grade LEAP scores to be linked to the communities where the students lived and grew up during childhood development because advancing years, moving, and other events are expected to gradually change the student classroom composition. The 32,741 test scores are derived from the 1999 administration of the LEAP test (Louisiana Department of Education, 2001). The four LEAP tests involved English Language Arts (ELA), Social Studies (SOC), Mathematics (MAT), and Science (SCI) and were administered to 4th grade students. The scoring frequencies of students from each school were available for five different categories of achievement designated as Advanced (A), Proficient (P), Basic (B), Approaching Basic (AB), and Unsatisfactory (U). The test scores in these five categories of the four LEAP tests for 111 elementary schools in metropolitan New Orleans provide the raw data for evaluating the learning response.

The New Orleans metropolitan area consists of 286 census tracts (US Census Bureau, 2003). Geographic Information Systems (GIS) techniques were used to assemble attendance district data, LEAP score data, census tract data, and soil metal data for each census tract with public elementary schools in New Orleans. Figure 3.2 shows the location of the elementary schools for the assembled LEAP score database and the soil MMA database of metropolitan New Orleans. The MMA map is based on kriging of census tract centroids with their assigned MMA soil values. The relatively small MMA soil values in the central business district of New Orleans are a consequence of open soil being removed, replaced, and paved over. Note the large MMA soil values in the first ring of inner-city communities and the reduction of MMA soil values toward the suburban communities in the outer parts of the city.

TABLE 3.18. Listings of minimum ($P_{0.00}$), first quartile ($P_{0.25}$), median ($P_{0.50}$), third quartile ($P_{0.75}$), and maximum ($P_{1.00}$) amounts in mg/kg for nine soil metals and MMA.

Soil metal	Quantile				
	$P_{0.00}$	$P_{0.25}$	$P_{0.50}$	$P_{0.75}$	$P_{1.00}$
Pb	6.2	37.0	81.0	293.5	1,164.0
Zn	22.8	75.5	159.9	323.1	874.5
Cd	0.3	1.5	2.4	3.3	5.2
Ni	2.6	6.3	8.1	9.7	13.6
Mn	72.3	105.6	132.3	157.7	229.3
Cu	4.6	9.8	19.0	29.0	53.0
Cr	0.1	1.3	2.0	3.3	6.7
Co	1.3	3.3	4.2	5.4	7.0
V	1.0	3.1	4.0	4.8	7.8
MMA	127.4	233.4	418.3	841.3	2,282.5

3.7.2 Results

Table 3.18 lists the minimum ($P_{0.00}$), first quartile ($P_{0.25}$), median ($P_{0.50}$), third quartile ($P_{0.75}$), and maximum ($P_{1.00}$) values in mg/kg for nine sampled heavy metals (Pb, Zn, Cd, Ni, Mn, Cu, Cr, Co, V) and the Multiple Metal Accumulations (MMA) for the 111 school attendance districts. Specifically, the MMA value is the simple sum of the nine individual metal values in mg/kg.

Table 3.19 lists the pairwise Pearson product-moment correlations among the nine metals for the 111 school attendance districts. Note that correlations between the individual metals and the MMA are generally stronger than the correlations between individual metals. Alternative linear combinations of these nine individual metals would yield stronger results than those obtained for the simply-defined MMA.

For the statistical analysis, the 111 school attendance districts were divided into three groups of equal size ($n_1 = n_2 = n_3 = 37$) based on the ordered MMA soil values categorized into Low ($P_{0.33}$ and below), Middle ($P_{0.34}$ to $P_{0.66}$), and High ($P_{0.67}$ and above) MMA soil groups. The locations of the Low, Middle, and High MMA soil groups were compared in a five-dimensional space based on the five student score proportions of each school (A, P, B, AB, and U) for each of the four LEAP tests: ELA, SOC, MAT, and SCI. Table 3.20 contains the ELA, SOC, MAT, and SCI test distributions of student score proportions for the Low, Middle, and High MMA soil groups.

Because it is not possible to order data values in a five-dimensional space, the data values are ordered according to the MMA soil values within each of the Low, Middle, and High MMA soil groups. Inspection of Table 3.20 reveals that for ELA, SOC, MAT, and SCI, the proportion of students

TABLE 3.19. Pairwise correlations of nine soil metals and MMA for 111 school attendance districts in metropolitan New Orleans.

Soil metal	Soil metal and MMA								
	Zn	Cd	Ni	Mn	Cu	Cr	Co	V	MMA
Pb	0.88	0.58	0.44	0.40	0.83	0.82	0.49	0.52	0.97
Zn		0.72	0.64	0.43	0.90	0.88	0.65	0.59	0.96
Cd			0.82	0.45	0.76	0.74	0.90	0.56	0.67
Ni				0.55	0.70	0.73	0.91	0.74	0.57
Mn					0.58	0.54	0.50	0.76	0.50
Cu						0.89	0.68	0.70	0.90
Cr							0.74	0.70	0.89
Co								0.66	0.60
V									0.61

TABLE 3.20. Proportions of advanced (A), proficient (P), basic (B), approaching basic (AB), and unsatisfactory (U) scores for low, middle, and high soil MMA amounts for English language arts (ELA), social studies (SOC), mathematics (MAT), and science (SCI) 4th grade LEAP tests.*

	LEAP score categories					
Tests	A	P	B	AB	U	(n)
MMA and ELA						
Low	0.0172	0.1199	0.3768	0.2579	0.2282	(3,195)
Middle	0.0074	0.0971	0.3063	0.2497	0.3394	(2,687)
High	0.0030	0.0272	0.1955	0.2598	0.5145	(2,317)
MMA and SOC						
Low	0.0047	0.1025	0.3991	0.2241	0.2696	(3,182)
Middle	0.0026	0.0488	0.2761	0.2329	0.4396	(2,684)
High	0.0004	0.0056	0.1577	0.2210	0.6153	(2,308)
MMA and MAT						
Low	0.0163	0.0964	0.3389	0.2205	0.3279	(3,184)
Middle	0.0086	0.0599	0.2626	0.2187	0.4504	(2,689)
High	0.0009	0.0117	0.1748	0.1977	0.6150	(2,317)
MMA and SCI						
Low	0.0085	0.0829	0.3849	0.3047	0.2190	(3,183)
Middle	0.0034	0.0499	0.2587	0.3165	0.3716	(2,686)
High	0.0000	0.0069	0.1217	0.3123	0.5591	(2,309)

*Number of 4th grade students (n) is given in parentheses.

TABLE 3.21. MRPP LEAP test Pearson type III P-values listed for data values by the soil values of each individual metal along with MMA LEAP test Pearson type III P-values for comparison.

Soil	LEAP test			
metal	ELA	SOC	MAT	SCI
Pb	0.17×10^{-6}	0.19×10^{-7}	0.41×10^{-5}	0.30×10^{-7}
Zn	0.18×10^{-6}	0.34×10^{-8}	0.79×10^{-6}	0.20×10^{-8}
Cd	0.96×10^{-6}	0.15×10^{-6}	0.14×10^{-5}	0.35×10^{-6}
Ni	0.74×10^{-4}	0.39×10^{-4}	0.16×10^{-4}	0.15×10^{-4}
Mn	0.65×10^{-6}	0.24×10^{-6}	0.15×10^{-6}	0.15×10^{-6}
Cu	0.19×10^{-7}	0.25×10^{-8}	0.47×10^{-6}	0.70×10^{-9}
Cr	0.23×10^{-7}	0.39×10^{-9}	0.64×10^{-7}	0.23×10^{-9}
Co	0.21×10^{-5}	0.58×10^{-8}	0.42×10^{-6}	0.66×10^{-7}
V	0.93×10^{-5}	0.65×10^{-6}	0.27×10^{-4}	0.43×10^{-6}
MMA	0.57×10^{-7}	0.29×10^{-8}	0.41×10^{-6}	0.17×10^{-8}

classified as A, P, and B consistently decreases with increasing MMA, the proportion of students classified as U increases with increasing MMA, and the proportion of students classified as AB are not consistent in order as these proportions contain the reversal values between A, P, B, and U. The MRPP P-values for the separation differences in the Low, Middle, and High MMA soil groups in the five-dimensional data space are 0.57×10^{-7}, 0.29×10^{-8}, 0.41×10^{-6}, and 0.17×10^{-8} for ELA, SOC, MAT, and SCI, respectively. In addition, analogous MRPP LEAP test Pearson type III P-values are listed in Table 3.21 with the data values ordered by the soil values of each metal; for comparison, the MMA LEAP test Pearson type III P-values are also included. The strongest results interestingly occur for Cr, Cu, Zn, and MMA rather than Pb as might be anticipated. Calculation of exact P-values is prohibitive since they require

$$M = \frac{111!}{37!^3} \doteq 6.761 \times 10^{50}$$

equally-likely distinct arrangements. Moreover, resampling approximate P-values were not obtained since they require at least 10^{10} randomly obtained arrangements to estimate the exact P-values for some cases. Consequently, the Pearson type III approximate P-values were obtained for all cases.

3.7.3 Alternative Analyses

The experimental units of the previous analyses are based on 111 elementary schools where the experimental response for each elementary school is the proportion of 4th grade students in each of the five LEAP score categories. In contrast, the experimental units of alternative analyses can

TABLE 3.22. Frequencies of advanced (A), proficient (P), basic (B), approaching basic (AB), and unsatisfactory (U) scores for low, middle, and high soil MMA amounts for English language arts (ELA), social studies (SOC), mathematics (MAT), and science (SCI) 4th grade LEAP tests.

	LEAP score categories				
Tests	A	P	B	AB	U
ELA					
Low	55	383	1,204	824	729
Middle	20	261	823	671	912
High	7	63	453	602	1,192
SOC					
Low	15	326	1,270	713	858
Middle	7	131	741	625	1,180
High	1	13	364	510	1,420
MAT					
Low	52	307	1,079	702	1,044
Middle	23	161	706	588	1,211
High	2	27	405	458	1,425
SCI					
Low	27	264	1,225	970	697
Middle	9	134	695	850	998
High	0	16	281	721	1,291

TABLE 3.23. Alternative MRPP LEAP test Pearson type III P-values listed for data values ordered by soil values of each individual metal along with MMA LEAP test Pearson type III P-values for comparison.

Soil metal	LEAP test			
	ELA	SOC	MAT	SCI
Pb	0.6×10^{-113}	0.6×10^{-152}	0.7×10^{-97}	0.1×10^{-152}
Zn	0.2×10^{-129}	0.4×10^{-200}	0.6×10^{-123}	0.4×10^{-192}
Cd	0.4×10^{-118}	0.3×10^{-170}	0.9×10^{-108}	0.2×10^{-151}
Ni	0.2×10^{-89}	0.4×10^{-136}	0.2×10^{-86}	0.1×10^{-124}
Mn	0.5×10^{-96}	0.5×10^{-124}	0.1×10^{-99}	0.5×10^{-121}
Cu	0.2×10^{-140}	0.2×10^{-192}	0.3×10^{-115}	0.6×10^{-194}
Cr	0.4×10^{-159}	0.8×10^{-247}	0.2×10^{-166}	0.1×10^{-233}
Co	0.5×10^{-120}	0.9×10^{-191}	0.3×10^{-129}	0.3×10^{-177}
V	0.1×10^{-76}	0.1×10^{-112}	0.1×10^{-61}	0.6×10^{-110}
MMA	0.1×10^{-120}	0.1×10^{-171}	0.2×10^{-107}	0.4×10^{-175}

be based on the number of 4th grade students in each of the five LEAP score categories (i.e., $r = 5$), where each experimental response consists of a 1 in the category in which a student is classified and a 0 in each of the remaining four categories. The number of 4th grade students test scores for ELA, SOC, MAT, and SCI were 8,199, 8,174, 8,190, and 8,178, respectively. Because these numbers are much larger than 111, substantially stronger results (i.e., smaller P-values) are anticipated for the alternative analyses. The Low, Middle, and High soil metal amounts partitions (i.e., $g = 3$) for the alternative analyses are the same as the previous analyses. Note that these alternative analyses are described in Section 3.2.2 with

$$C_i = \frac{n_i}{K},$$

where $K = N$. Table 3.22 contains the specific MMA frequency data used in these alternative MRPP analyses.

Exact P-values are obviously impossible to compute for these alternative analyses. For example, the number of equally-likely arrangements for the MMA and ELA combination is

$$M = \frac{8,199!}{(3,195!)(2,687!)(2,317!)} \doteq 1.495 \times 10^{3,877}.$$

Table 3.23 contains the alternative MRPP LEAP test Pearson type III P-values that correspond to the P-values given in Table 3.21 for the previous analyses. While all the inferential results in Table 3.23 are exceedingly strong, the strongest results once again occur for Cr, Cu, Zn, and MMA in an ordering that is roughly consistent with the previous results where the 111 elementary schools were the experimental units. The results are so spectacularly strong that it is difficult to believe that other urban areas in the world do not suffer from a similar environmental problem. As shown in Section 2.5, heavy metal contamination in urban areas is not an isolated situation. Since this study is based on real data, the results imply that the inherent mental capacities of a large proportion of children around the world are reduced as a consequence of environmental contamination.

4
Description of MRBP

The analysis of data obtained from balanced randomized block designs is an important part of experimental research. In this chapter, permutation versions of univariate and multivariate balanced randomized block analyses, based on Euclidean distances, are presented. Methods for obtaining exact and approximate resampling and Pearson type III P-values are described. Rank and binary transformations for randomized block designs are discussed, and power comparisons are provided for a variety of univariate rank tests. A measure of agreement based on randomized blocks is developed and extended to various levels of measurement, multiple observers, and multivariate analyses.

As a motivation for multivariate randomized block permutation procedures (MRBP), consider samples of bg independent random variables x_{ij} with cumulative distribution functions $F_i(x + \beta_j)$ for $i = 1, ..., g$ and $j = 1, ..., b$, respectively, where g is the number of treatments and b is the number of blocks. For simplicity, assume that x_{ij} is from a normal distribution with mean $\mu_i + \beta_j$ and variance σ^2 ($i = 1, ..., g$ and $j = 1, ..., b$). To test the null hypothesis of no differences among treatments, one tests H_0: $\mu_1 = \cdots = \mu_g$ versus H_1: $\mu_i \neq \mu_j$ for some $i \neq j$ using the F statistic given by

$$F = \frac{MS_{Treatment}}{MS_{Error}},$$

where

$$MS_{Treatment} = \frac{1}{g-1} SS_{Treatment},$$

$$SS_{Treatment} = b \sum_{i=1}^{g} (\bar{x}_{i.} - \bar{x}_{..})^2,$$

$$MS_{Error} = \frac{1}{(b-1)(g-1)} SS_{Error},$$

$$SS_{Error} = SS_{Total} - SS_{Blocks} - SS_{Treatment},$$

$$SS_{Blocks} = g \sum_{j=1}^{b} (\bar{x}_{.j} - \bar{x}_{..})^2,$$

$$SS_{Total} = \sum_{i=1}^{g} \sum_{j=1}^{b} (x_{ij} - \bar{x}_{..})^2,$$

$$\bar{x}_{i.} = \frac{1}{b} \sum_{j=1}^{b} x_{ij},$$

for $i = 1, ..., g,$

$$\bar{x}_{.j} = \frac{1}{g} \sum_{i=1}^{g} x_{ij},$$

for $j = 1, ..., b,$ and

$$\bar{x}_{..} = \frac{1}{bg} \sum_{i=1}^{g} \sum_{j=1}^{b} x_{ij}.$$

Under H_0, the distribution of F is known to be Snedecor's F distribution with $g - 1$ degrees-of-freedom (df) in the numerator and $(b-1)(g-1)$ df in the denominator. If x_{ij} is not from a normal distribution, then the distribution of statistic F does not follow Snedecor's F distribution. However, the F statistic is a reasonable measure of how consistent or inconsistent the data are with H_0. The F statistic compares the between-treatment variability with the error variability, i.e., within-treatment variability corrected for block differences. If the treatment variability is much larger than the error variability, then this can be interpreted as evidence against H_0. The critical value of F to reject H_0 depends on the distribution of F under the null hypothesis that $F_i(x + \beta_j) = F_0(x + \beta_j)$ for $i = 1, ..., g$ and $j = 1, ..., b$. The analogous Fisher–Pitman permutation test involves the conditional distribution of F given the sets of order statistics $x_{1j,g} \leq \cdots \leq x_{gj,g}$ for $j = 1, ..., b$. Under the null hypothesis that $F_i(x + \beta_j) = F_0(x + \beta_j)$ for $i = 1, ..., g$ and $j = 1, ..., b$, every assignment of $x_{1j}, ..., x_{gj}$ to the $g!$ ordered positions occurs with equal probability $1/g!$ for $j = 1, ..., b$. Thus, the conditional distribution of F given $x_{1j,g} \leq \cdots \leq x_{gj,g}$ does not depend on $F_0(x + \beta_j)$ for $j = 1, ..., b$ and can be explicitly calculated by enumerating the

$$M = (g!)^b$$

assignments and calculating the value of F corresponding to each assignment, i.e., a reference distribution of M equally-likely values of F. If F_o is the calculated value of F associated with the observed data, then the significance probability under H_0 is the proportion of the M values of F comprising the reference distribution equal to or greater than F_o. This procedure yields a conditionally exact significance test that is distribution-free, i.e., does not depend on $F_0(x + \beta_j)$ for $j = 1, ..., b$. MRBP is based on this concept and an alternative representation of the F statistic is given by

$$F = \frac{(b-1)\left[2SS_{Total} - g(b-1)\delta\right]}{g(b-1)\delta - 2SS_{Blocks}},$$

where

$$\delta = \frac{1}{g\binom{b}{2}} \sum_{i=1}^{g} \sum_{j<k} (x_{ij} - x_{ik})^2$$

(Mielke and Iyer, 1982). Because both SS_{Total} and SS_{Blocks} are invariant under all M assignments, δ may be used as a test statistic that is equivalent to F. Since large values of F correspond to small values of δ, the P-value of this test is

$$P(\delta \le \delta_o \,|\, x_{1j,g} \le \cdots \le x_{gj,g})$$

for $j = 1, ..., b$, where δ_o is the value of δ that corresponds to F_o. Thus, the Fisher–Pitman permutation test for randomized blocks may utilize either δ or F.

Given that the data values are points in a data space, the statistic δ is based on the "interpoint" squared distances of data belonging to the same treatment group. After adjusting for block differences, this feature is indicated by data values exhibiting clumping within treatment groups relative to all other possible within-block permutations of the data values. Variations of δ lead to natural and meaningful generalizations that might otherwise be unanticipated. Since the key feature of δ is the interpoint squared distance $(x_i - x_j)^2$, generalizations occur by replacing $(x_i - x_j)^2$ with Δ_{ij}, where Δ_{ij} is any other measure of separation between x_i and x_j, such as $|x_i - x_j|$. As with the MRPP statistic, Δ_{ij} is a symmetric nonnegative distance function, which may be a metric. Furthermore, δ extends itself to multivariate data far more naturally than F. These properties lead to the use of δ, the MRBP statistic, as a test of H_0.

4.1   General Formulation of MRBP

Suppose a number of observed fields are compared to corresponding fields generated by one or more numerical models. Let the observed phenomena and the one or more numerical model predictions of these phenomena be termed "blocks," i.e., the first block represents the observed phenomena and the remaining $b - 1$ blocks represent the $b - 1$ numerical model predictions of these phenomena for a total of b blocks. Also, let r denote the number of commensurate response measurements (vector size) from each phenomenon and let g denote the number of phenomena, which will be termed "treatments." Suppose $x'_{ij} = (x_{1ij}, ..., x_{rij})$ is the vector of r response measurements associated with the ith treatment and jth block. Then, the MRBP statistic is given by

$$\delta = \left[g \binom{b}{2} \right]^{-1} \sum_{i=1}^{g} \sum_{j<k} \Delta(x_{ij}, x_{ik}),$$

where $\sum_{j<k}$ is the sum over all j and k such that $1 \leq j < k \leq b$ and $\Delta(x, y)$ is the symmetric distance function value of the two points (r-dimensional vectors) $x' = (x_1, ..., x_r)$ and $y' = (y_1, ..., y_r)$ in the r-dimensional Euclidean space. The choice of symmetric distance functions considered here is given by

$$\Delta(x, y) = \left[\sum_{i=1}^{r} (x_i - y_i)^2 \right]^{v/2}, \tag{4.1}$$

where $v > 0$ (note that $v = 1$ yields ordinary Euclidean distance). Although the truncation constant, B, discussed in Section 2.2 is omitted from Expression (4.1), some applications may find the truncation constant to be very useful. The null hypothesis (H_0) states that the distribution of δ assigns an equal probability to each of the

$$M = (g!)^b$$

possible allocations of the g r-dimensional response measurements to the g treatment positions within each of the b blocks. Consequently, the collection of r response measurements within each block yields g r-dimensional exchangeable random variables under H_0. The δ statistic compares the within-group clumping of response measurements against the model specified by random allocation under H_0. The initial presentations and theoretical developments of MRBP are given in Brockwell and Mielke (1984), Brown (1982), Mielke (1984, 1986), Mielke and Berry (1982), and Mielke and Iyer (1982).

The exact MRBP P-values are analogous to the exact MRPP P-values described in Section 2.3. Like MRPP, the calculation of exact MRBP P-values becomes unreasonable when M exceeds, say, 10^9, e.g., $b = 6$ and $g = 5$ yield $M = 2.99 \times 10^{12}$, and $b = 3$ and $g = 8$ yield $M = 6.55 \times 10^{13}$. Thus, resampling and Pearson type III approximations are just as essential for MRBP as they are for MRPP (see Section 2.3). A resampling approximation is based on L independent realizations of δ. Since each realization of δ requires a constant multiple of gb^2 operations, a resampling P-value requires a constant multiple of Lgb^2 operations. Alternatively, a Pearson type III approximation depends on the exact mean, variance, and skewness of δ under H_0. However, the following efficient computational expressions for μ, σ^2, and γ pertain to MRBP. If

$$\Delta(i, s; j, t) = \Delta(x_{is}, x_{jt})$$

and

$$D(i, s; j, t) = \Delta(i, s; j, t) - g^{-1} \sum_{m=1}^{g} \Delta(m, s; j, t) - g^{-1} \sum_{n=1}^{g} \Delta(i, s; n, t)$$

$$+ g^{-2} \sum_{m=1}^{g} \sum_{n=1}^{g} \Delta(m, s; n, t),$$

then, μ, σ^2, and γ are conveniently expressed as

$$\mu = \left[g^2 \binom{b}{2} \right]^{-1} \sum_{s<t} \sum_{i=1}^{g} \sum_{j=1}^{g} \Delta(i, s; j, t),$$

$$\sigma^2 = \left[g \binom{b}{2} \right]^{-2} \frac{1}{g-1} \sum_{s<t} \sum_{i=1}^{g} \sum_{j=1}^{g} \left[D(i, s; j, t) \right]^2,$$

and

$$\gamma = \frac{\kappa_3}{\sigma^3},$$

using the definition of κ_3 given by

$$\kappa_3 = \left[g \binom{b}{2} \right]^{-3} \frac{1}{g-1} \left[H(g) + L(b) \right],$$

where $g \geq 2$, $b \geq 2$, and wherein (1) $H(g) = 0$ if $g = 2$, and

$$H(g) = \frac{g}{g-2} \sum_{s<t} \sum_{i=1}^{g} \sum_{j=1}^{g} \left[D(i, s; j, t) \right]^3$$

if $g \geq 3$, and (2) $L(b) = 0$ if $b = 2$, and

$$L(b) = \frac{6}{g-1} \sum_{s<t<u} \sum_{i=1}^{g} \sum_{j=1}^{g} \sum_{k=1}^{g} D(i, s; j, t) D(i, s; k, u) D(j, t; k, u)$$

if $b \geq 3$ ($\sum_{s<t<u}$ denotes the sum over all s, t, and u such that $1 \leq s < t < u \leq b$). Therefore, a Pearson type III P-value requires a constant multiple of $g^3 b^3$ operations. The resampling and Pearson type III approximation comparisons described in Section 2.3 for MRPP also pertain to MRBP.

Here, the execution time of a Pearson type III approximation is roughly $g^2 b/L$ that of a resampling approximation. The Pearson type III P-value program was given by Iyer et al. (1983).

The chance-corrected agreement measure given by

$$\Re = 1 - \frac{\delta}{\mu} \qquad (4.2)$$

estimates the composite measurement of agreement among blocks for all treatments. As an example, perfect agreement between the observed data and the results of a numerical model implies that the observed and model predicated data sets (blocks) are identical for each event among the number of events (treatments) in question. As with the chance-corrected within-group agreement measure in Section 2.3, the values of $\Re$ range from negative values to 1 when perfect agreement is achieved, $E[\Re \mid H_0] = 0$, and either agreement or disagreement is implied by $\Re > 0$ or $\Re < 0$, respectively. As noted in Section 2.3, large data sets can yield small positive values of $\Re$ with very small P-values, and small data sets can yield relatively large positive values of $\Re$ with fairly large P-values. Although P-values are highly dependent on sample size, this sample size dependence does not hold for the agreement measure $\Re$. Incidentally, special cases of $\Re$ include the classical Pearson correlation coefficient (which differs by, at most, a constant multiple) and Spearman's rank-order correlation coefficient (Mielke, 1984). Although $\Re$ (initially termed ρ) was suggested by Mielke (1984), a more recent discussion by Berry and Mielke (1988b) demonstrates that $\Re$ includes a wide variety of agreement measures as special cases. As noted in Section 2.3.5 for MRPP, $\Re$ is also a recommended measure of effect size for MRBP.

A major point noted by Mielke and Iyer (1982) involves aligning blocks prior to an MRBP analysis. For example, if the response measurement medians of each block are subtracted from the corresponding response measurements of each block, then the adjusted response measurement medians are said to be aligned to zero for all blocks. Since the permutation structure of this MRBP analysis is not affected by block alignment, the exchangeability of response measurements within blocks is maintained. Consider the following univariate data, where $r = 1$, $b = 2$, and $g = 3$: $x_{111} = 4$, $x_{112} = 2$, $x_{113} = 3$, $x_{121} = 9$, $x_{122} = 7$, and $x_{123} = 8$. If $v = 1$, then $\delta_0 = 5$ and also the statistic δ is 5 for all permutations of values within blocks, i.e., the P-value of δ_0 is 1 without alignment. The median values for blocks 1 and 2 are 3 and 8, respectively. If the median value is subtracted from the values of each block, then the aligned data are $y_{111} = 1$, $y_{112} = -1$, $y_{113} = 0$, $y_{121} = 1$, $y_{122} = -1$, and $y_{123} = 0$. If $v = 1$, then $\delta_0 = 0$ and statistic δ is 0, 2/3, and 4/3 with probabilities of 1/6, 1/3, and 1/2, respectively (the P-value of δ_0 is 1/6 with alignment). If y_{kij} represents an aligned set of data, then $x_{kij} = y_{kij}/\phi_k$, where

$$\phi_k = \left[\sum_{i_1=1}^{g} \sum_{i_2=1}^{g} \sum_{j_1<j_2} \left| y_{ki_1j_1} - y_{ki_2j_2} \right|^v \right]^{1/v}$$

for $k = 1, ..., r$. These commensurate data have the desired property that

$$\sum_{i_1=1}^{g} \sum_{i_2=1}^{g} \sum_{j_1<j_2} \left| x_{ki_1j_1} - x_{ki_2j_2} \right|^v = 1$$

for $k = 1, ..., r$ and any $v > 0$. If $v = 1$, then the commensuration is Euclidean commensuration. If a single object is not assigned to each block by treatment combination as required for MRBP, then an approximate analysis based on MRPP may be accomplished after (1) aligning all blocks, (2) making the data commensurate for each response when $r > 1$, and (3) collapsing the data over blocks (Mielke and Iyer, 1982). Specifically, suppose that $m_{ij} \geq 0$ objects are contained in the ith treatment and jth block combination for $i = 1, ..., g+1$ and $j = 1, ..., b$, where the $(g+1)$-st treatment is analogous to the excess group of MRPP. Then, $N_j = \sum_{i=1}^{g+1} m_{ij}$ is the number of objects in the jth block $(j = 1, ..., b)$ and $n_i = \sum_{j=1}^{b} m_{ij}$ is the number of objects in the ith treatment, where $n_i \geq 2$ for $i = 1, ..., g$ and $n_{g+1} \geq 0$. The total number of permutations in this generalized MRBP context is

$$M' = \prod_{j=1}^{b} \left(\frac{N_j!}{\prod_{i=1}^{g+1} m_{ij}!} \right).$$

If the blocks are aligned and collapsed, then the total number of permutations in the resulting MRPP context is

$$M'' = \frac{N!}{\prod_{i=1}^{g+1} n_i!}.$$

Since the permutation structures associated with M' and M'' are different, the MRPP of the align and collapse procedure is an approximation of the generalized MRBP.

4.2 Permutation Randomized Block Analysis of Variance

In this section, the relation between δ and the classical F statistic for testing the null hypothesis of a randomized block design is described. If $v = 2$ and

$r = 1$, then the functional relation between F and δ is given by

$$F = \frac{(b-1)\,[2SS_T - g(b-1)\delta]}{g(b-1)\delta - 2SS_B},$$

where the corrected total sum of squares is given by

$$SS_T = \sum_{i=1}^{g} \sum_{j=1}^{b} x_{ij}^2 - SS_M,$$

the block sum of squares is given by

$$SS_B = \frac{1}{g} \sum_{j=1}^{b} \left(\sum_{i=1}^{g} x_{ij} \right)^2 - SS_M,$$

and

$$SS_M = \frac{1}{bg} \left(\sum_{i=1}^{g} \sum_{j=1}^{b} x_{ij} \right)^2.$$

Thus, F and δ are equivalent under the null hypothesis since SS_T and SS_B are invariant relative to the $(g!)^b$ permutations of the response measurements. For this and other cases involving univariate responses, the response measurement subscript is omitted, i.e., $x_{1ij} = x_{ij}$.

Let R denote the ordinary Pearson product-moment correlation coefficient. If $v = 2$, $b = 2$, and $r = 1$, then the functional relation between R and δ is given by

$$R = \frac{\mu - \delta}{2S_1 S_2},$$

where

$$R = \frac{1}{gS_1 S_2} \sum_{i=1}^{g} (x_{i1} - \bar{x}_1)(x_{i2} - \bar{x}_2),$$

$$\mu = S_1^2 + S_2^2 + (\bar{x}_1 - \bar{x}_2)^2,$$

$$\bar{x}_j = \frac{1}{g} \sum_{i=1}^{g} x_{ij},$$

and

$$S_j^2 = \frac{1}{g} \sum_{i=1}^{g} (x_{ij} - \bar{x}_j)^2$$

for $j = 1$ and 2. Then, R and δ are equivalent under the null hypothesis because $\bar{x}_1$, $\bar{x}_2$, S_1, and S_2 are invariant relative to the $(g!)^2$ permutations of the response measurements. If $(x_{11}, ..., x_{g1})$ is one of the $g!$ permutations of $(x_{12}, ..., x_{g2})$, then $\mu = 2S_1S_2$ and $R = \Re$ of Expression (4.2). If $g = 2$, $r = 1$, $x_{1j} = -x_{2j} = x_j$, and $|x_j| > 0$ for $j = 1, ..., b$, then the test based on δ is equivalent to the permutation version of either the matched-pair or one-sample t test.

For comparison, the chance-corrected agreement measure between n pairs of values (x_i, y_i), for $i = 1, ..., n$, is given by

$$\Re = 1 - \frac{\delta}{\mu},$$

where

$$\delta = n^{-1} \sum_{i=1}^{n} |x_i - y_i|$$

and

$$\mu = n^{-2} \sum_{i=1}^{n} \sum_{j=1}^{n} |x_i - y_i|.$$

Specifically, δ is the simple version of the MRBP statistic where $v = 1$, $b = 2$, and $r = 1$, i.e., there are only two blocks and μ is the expected value of δ under H_0 that each of the $n!$ orderings of $x_1, ..., x_n$ relative to a fixed ordering of $y_1, ..., y_n$ are equally likely. As defined, $-1 \leq \Re \leq +1$, $\Re = +1$ implies perfect agreement, $\Re > 0$ implies agreement, and $\Re \leq 0$ implies no agreement. Thus, the closer $\Re$ is to $+1$, the higher the agreement. While $R \geq -1$ when $n = 2$, $\Re > -1$ when $n \geq 3$. If $\Re_o$ is the observed value of $\Re$, then the probability that $\Re \geq \Re_o$ under H_0 is the P-value in question. Also, $\Re$ has advantages over the Pearson product-moment correlation coefficient, R, since (1) $\Re$ is a measure of agreement rather than a measure of linearity and (2) $\Re$ is far more stable (i.e., robust) than R since it is based on ordinary Euclidean distances rather than squared Euclidean distances.

4.3   Rank and Binary Data

Let the g treatment responses for each of the b block and r response measurement combinations be replaced with their corresponding rank-order statistics, i.e., permutations of $1, ..., g$. Although data-related information is lost with this transformation, this approach simultaneously aligns and makes commensurate the resulting randomized block data. If $v = 1$ and $r = 1$, then statistic δ is equivalent to an extension of the Spearman (1904, 1906) footrule statistic, $\Re = 1 - \delta/\mu$, from $b = 2$ to any $b \geq 2$. If $v = 1$, $r = 1$, $b \geq 2$, $g \geq 2$, and there are no tied response values within blocks, then the mean, variance, and skewness of δ are given by

$$\mu = \frac{g^2 - 1}{3g},$$

$$\sigma^2 = \frac{2(g+1)(2g^2+7)}{45g^2b(b-1)},$$

and

$$\gamma = -\frac{(g+2)(2g^2+31)\Theta(g) + (8g^4+29g^2+71)(b-2)/(g-1)}{[49(g+1)(2g^2+7)^3b(b-1)/40]^{1/2}},$$

respectively, where $\Theta(g) = 0$ or 1 if $g = 2$ or $g \geq 3$, respectively (Mielke, 1984). Also, if $v = 2$, $r = 1$, and $b \geq 2$, then statistic δ is equivalent to the Friedman (1937) two-way analysis-of-variance statistic, also termed the Kendall coefficient of concordance (Kendall and Smith, 1939; Wallis, 1939). If $v = 2$, $r = 1$, $b \geq 2$, $g \geq 2$, and there are no tied response values within blocks, then the mean, variance, and skewness of δ are given by

$$\mu = \frac{g^2-1}{6},$$

$$\sigma^2 = \frac{(g+1)(g^2-1)}{18b(b-1)},$$

and

$$\gamma = -\left[\frac{8(b-2)^2}{(g-1)b(b-1)}\right]^{1/2},$$

respectively (Mielke, 1984). For the special case of the Friedman (1937) two-way analysis-of-variance statistic when $b = 2$, $\Re = 1 - \delta/\mu$ is the Spearman (1904, 1906) rank order correlation coefficient or ρ statistic. In addition to the previously mentioned statistics, the present approach includes most any type of rank function, i.e., $f(i)$ for $i = 1, ..., g$. Furthermore, adjustments for tied response values within any block may be accomplished in any manner desired since MRBP handles all types of data. Finally, multivariate extensions ($r \geq 2$) for any of the present rank function techniques are trivial since MRBP is inherently a multivariate procedure.

If the x_{kij} values are replaced with 0 and 1 binary values, then δ is equivalent to the multivariate version of the Cochran (1950) Q statistic. Cochran's (1950) Q test for the equality of matched proportions is widely used in social science research. The test can be viewed as an extension of the McNemar (1947) test to three or more treatment conditions. As an example application, suppose that $b \geq 2$ subjects are observed in a situation where each subject performs individually under each of $g \geq 2$ different experimental conditions. Each subject is assigned the treatment conditions in a random order and, within each condition, each of the b subjects performs one of a set of g motor skill tasks. If the task is completed in a fixed time period, the performance is scored as a success (1) and as a failure (0) otherwise. The research interest of the experimenter is to evaluate whether the motor skill tasks are of equal difficulty for the subjects, i.e., whether the true proportion of successes is constant over the g conditions.

If $r = 1$ and p_j denotes the proportion of 1s $(0 \leq p_j \leq 1)$ in the jth block $(j = 1, ..., b)$, then δ is equivalent to the Cochran (1950) Q statistic, and the exact mean, variance, and skewness of δ are given by

$$\mu = \frac{2}{b(b-1)} \left[\left(\sum_{j=1}^{b} p_j \right) \left(b - \sum_{j=1}^{b} p_j \right) - A_1 \right],$$

$$\sigma^2 = \frac{8}{b^2(b-1)^2 (g-1)} \left(A_1^2 - A_2 \right),$$

and

$$\gamma = - \left(\frac{8}{g-1} \right)^{1/2}$$

$$\times \frac{A_1^3 - 3A_1 A_2 + 2A_3 + \{(g-1) \left(B_1^2 - B_2 \right) / [2(g-2)]\} \Theta(g)}{\left(A_1^2 - A_2 \right)^{3/2}},$$

respectively, where

$$A_h = \sum_{j=1}^{b} \left[p_j(1 - p_j) \right]^h,$$

$$B_h = \sum_{j=1}^{b} \left[p_j(1 - p_j)(1 - 2p_j) \right]^h,$$

and $\Theta(g) = 1$ if $g \geq 3$; in the equation for γ, the expression in braces is omitted if $g = 2$ (Mielke and Berry, 1995). The special case of δ involving $g = 2$ is equivalent to the McNemar (1947) measure of change. The identity relating the Q and δ statistics is given by

$$Q = \frac{g-1}{2A_1} \left[2 \left(\sum_{j=1}^{b} p_j \right) \left(b - \sum_{j=1}^{b} p_j \right) - b (b-1) \delta \right].$$

This identity, together with the exact mean, variance, and skewness of δ, yields the nonasymptotic distribution of Q. The asymptotic distribution of Q is the χ^2 distribution with $g - 1$ df.

A procedure closely related to the test based on the Cochran (1950) Q statistic is useful when b is small and g is large. This procedure is the exact solution of a matrix occupancy problem (Mielke and Berry, 1996a; Mielke and Siddiqui, 1965).[1] If $r = 1$ and the $x_{1ij} = x_{ij}$ values again involve 0 and 1 binary values, let

$$R_j = \sum_{i=1}^{g} x_{ij}$$

denote the fixed total of the jth block ($j = 1, ..., b$), let

$$T = \prod_{j=1}^{b} \binom{g}{R_j}$$

denote the number of distinct $g \times b$ matrices, and let $w = \min(R_1, ..., R_b)$. Under H_0, each of the T distinguishable configurations of 0s and 1s occurs with equal probability. If U_k is the number of distinct configurations where exactly k treatments are filled with 1s, then

$$U_w = \binom{g}{w} \prod_{j=1}^{b} \binom{g-w}{R_j-w}$$

and

$$U_k = \binom{g}{k} \left[\prod_{j=1}^{b} \binom{g-k}{R_j-k} - \sum_{i=k+1}^{w} \binom{g-k}{i-k} \frac{U_i}{\binom{g}{i}} \right], \tag{4.3}$$

where $0 \le k \le w - 1$. Setting $k = 0$ in Expression (4.3) implies that

$$T = \sum_{k=0}^{w} U_k$$

and the exact P-value of observing s or more treatments completely filled with 1s is given by

$$P\text{-value} = \frac{1}{T} \sum_{k=s}^{w} U_k,$$

where $0 \le s \le w$. Eicker et al. (1972) describe extensions of this matrix occupancy problem that include cases such as the number of treatments that are filled with at least $n \le b$ 1s.

Mantel (1974) noted that the matrix occupancy problem solution given by Mielke and Siddiqui (1965) was also the solution for a subsequently discussed "committee problem" (Gittlesohn, 1969; Mantel and Pasternack,

---

[1]Adapted and reprinted with permission of Perceptual and Motor Skills from P.W. Mielke, Jr. and K.J. Berry. An exact solution to an occupancy problem: a useful alternative to Cochran's Q test. *Perceptual and Motor Skills*, 1996, 82, 91–95. Copyright © 1996 by Perceptual and Motor Skills.

TABLE 4.1. Successes (1) and failures (0) of $b = 6$ subjects on a series of $g = 8$ treatments.

Subject	Treatment condition								R_i
	1	2	3	4	5	6	7	8	
1	0	1	1	1	0	0	1	0	4
2	1	1	1	0	0	1	1	1	6
3	0	1	0	1	1	0	1	1	5
4	1	1	1	1	0	1	1	1	7
5	0	1	1	0	0	0	1	1	4
6	1	1	1	1	0	1	1	0	6
C_j	3	6	5	4	1	3	6	4	

1968; Sprott, 1969; White, 1971). Whereas the matrix occupancy problem considers b subjects and g treatments, and scores a success by a subject for a specific treatment as a 1 and a failure as a 0, the committee problem considers b committees and g individuals, and scores a 1 if an individual is not a member of a specific committee and 0 otherwise. Since the committee problem is concerned with the number of individuals belonging to no committees, this is equivalent to the matrix occupancy problem's concern with the number of treatments associated with successes among all subjects.

The following two examples compare Cochran's Q (1950) test to the matrix occupancy problem solution for entirely different data sets. Since $C_j = gp_j$ is the number of 1s in the jth block ($j = 1, ..., b$), it is convenient to use the C_js instead of the p_js in these examples. The first example is from Mantel (1974), and the second example is constructed to illustrate a typical long-term longitudinal study of the type initially considered in Mielke and Siddiqui (1965).

4.3.1   Example 1

Consider an experiment with $b = 6$ subjects and $g = 8$ treatment conditions (Mantel, 1974). The data are summarized in Table 4.1. The R_i (subject total) values are $\{4, 6, 5, 7, 4, 6\}$ for $i = 1, ..., b$, and s, the number of observed treatment columns filled with 1s, is two, i.e., treatment conditions 2 and 7. The exact occupancy test P-value of observing $s \geq 2$ is 0.9077×10^{-1}. Treatment marginals are required to compute Cochran's Q test and the nonasymptotic version of the Q test (Mielke and Berry, 1995). Let C_j be the observed total number of successes (1s) for the jth treatment condition ($j = 1, ..., g$). The values of C_j for these data are $\{3, 6, 5, 4, 1, 3, 6, 4\}$ and are given in Table 4.1. Cochran's Q test for this data set yields $Q = 14.3590$, a resampling approximate P-value of 0.4236×10^{-1} with $L = 1,000,000$, an asymptotic approximate P-value of 0.4515×10^{-1}, and a nonasymptotic Pearson type III approximate P-value of 0.3094×10^{-1}.

Both Cochran's Q test and the nonasymptotic version of the Q test reject H_0 at the customary $\alpha = 0.05$ level of significance, whereas the exact occupancy test yields a P-value of 0.9077×10^{-1}.

The differences in the P-values are primarily due to different interpretations of treatment effects considered by each test. Cochran's Q test and the nonasymptotic version of the Q test take into consideration all $g = 8$ treatment conditions in Table 4.1, considering the success of even a single subject as evidence of the effectiveness of that treatment condition. On the other hand, the exact occupancy test considers a treatment condition as effective only if all b subjects score a success.

4.3.2   Example 2

Consider a long-term longitudinal study where $b = 4$ subjects are observed daily for $g = 140$ days. The R_i (subject total) values are $\{23, 16, 12, 31\}$ for $i = 1, ..., b$, and s, the number of observed treatment columns filled with 1s, is equal to 3. The exact occupancy test P-value of $s \geq 3$ is 0.1073×10^{-4}. The values for C_j consisted of $C_j = 4$ for three treatments, $C_j = 1$ for 70 treatments, and $C_j = 0$ for 67 treatments. In contrast to the previous example, Cochran's Q test for these data yields $Q = 141.9858$, a resampling approximate P-value of 0.4594 with $L = 100,000$, an asymptotic approximate P-value of 0.4138, and a nonasymptotic Pearson type III approximate P-value of 0.4004, whereas the exact occupancy test yields a P-value of 0.1073×10^{-4}.

4.3.3   Multiple Binary Category Choices

Consider the extension of Cochran's Q when $r > 1$ and each of the r values can be 1 or 0 (Berry and Mielke, 2003b). Thus, the analysis of these multivariate data is an obvious application of MRBP. The following paragraph motivates the problem.

Many types of research include multiple-response questions wherein subjects mark all applicable categories. For example, patients may be asked to select from a list and check all illnesses they have had in the past five years, employees may be asked to select names of close friends from a list of co-workers, faculty may be asked to indicate to which journals they subscribe, or subjects may be asked to select from a list the recreational sites they have visited in the past year.

The longitudinal analysis of multiple category choices may be conceptualized as a binary argument problem in which b subjects choose any or all of r presented categories and the responses for each subject are coded 1 if the category is selected and 0 otherwise. The same or matched subjects are assessed at g time periods and the multiple binary responses over the g trials are compared.

The null hypothesis (H_0) of no differences in the response structures over the g trials specifies that each of the

$$M = (g!)^b$$

possible allocations of the b r-dimensional response measurements to the g trials is equally likely. Under H_0, the permutation distribution of δ assigns equal probabilities to the resulting M values of δ. Because small values of δ imply a concentration of similar scores over the g trials, H_0 is rejected when the observed value of δ, δ_o, is small.

Example

Consider an example in which b subjects are compared on r binary responses over g trials, and each subject is allowed to select any one of the 2^r possible arrangements of categorical responses.[2] Specifically, consider $b = 12$ adolescent subjects who have been diagnosed as clinically depressed with childhood-onset dysthymia. Presented with a list of $r = 14$ symptoms (Kovacs et al., 1994; Mondimore, 2002, p. 46), a trained clinical psychologist assesses and records any and all symptoms experienced by each subject in the past month. Table 4.2 lists the $r = 14$ response categories and the pretreatment vectors of observed binary responses from the $2^{14} = 16{,}384$ possible response arrangements, where a 1 indicates the symptom was recorded and a 0 indicates that a symptom was not recorded. Table 4.2 provides the baseline values for evaluation of the intervention. After counseling by a clinical psychologist for a period of six months, the subjects are again evaluated and the symptoms recorded. The posttreatment results are given in Table 4.3. Finally, a follow-up evaluation six months after the termination of treatment yields the results listed in Table 4.4. The H_0 specifies no differences among the binary multiple responses over the $g = 3$ assessments.

The exact permutation analysis based on $(g!)^{b-1} = 6^{11} = 362{,}797{,}056$ arrangements yields $\delta_o = 2.3413$ with an exact P-value of 0.0020. To reduce computations, the exact test is based on $(g!)^{b-1}$ rather than $M = (g!)^b$ arrangements since the ordered responses of one subject may be held fixed relative to the other $b-1$ subjects. The resampling permutation procedure based on $L = 1{,}000{,}000$ resamplings yields an approximate P-value of 0.0021. Finally, the Pearson type III moment approximation permutation analysis yields an approximate P-value of 0.0042. In all three analyses, there is a low probability that the differences in symptoms over the three assessments can be attributed to chance under H_0.

---

[2] Adapted and reprinted with permission of Psychological Reports from K.J. Berry and P.W. Mielke, Jr. Longitudinal analysis of data with multiple binary category choices. *Psychological Reports*, 2003, 93, 127–131. Copyright © 2003 by Psychological Reports.

TABLE 4.2. Baseline longitudinal multiple binary data.

Symptom	A	B	C	D	E	F	G	H	I	J	K	L
Depressed or sad mood	1	1	1	1	1	1	0	1	1	1	1	1
Feeling unloved	0	1	1	0	1	1	1	0	1	1	0	0
Feeling friendless	0	1	0	0	1	1	0	0	1	0	0	1
Irritability	1	1	0	1	0	0	1	1	0	1	1	0
Anger	1	0	1	1	1	0	1	1	0	1	0	1
Anhedonia	0	0	0	0	1	0	0	0	0	0	0	1
Guilty feelings	0	0	0	1	0	0	1	0	0	0	0	0
Social withdrawal	0	0	0	0	0	0	0	1	0	0	0	0
Impaired concentration	0	1	1	0	1	1	0	0	0	1	0	0
Thoughts of wanting to die	0	1	0	0	1	0	0	0	0	0	0	0
Reduced sleep	1	0	0	0	0	0	0	0	1	0	1	0
Reduced appetite	0	0	1	0	0	0	0	0	0	0	0	0
Fatigue	0	1	0	0	1	0	0	0	0	1	0	0
Disobedience	1	0	0	1	1	0	0	1	1	0	1	1

TABLE 4.3. Posttreatment longitudinal multiple binary data.

Symptom	A	B	C	D	E	F	G	H	I	J	K	L
Depressed or sad mood	1	0	1	1	1	1	0	1	0	1	1	1
Feeling unloved	0	1	0	0	1	1	0	0	1	1	0	0
Feeling friendless	0	1	0	0	1	1	0	0	1	0	0	1
Irritability	1	1	0	1	0	0	1	1	0	1	1	0
Anger	1	0	1	1	1	0	1	1	0	1	0	1
Anhedonia	0	1	0	0	1	0	0	0	1	0	0	1
Guilty feelings	0	0	0	1	0	0	1	0	0	0	0	0
Social withdrawal	0	0	0	0	0	0	0	1	0	0	0	0
Impaired concentration	0	0	1	0	0	1	0	0	0	1	0	0
Thoughts of wanting to die	0	1	0	0	1	0	0	0	0	0	1	0
Reduced sleep	1	0	0	0	0	0	0	0	0	0	1	0
Reduced appetite	0	0	1	0	0	0	1	0	0	0	0	0
Fatigue	0	1	0	0	1	0	0	0	0	1	0	0
Disobedience	1	0	0	1	1	0	0	0	0	0	1	1

TABLE 4.4. Follow-up longitudinal multiple binary data.

Symptom	A	B	C	D	E	F	G	H	I	J	K	L
Depressed or sad mood	1	0	1	0	1	1	0	1	0	1	1	0
Feeling unloved	0	0	0	0	1	1	0	0	1	1	0	0
Feeling friendless	0	1	0	0	1	1	0	0	1	0	0	1
Irritability	1	1	0	1	0	0	0	1	0	1	1	0
Anger	1	0	1	1	1	0	1	1	0	1	0	1
Anhedonia	0	1	0	0	1	0	0	0	1	0	0	1
Guilty feelings	0	0	0	1	0	0	0	0	0	0	0	0
Social withdrawal	0	0	0	0	0	0	0	1	0	0	0	0
Impaired concentration	0	1	1	0	1	1	0	0	0	1	0	0
Thoughts of wanting to die	0	1	0	0	1	0	0	0	0	0	1	0
Reduced sleep	1	0	0	0	0	0	0	0	0	0	1	0
Reduced appetite	0	0	1	0	0	0	1	0	0	0	0	0
Fatigue	0	1	0	0	0	0	0	0	0	1	0	0
Disobedience	1	0	0	1	1	0	0	1	0	0	1	1

4.4 One-Sample and Matched-Pair Designs

For the one-sample design, w_{kj} denotes the kth of r responses from the jth of b blocks and μ_k denotes the hypothesized centering value of the kth response under the null hypothesis (H_0). Within this MRBP setting, $y_{k1j} = w_{kj} - \mu_k = -y_{k2j}$ for $k = 1, ..., r$ and $j = 1, ..., b$ yield the aligned values for a one-sample design analysis. If a matched-pair design is in question, then w_{k1j} and w_{k2j} denote the kth of r responses from the jth of b blocks for the first and second treatments, respectively. Under H_0, the matched-pair design specifies that w_{k1j} and w_{k2j} have a common distribution for each combination of $k = 1, ..., r$ and $j = 1, ..., b$. In the context of MRBP, $y_{k1j} = w_{k1j} - w_{k2j} = -y_{k2j}$ for $k = 1, ..., r$ and $j = 1, ..., b$ and yield the aligned values for a matched-pair design analysis.

When $r = 1$, the MRBP statistic may be conveniently expressed as

$$\delta = \binom{b}{2}^{-1} \sum_{i<j} |x_i - x_j|^v,$$

where $x_i = d_i z_i$, $d_i = |y_{11i}|$, z_i is either $+1$ or -1, H_0 specifies that

$$P(z_i = 1) = P(z_i = -1) = 0.5$$

for $i = 1, ..., b$, $v > 0$, and the sum is over all $\binom{b}{2}$ combinations of the integers from 1 to b. The mean, variance, and skewness of δ under H_0 are given by

$$\mu = \frac{A}{b(b-1)},$$

$$\sigma^2 = \frac{B}{[b(b-1)]^2},$$

and

$$\gamma = -\frac{6C}{B^{3/2}},$$

respectively, where

$$A = \sum_{i<j}(a_{ij}+b_{ij}),$$

$$B = \sum_{i<j}(a_{ij}-b_{ij})^2,$$

$$C = \sum_{i<j<k}(a_{ij}-b_{ij})(a_{ik}-b_{ik})(a_{jk}-b_{jk}),$$

$$a_{ij} = |d_i+d_j|^v,$$

$$b_{ij} = |d_i-d_j|^v,$$

and the sums are respectively over all $\binom{b}{2}$ and $\binom{b}{3}$ combinations of the integers from 1 to b. Specifically, $d_i = |y_{11i}|$ and $v = 1$ yield a matched-pair/one-sample permutation test satisfying the congruence principle (Mielke, 1984, 1985, 1986, 1991; Mielke and Berry, 1983, 2000a). Also, $d_i = |y_{11i}|$ and $v = 2$ yield the permutation version of the classical Fisher–Pitman matched-pair/one-sample t test where

$$\delta(t^2+b-1) = 2\sum_{i=1}^{b}d_i^2$$

relates δ and test statistic t. Alternative choices of the positive constant d_i (termed a score) yield a variety of well-known permutation procedures. For an initial example, $d_i = 1/2$ yields a variation of δ, say δ^*, which is equivalent to the sign test since

$$b(b-1)\delta^* = 2H(b-H)$$

relates δ^* and the number of positive signs (H). In this case, the expressions μ, σ^2, and γ reduce to

$$\mu = \tfrac{1}{2},$$

$$\sigma^2 = [2b(b-1)]^{-1},$$

and

$$\gamma = -4(b-2)/[2b(b-1)]^{1/2}.$$

As a further example, let $\delta_{s,v}$ denote the present MRBP statistic where $d_i = r_i^s$ ($i = 1, ..., b$), $r_1, ..., r_b$ are the rank-order statistics associated with $|y_{111}|, ..., |y_{11b}|$, and there are no ties. An extended class of rank-order statistics based on $\delta_{s,2}$ has been considered (Mielke and Berry, 1976). Although $\delta_{1,2}$ is equivalent to the two-sided Wilcoxon matched-pair rank test statistic (Wilcoxon, 1945), simulated power comparisons indicate that $\delta_{1,1}$ and $\delta_{2,1}$ are superior to $\delta_{1,2}$ for many applications involving location alternatives (Mielke and Berry, 1982). The following reduced values of μ, σ^2, and γ have been obtained for $\delta_{1,1}$, $\delta_{2,1}$, and $\delta_{1,2}$. The values for $\delta_{1,1}$ are given by

$$\mu = \frac{2(b+1)}{3},$$

$$\sigma^2 = \frac{b+1}{3(b-1)},$$

and

$$\gamma = -\frac{2(4b^2 - 5b - 6)[3(b-1)]^{1/2}}{5b^2(b+1)^{1/2}}.$$

The values for $\delta_{2,1}$ are given by

$$\mu = \frac{(b+1)(3b+2)}{6},$$

$$\sigma^2 = \frac{(b+1)(2b^2 - 3)}{15(b-1)},$$

and

$$\gamma = -\frac{(b-2)(14b^5 - 17b^4 - 64b^3 + 37b^2 + 72b - 6)}{7b^2 \left[(b^2 - 1)(2b^2 - 3)^3 / 15\right]^{1/2}}.$$

Finally, the values for $\delta_{1,2}$ are given by

$$\mu = \frac{(b+1)(2b+1)}{3},$$

$$\sigma^2 = \frac{2(b+1)(4b^2 - 1)(5b + 6)}{45b(b-1)},$$

and

$$\gamma = -\frac{2(2b^2 - 7b + 6)(35b^2 + 91b + 60)}{7 \left[b(b^2 - 1)(4b^2 - 1)(5b + 6)^3 / 10\right]^{1/2}}.$$

TABLE 4.5. Estimated significance levels for 1,000,000 simulated samples of size $n = 20$ and $n = 80$ based on the Pearson type III distribution critical values.

	$n = 20$				$n = 80$			
α	δ^*	$\delta_{1,1}$	$\delta_{2,1}$	$\delta_{1,2}$	δ^*	$\delta_{1,1}$	$\delta_{2,1}$	$\delta_{1,2}$
0.100	0.1154	0.1001	0.1008	0.1055	0.0931	0.0996	0.0995	0.1013
0.020	0.0119	0.0213	0.0221	0.0217	0.0182	0.0198	0.0199	0.0201
0.002	0.0026	0.0019	0.0019	0.0020	0.0023	0.0020	0.0019	0.0019

TABLE 4.6. Estimated powers for 100,000 simulated samples for size $n = 20$ and $n = 80$ against location shifts of 0.6σ for $n = 20$ and 0.3σ for $n = 80$.

Distribution	α	$n = 20$				$n = 80$			
		δ^*	$\delta_{1,1}$	$\delta_{2,1}$	$\delta_{1,2}$	δ^*	$\delta_{1,1}$	$\delta_{2,1}$	$\delta_{1,2}$
Laplace	0.100	0.885	0.898	0.862	0.888	0.932	0.944	0.908	0.930
	0.020	0.570	0.705	0.645	0.683	0.786	0.814	0.736	0.783
	0.002	0.357	0.357	0.293	0.341	0.537	0.541	0.435	0.496
Logistic	0.100	0.780	0.841	0.835	0.851	0.767	0.864	0.860	0.869
	0.020	0.408	0.608	0.599	0.612	0.515	0.659	0.654	0.668
	0.002	0.222	0.263	0.245	0.267	0.255	0.354	0.347	0.359
Normal	0.100	0.703	0.796	0.812	0.819	0.675	0.812	0.829	0.829
	0.020	0.323	0.541	0.564	0.563	0.407	0.576	0.604	0.604
	0.002	0.161	0.210	0.212	0.223	0.177	0.278	0.300	0.297
Uniform	0.100	0.505	0.725	0.834	0.770	0.453	0.764	0.893	0.803
	0.020	0.166	0.439	0.581	0.492	0.212	0.488	0.680	0.563
	0.002	0.068	0.134	0.194	0.160	0.067	0.193	0.352	0.259
U-shaped	0.100	0.151	0.638	0.870	0.631	0.096	1.000	1.000	0.970
	0.020	0.020	0.323	0.604	0.355	0.019	0.986	1.000	0.887
	0.002	0.005	0.067	0.253	0.082	0.002	0.759	0.990	0.673

4.4.1   Comparisons Among Univariate Rank Tests

Power comparisons among δ^*, $\delta_{1,1}$, $\delta_{2,1}$, and $\delta_{1,2}$ are given in Tables 4.5 and 4.6. Estimated significance levels based on the Pearson type III approximation involving 1,000,000 simulated samples of size $n = 20$ and $n = 80$ are given in Table 4.5, where the specified α values are 0.1, 0.02, and 0.002. Because of computer limitations at the time, Mielke and Berry (1982) originally presented analogous significance levels based on only 20,000 simulated samples.

Estimated powers based on the Pearson type III approximation involving 100,000 simulated samples of size $n = 20$ and $n = 80$ for location shifts are given in Table 4.6 for the Laplace (double exponential), logistic, normal, uniform, and a U-shaped distribution when the specified α values are 0.1,

0.02, and 0.002. The density function of the U-shaped distribution is $1.5x^2$ if $-1 < x < 1$ and zero elsewhere. The location shifts are 0.6σ when $n = 20$ and 0.3σ when $n = 80$, where σ is the standard deviation of the distribution in question. Analogous power results were also presented by Mielke and Berry (1982), based on only 300 simulated samples.

A feature of Table 4.5 that affects the corresponding results in Table 4.6 is the existence of low estimated significance levels for the two cases of δ^* involving $\alpha = 0.02$ with $n = 20$ and $\alpha = 0.002$ with $n = 80$. Except for the Laplace distribution where the sign test is known to be asymptotically optimal, δ^* has (1) lower power relative to $\delta_{1,1}$, $\delta_{2,1}$, and $\delta_{1,2}$ for the logistic and normal distributions and (2) exceedingly low power relative to $\delta_{1,1}$, $\delta_{2,1}$, and $\delta_{1,2}$ for the uniform and U-shaped distributions. Whereas $\delta_{1,1}$ has the highest power for the Laplace distribution and is second in power only to $\delta_{1,2}$ for the logistic distribution where $\delta_{1,2}$ is known to be asymptotically optimal, $\delta_{1,1}$ has lower power than $\delta_{2,1}$ and $\delta_{1,2}$ for the normal, uniform, and U-shaped distributions. Interestingly, in Table 4.6, $\delta_{2,1}$ and $\delta_{1,2}$ appear tied in having the highest power for the normal distribution. However, $\delta_{2,1}$ has much higher power than $\delta_{1,2}$ for the uniform and U-shaped distributions. Note that the asymptotic optimality associated with δ^* and $\delta_{1,2}$ only pertains to linear rank tests where $v = 2$ (e.g., Mielke and Sen, 1981). This concept of asymptotic optimality is not relevant for small sample sizes or $v \neq 2$. Obviously, other choices of $\delta_{s,v}$ will attain greater power than $\delta_{1,1}$, $\delta_{2,1}$, and $\delta_{1,2}$ for the distributions considered here.

4.4.2 Multivariate Tests

If $r \geq 2$ and b subjects are associated with a multivariate pretreatment and posttreatment matched-pairs permutation test, let $(w_{11j}, ..., w_{r1j})$ and $(w_{12j}, ..., w_{r2j})$ denote r-dimensional row vectors with elements comprised of the r measurements on the jth subject from the pretreatment and posttreatment, respectively, where $j = 1, ..., b$. Let

$$y_{1j} = \begin{pmatrix} y_{11j} \\ \vdots \\ y_{r1j} \end{pmatrix},$$

where $y_{k1j} = w_{k1j} - w_{k2j}$ for $k = 1, ..., r$, be the r-dimensional column vector of differences between pretreatment and posttreatment measurements for the jth subject, and let $y_{2j} = -y_{1j}$ be the r-dimensional origin reflection of y_{1j} ($j = 1, ..., b$). The probability (P), under the null hypothesis (H_0) of the matched-pair experiment, is $P(y_{1j}) = P(y_{2j}) = 0.5$, for $j = 1, ..., b$. Consider the test statistic given by

$$\delta = \binom{b}{2}^{-1} \sum_{m<n} \Delta(y_{1m}, y_{1n}),$$

where

$$\Delta\left(y_{1m}, y_{1n}\right) = \left[\left(y_{1m} - y_{1n}\right)'\left(y_{1m} - y_{1n}\right)\right]^{1/2}$$

is the r-dimensional Euclidean distance between the mth and nth subjects' differences, and the sum $\sum_{m<n}$ is over all m and n such that $1 \leq m < n \leq b$. This approach includes the multivariate one-sample permutation test in which $y_{kj} = x_{kj} - \mu_k$ for $k = 1, ..., r$, where $(x_{1j}, ..., x_{rj})$ denotes the r-dimensional row vector with elements comprised of the r measurements for the jth subject $(j = 1, ..., b)$, and $(\mu_1, ..., \mu_r)$ is the r-dimensional row vector of the r hypothesized central values under H_0.

If the r response measurements are in different units, then it is recommended that the measurements be made commensurate, i.e., standardized to a common unit of measurement. The replacement of y_{kij} with $y_{kij}^* = y_{kij}/\phi_k$, where

$$\phi_k = \sum_{i_1=1}^{2} \sum_{i_2=1}^{2} \sum_{m<n} |y_{ki_1m} - y_{ki_2n}|$$

for $k = 1, ..., r$ and $1 \leq m < n \leq b$, ensures that each response measurement makes a similar contribution in the r-dimensional Euclidean space since

$$\sum_{i_1=1}^{2} \sum_{i_2=1}^{2} \sum_{m<n} |y_{ki_1m}^* - y_{ki_2n}^*| = 1$$

for $k = 1, ..., r$ (Mielke et al., 1996b). This commensuration is invariant relative to any permutation under H_0 and is termed Euclidean commensuration (Berry and Mielke, 1992).

Hotelling's multivariate matched-pair T^2 test statistic (Anderson, 1958, pp. 101–108; Hotelling, 1931) is given by

$$T^2 = b\,\bar{y}_1'\,\mathbf{S}_y^{-1}\,\bar{y}_1,$$

where $\mathbf{S}_y$ is an $r \times r$ matrix given by

$$\mathbf{S}_y = \frac{1}{b-1} \sum_{j=1}^{b} \left(y_{1j} - \bar{y}_1\right)\left(y_{1j} - \bar{y}_1\right)',$$

and

$$\bar{y}_1 = \frac{1}{b} \sum_{j=1}^{b} y_{1j}.$$

If the observed value of δ is δ_o, then the exact P-value is given by $P(\delta \leq \delta_o \,|\, H_0)$, i.e., the proportion of the 2^b possible δ values that are less than or equal to δ_o. If the observed value of T^2 is T_o^2, then the analogous exact P-value is given by $P(T^2 \geq T_o^2 \,|\, H_0)$, i.e., the proportion of the

2^b possible T^2 values that are greater than or equal to T_o^2. When b is large (e.g., $b > 20$ since $2^{20} = 1,048,576$), then a method to approximate the P-value is essential. One such method involves calculating the first three exact cumulants of δ under H_0, equating the obtained exact cumulants of δ to the corresponding three cumulants that characterize the Pearson type III distribution, and obtaining an approximate P-value by numerically integrating the resulting Pearson type III distribution (Mielke, 1984, 1991). The first three exact cumulants of δ under H_0 are given by

$$\kappa_1 = \mu = \left[2b(b-1)\right]^{-1} \sum_{m<n} \sum_{i=1}^{2} \sum_{j=1}^{2} \Delta\left(y_{im}, y_{jn}\right),$$

$$\kappa_2 = \sigma^2 = \left[b(b-1)\right]^{-2} \sum_{m<n} \sum_{i=1}^{2} \sum_{j=1}^{2} \left[D(i,m;j,n)\right]^2,$$

and

$$\kappa_3 = \sigma^3\gamma = 6\left[b(b-1)\right]^{-3}$$

$$\times \sum_{l<m<n} \sum_{i=1}^{2} \sum_{j=1}^{2} \sum_{k=1}^{2} D(i,l;j,m)D(i,l;k,n)D(j,m;k,n),$$

where

$$D(i,m;j,n) = \Delta\left(y_{im}, y_{jn}\right) - \frac{1}{2}\sum_{i=1}^{2} \Delta\left(y_{im}, y_{jn}\right)$$

$$- \frac{1}{2}\sum_{j=1}^{2} \Delta\left(y_{im}, y_{jn}\right) + \frac{1}{4}\sum_{i=1}^{2} \sum_{j=1}^{2} \Delta\left(y_{im}, y_{jn}\right),$$

and μ, σ^2, and γ are the exact mean, variance, and skewness of δ, respectively, under H_0. The use of higher order cumulants (i.e., κ_h where $h \geq 4$) has yielded Tchebyshev–Markov bounds for P-values (Iyer et al., 2002). While the permutation test is applicable to any combination of $r \geq 1$ and b (although $b \geq 10$ might be desired simply to ensure at least $2^{10} = 1024$ permutations), any application of the T^2 test under its null hypothesis with the assumption of multivariate normality requires that $\min(r, b-r) \geq 1$ since the distribution of the modified statistic given by

$$\frac{(b-r)T^2}{(b-1)r}$$

is Snedecor's F distribution with r df in the numerator and $b-r$ df in the denominator.

TABLE 4.7. Pretraining scores assigned by $r = 13$ judges to writing samples of $b = 11$ students.

Judge	Student 1	2	3	4	5	6	7	8	9	10	11
1	1	6	1	1	8	1	5	8	6	3	1
2	3	4	6	2	8	3	6	9	9	7	3
3	1	6	2	3	7	3	3	5	5	2	4
4	2	5	5	1	8	2	4	7	8	6	4
5	3	6	5	2	8	2	3	5	9	4	2
6	0	4	3	0	8	0	3	9	7	3	0
7	1	5	0	1	7	0	1	2	8	5	1
8	5	8	4	0	2	0	2	10	2	2	0
9	1	7	2	5	9	2	6	6	9	6	3
10	2	3	2	0	6	1	5	7	5	3	3
11	1	5	2	1	7	1	2	8	8	7	4
12	0	4	1	0	9	0	2	5	3	2	1
13	4	9	2	2	5	3	3	9	8	4	3

Example

The data are from a study in which students majoring in mathematics education were enrolled in a course on teaching discrete mathematics to secondary school students (Mielke et al., 1996b).[3] One of the objectives of the course was to enhance the skills of the prospective teachers in writing in the discipline of mathematics. On the first day of the course, the students were given a mathematics writing exercise. The same exercise was repeated on the last day of the semester-long course. A total of 11 students completed both writing exercises. The paired, but randomly arranged, pretraining and posttraining writing samples of the 11 students were presented blindly to 13 experienced teachers of mathematics and language arts for grading. Each of the 13 judges scored each of the 22 writing samples on a scale from 0 to 10. The pretraining grades are given in Table 4.7, and the posttraining grades are given in Table 4.8. Analyses for two cases are considered.

Case 1. The first analysis blocks on the $b = 11$ students and compares the pretraining and posttraining grades of the $r = 13$ judges. This analysis evaluates the following question: Are the judges consistent in their grading or are there significant pretraining/posttraining differences in grading among the judges?

---

[3]Adapted and reprinted with permission of Psychological Reports from P.W. Mielke, Jr., K.J. Berry, and C.O. Neidt. A permutation test for multivariate matched-pair analyses: comparisons with Hotelling's multivariate matched-pair T^2 test. *Psychological Reports*, 1996, 78, 1003–1008. Copyright © 1996 by Psychological Reports.

TABLE 4.8. Posttraining scores assigned by $r = 13$ judges to writing samples of $b = 11$ students.

Judge	Student										
	1	2	3	4	5	6	7	8	9	10	11
1	9	5	3	1	8	1	7	6	6	4	5
2	8	5	5	2	9	2	6	6	7	5	5
3	5	6	2	3	3	3	6	8	7	5	8
4	7	6	3	2	9	4	5	6	6	4	7
5	8	7	4	2	8	4	7	8	6	3	5
6	6	7	2	0	6	0	5	7	6	5	4
7	5	5	2	1	5	3	5	5	4	0	7
8	4	9	6	0	3	3	10	8	5	3	5
9	9	5	5	7	8	3	8	8	8	7	8
10	4	4	1	0	4	3	4	5	6	6	6
11	6	3	3	2	9	2	9	7	7	5	9
12	6	2	3	1	5	1	6	9	6	5	6
13	9	6	4	4	7	6	9	7	6	7	5

The multivariate permutation test based on Euclidean commensuration yields an exact P-value of $182/2048 = 0.8887 \times 10^{-1}$, a resampling P-value of 0.8851×10^{-1} with $L = 1,000,000$, and the Pearson type III approximate P-value of 0.7242×10^{-1}. Because the $\mathbf{S}_y$ matrix is singular in this context, the T^2 test is not defined. The df in the denominator of the F distribution is negative, i.e., $b - r = 11 - 13 = -2$. Obviously, this is a serious limitation of the T^2 test.

Case 2. The second analysis blocks on the $b = 13$ judges and compares the pretraining and posttraining grades of the $r = 11$ students. This analysis evaluates the following question: Did the coursework result in significant pretraining/posttraining differences in writing among the students? The multivariate permutation test based on Euclidean commensuration yields an exact P-value of $2/8,192 = 0.2441 \times 10^{-3}$, a resampling P-value of 0.2480×10^{-3} with $L = 1,000,000$, and the Pearson type III P-value of 0.1939×10^{-3}. The permutation version of the T^2 test under H_0 that $P(y_{1j}) = P(y_{2j}) = 0.5$ for $j = 1, ..., 13$ yields an exact P-value of $634/8,192 = 0.7739 \times 10^{-1}$, and the T^2 test yields a P-value of 0.8193×10^{-1} under the assumption of multivariate normality.

The results of the analysis of the data for Case 1 indicate that the T^2 test is undefined for $r \geq b$. However, the multivariate permutation test employing Euclidean commensuration is unaffected by this constraint. The results of the analysis of the data for Case 2 indicate that the T^2 test yields results that differ substantially from the results of the multivariate permutation test based on Euclidean commensuration when $2 \leq r < b$.

Although the analyses of the present examples indicate that substantial advantages exist for the multivariate permutation test based on Euclidean commensuration, other data sets will indicate advantages for the T^2 test. Not only is the multivariate permutation test applicable to situations where the T^2 test cannot be used, it may be more discriminating than the classical Hotelling multivariate matched-pair T^2 test as with the two-sample case (see Section 2.11).

4.5   Measurement of Agreement

A number of statistical research problems require the measurement of agreement, rather than association or correlation, between two or more observers, raters, or judges. This is to say that a researcher is more interested in the extent to which a set of measurements are identical (i.e., agree) than the extent to which one set of measurements is a function (usually linear) of another set of measurements, i.e., correlated. A universal measure of both agreement and/or effect size (see Section 3.1) should, as a minimum, embody the following seven basic attributes (Berry and Mielke, 1988b).[4]

First, a measure of agreement should be corrected for chance, i.e., any agreement coefficient should reflect the amount of agreement in excess of what would be expected by chance. Several investigators have advocated chance-corrected measures of agreement, including Brennan and Prediger (1981), Cicchetti et al. (1985), Conger (1985), and Krippendorff (1970a). Although some investigators have argued against chance-corrected measures (Armitage et al., 1966; Goodman and Kruskal, 1954), supporters of chance-corrected measures of agreement far outweigh detractors.

Second, a measure of agreement possesses an added advantage if it is directly applicable to the assessment of reliability (Bartko, 1966, 1976; Bartko and Carpenter, 1976; Krippendorff, 1970b).

Third, a number of investigators have commented on the simplicity of Euclidean distance for measures of agreement. They have emphasized that the squaring of differences between scale values is questionable at best, while acknowledging that squared differences allow for conventional interpretations of coefficients (Fleiss and Cohen, 1973; Krippendorff, 1970a).

Fourth, every measure of agreement should have a statistical basis (Bartko and Carpenter, 1976). A measure of agreement without a proper test of significance is severely limited in application to practical research situations. Although asymptotic tests of significance are interesting and useful under large sample conditions, they are limited in their practical utility.

---

[4]Adapted and reprinted with permission of Sage Publications, Inc. from K.J. Berry and P.W. Mielke, Jr. A generalization of Cohen's kappa agreement measure to interval measurement and multiple raters. *Educational and Psychological Measurement*, 1988, 48, 921–933. Copyright © 1988 by Sage Publications, Inc.

Fifth, a measure of agreement that analyzes multivariate data has a decided advantage over other (i.e., univariate) measures of agreement. Thus, if one observer locates a group of subjects in an r-dimensional data space, a multivariate measure of agreement can ascertain the degree to which a second observer locates the same subjects in the same data space.

Sixth, a measure of agreement should be able to analyze data at any level of measurement. Cohen's (1960) kappa is a measure of agreement for the nominal level of measurement. Although extensions of Cohen's kappa measure of agreement to incompletely ranked data (Iachan, 1984) and to continuous nominal data (Conger, 1985) have been presented, a measure of agreement suitable for any level of measurement is desirable.

Seventh, a measure of agreement should be able to evaluate information from more than two observers. Williams (1976b) has presented a measure that is limited to comparisons of the joint agreement of several observers with another observer singled out as being of special interest. Landis and Koch (1977) have considered agreement among several observers in terms of a majority opinion. Light (1971) has focused on an extension of Cohen's (1960) kappa measure to multiple observers that is based on the average of all pairwise kappas. The measure proposed by Fleiss (1971) is dependent on the average proportion of observers who agree on the classification of each observation. The limitation in Williams (1976b) appears to be overly restrictive, and the formulation by Landis and Koch (1977) becomes computationally prohibitive if either the number of observers or the number of response categories is large. The extension of kappa proposed by Fleiss (1971) does not reduce to Cohen's kappa when the number of observers is two. Hubert (1977) and, especially, Conger (1980) have provided critical summaries of the problem of extending Cohen's (1960) kappa to multiple observers for categorical data.

4.5.1 Agreement Between Two Observers

The most popular measure of agreement between two observers is, without question, the chance-corrected measure of agreement proposed by Cohen (1960) and termed kappa (κ). Cohen's (1960) κ measures the agreement between two observers on the assignment to a set of discrete nominal categories.

Nominal Measurement

Assume that two observers independently classify each of g observations into one of r discrete, mutually exclusive, and exhaustive categories. The resulting classifications can be displayed on an r by r cross-classification, such as in Table 4.9, with proportions for cell entries. In the notation of

TABLE 4.9. Example of a 3 by 3 cross-classification.

Rows	Columns			Sum
	1	2	3	
1	P_{11}	P_{12}	P_{13}	$P_{1.}$
2	P_{21}	P_{22}	P_{23}	$P_{2.}$
3	P_{31}	P_{32}	P_{33}	$P_{3.}$
Sum	$P_{.1}$	$P_{.2}$	$P_{.3}$	$P_{..}$

Table 4.9, Cohen's (1960) κ is given by

$$\kappa = \frac{P_o - P_e}{1 - P_e},$$

where $P_o = \sum_{i=1}^{r} P_{ii}$, $P_e = \sum_{i=1}^{r} P_{i.} P_{.i}$, and $P_{..} = 1.0$. In this configuration, P_o is the observed proportion of observations on which two observers agree, P_e is the proportion of observations for which agreement is expected by chance, $P_o - P_e$ is the proportion of agreement beyond what is expected by chance, $1 - P_e$ is the maximum possible proportion of agreement beyond what is expected by chance, and the coefficient, κ, is the proportion of agreement between the two observers after chance agreement is removed (Berry and Mielke, 1988b).

For definitional purposes, let $\delta = 1 - P_o$ represent the observed proportion of disagreement and $\mu = 1 - P_e$ represent the expected proportion of disagreement. Substitution and simplification yields

$$\kappa = 1 - \frac{\delta}{\mu}.$$

Thus, κ may be interpreted as a ratio of measures of distance, or disagreement, between the two observers, where distance is measured by summing a series of zeros and ones (Light, 1971, p. 367). In this form, κ becomes a specific measure of agreement, $\Re$, based on the proximity of the classifications, which is measured by the Euclidean distance among the classifications of the two observers.

An alternative representation of Table 4.9 is presented in Table 4.10. The representation in Table 4.10 is constructed in the context of a multivariate randomized block design with g observations, $b = 2$ blocks (corresponding to the two observers), and the two polytomous variables of Table 4.9 represented by an r by 1 vector (x) where the ith element, corresponding to the ith of r categories, is set to $2^{-1/2}$ and where the remaining $r - 1$ elements of x are set to 0. The choice of the constant $(2^{-1/2})$ is to ensure that the distance between any two vectors will be 0 if the classifications agree and 1 if the classifications disagree.

TABLE 4.10. Example data in a multivariate randomized block representation.

Object	Block 1	Block 2
1	x_{11}	x_{12}
2	x_{21}	x_{22}
$\vdots$	$\vdots$	$\vdots$
g	x_{g1}	x_{g2}

TABLE 4.11. Example data set for nominal data with $g = 5$ objects, $b = 2$ observers, and $r = 3$ categories.

Observer 1	Observer 2 A	Observer 2 B	Observer 2 C
A	0	1	0
B	0	2	0
C	1	0	1

In this alternative representation (Berry and Mielke, 1988b), δ is given by

$$\delta = \frac{1}{g} \sum_{i=1}^{g} \Delta\left(x_{i1},\, x_{i2}\right),$$

where

$$\Delta\left(x_{i1},\, x_{i2}\right) = \left[\sum_{k=1}^{r} \left(x_{i1k} - x_{i2k}\right)^2\right]^{1/2},$$

and where x_{isk} denotes the kth element of vector x_{is} with $i = 1, ..., g$ (for objects 1 through g) and $s = 1, 2$ (for blocks 1 and 2). Then, μ is the expected proportion of disagreement, which is defined as

$$\mu = \frac{1}{g^2} \sum_{i=1}^{g} \sum_{j=1}^{g} \Delta\left(x_{i1},\, x_{j2}\right)$$

with

$$\Delta\left(x_{i1},\, x_{j2}\right) = \left[\sum_{k=1}^{r} \left(x_{i1k} - x_{j2k}\right)^2\right]^{1/2}.$$

The two representations are merely different mathematical formulations of the same structure. The advantage of the second method is that it simplifies extension and generalization to multiple observers and to higher levels of measurement.

To illustrate the equivalence of the two computational forms, consider the data in Table 4.11 where

$$\kappa = \frac{P_o - P_e}{1 - P_e} = \frac{0.6 - 0.36}{1.0 - 0.36} = 0.375.$$

Table 4.12 presents the same data in a multivariate randomized block representation. To illustrate the computation of $\Delta(x_{i1}, x_{i2})$, consider $i = 1$ (i.e., the first column of Table 4.12), where $\Delta(x_{11}, x_{12})$ is calculated as

$$\left[(2^{-1/2} - 0)^2 + (0 - 2^{-1/2})^2 + (0 - 0)^2 \right]^{1/2} = 1,$$

indicating disagreement on the classification of the first object: Observer 1 assigned object 1 to category "A" and Observer 2 assigned object 1 to category "B." Now, consider $i = 2$, where $\Delta(x_{21}, x_{22})$ is calculated as

$$\left[(0 - 0)^2 + (2^{-1/2} - 2^{-1/2})^2 + (0 - 0)^2 \right]^{1/2} = 0,$$

indicating agreement on the classification of the second object: Observer 1 and Observer 2 both assigned object 2 to category "B."

Completing the analysis leads to

$$\delta = \frac{1}{5} (1 + 0 + 0 + 1 + 0) = 0.40,$$

which is equal to $1 - P_o$, and

$$\mu = \frac{1}{25} (1 + 1 + \cdots + 1 + 0) = 0.64,$$

which is equal to $1 - P_e$. Finally,

$$\kappa = 1 - \frac{\delta}{\mu} = 1 - \frac{0.40}{0.64} = 0.375.$$

It should be noted that the choice of the constant $(2^{-1/2})$ to indicate inclusion in a category is completely arbitrary and any constant may be chosen. Although the values for δ and μ will be affected by the choice of the constant, the value for $\Re$ is independent of the units of measurement.

To illustrate this point, consider the recoded data listed in Table 4.13, where the value 1 is used to indicate membership in a category, instead of $2^{-1/2}$, and the value 0 indicates nonmembership. For these data, $\delta = 0.5657$, $\mu = 0.9051$, and

$$\kappa = 1 - \frac{0.5657}{0.9051} = 0.375.$$

Incidentally, exact, approximate resampling, and approximate normal analyses exist for the chance-corrected weighted kappa statistic (Berry et al., 2005; Mielke et al., 2005c). This statistic is a direct extension of Cohen's (1960) chance-corrected kappa statistic.

TABLE 4.12. Example data set for nominal data with $g = 5$ objects, $b = 2$ observers, and $r = 3$ categories in a multivariate randomized block representation.

| | Block | |
Object	1	2
1	$\begin{bmatrix} 2^{-1/2} \\ 0 \\ 0 \end{bmatrix}$	$\begin{bmatrix} 0 \\ 2^{-1/2} \\ 0 \end{bmatrix}$
2	$\begin{bmatrix} 0 \\ 2^{-1/2} \\ 0 \end{bmatrix}$	$\begin{bmatrix} 0 \\ 2^{-1/2} \\ 0 \end{bmatrix}$
3	$\begin{bmatrix} 0 \\ 2^{-1/2} \\ 0 \end{bmatrix}$	$\begin{bmatrix} 0 \\ 2^{-1/2} \\ 0 \end{bmatrix}$
4	$\begin{bmatrix} 0 \\ 0 \\ 2^{-1/2} \end{bmatrix}$	$\begin{bmatrix} 2^{-1/2} \\ 0 \\ 0 \end{bmatrix}$
5	$\begin{bmatrix} 0 \\ 0 \\ 2^{-1/2} \end{bmatrix}$	$\begin{bmatrix} 0 \\ 0 \\ 2^{-1/2} \end{bmatrix}$

Ordinal Measurement

Consider two rankings of g objects consisting of the first g integers, and let x_i and y_i for $i = 1, ..., g$ denote the first and second rankings, respectively. A measure of correlation between the two rankings that is common in social science research is Spearman's rank-order correlation coefficient, ρ, given by

$$\rho = 1 - \frac{6 \sum_{i=1}^{g} (x_i - y_i)^2}{g(g^2 - 1)}$$

(Spearman, 1904, 1906). An interesting and generally neglected alternative to Spearman's measure of rank correlation is Spearman's (1904, 1906) footrule, R. Spearman (1904, 1906) presented several coefficients for measuring the correlation between sets of ranked data, and it is not readily apparent exactly which coefficient he meant to be associated with the term "footrule" (Dineen and Blakesley, 1982; Lovie, 1995; Pearson, 1907).

TABLE 4.13. Recoded data set for nominal data with $g = 5$ objects, $b = 2$ observers (1, 2), and $r = 3$ categories (A, B, C).

	Observer					
	1			2		
Object	A	B	C	A	B	C
1	1	0	0	0	1	0
2	0	1	0	0	1	0
3	0	1	0	0	1	0
4	0	0	1	1	0	0
5	0	0	1	0	0	1

However,

$$R = 1 - \frac{3 \sum\limits_{i=1}^{g} |x_i - y_i|}{g^2 - 1}$$

is widely accepted as the formula for Spearman's footrule measure (Diaconis and Graham, 1977; Franklin, 1988; Kendall, 1962; Salama and Quade, 1990; Stuart, 1977; Ury and Kleinecke, 1979).

Spearman (1904, 1906) introduced the footrule (R) as an easy but precise method of measuring correlation between two rankings. Unlike other measures of rank correlation, the footrule does not norm properly between the limits of -1 and $+1$. Spearman's footrule attains a maximum value of $+1$ when no ties are present and x_i is identical to y_i for $i = 1, ..., g$. However, if $y_i = g - x_i + 1$, then $R = -0.5$ when g is odd and

$$R = -0.5 \left(1 + \frac{3}{g^2 - 1} \right)$$

when g is even (Kendall, 1962). Consequently, R does not attain a minimum value of -1 except for the uninteresting case when $g = 2$. Pearson (1907) criticized the footrule on this basis and Kendall (1962, p. 33) explicitly pointed to this apparent lack of proper norming as a "defect" in the footrule. Spearman, recognizing that negative values of R did not represent inverse correlation, actually suggested that "it is better to treat every correlation as positive" (Spearman, 1904, pp. 87–88). It can easily be shown that the footrule is a chance-corrected measure of agreement and not a measure of correlation because it takes the classic form of chance-corrected measures of agreement given by

$$R = 1 - \frac{\text{observed disagreement}}{\text{expected disagreement}}$$

(Krippendorff, 1970a, p. 140).

The expected value of a chance-corrected measure of agreement is zero under chance conditions, unity when agreement is perfect, and negative under conditions of disagreement. Thus, in the situation involving a complete inversion of the rankings, the deficiency in which the footrule does not norm to -1 is recast as a previously undocumented attribute of the footrule rather than a defect and places Spearman's footrule into the family of chance-corrected agreement measures, which include such well-known members as Scott's (1955) coefficient of intercoder agreement (π) and Cohen's (1960) coefficient of agreement (κ), both of which were designed for categorical data.

Spearman's (1904, 1906) footrule is limited to fully ranked data and does not accommodate tied ranks. Let

$$\delta = \frac{1}{g} \sum_{i=1}^{g} |x_i - y_i|,$$

$$\mu = \frac{1}{g^2} \sum_{i=1}^{g} \sum_{j=1}^{g} |x_i - y_i|,$$

and let

$$\Re = 1 - \frac{\delta}{\mu}$$

denote a general measure of the relationship between two sets of ranks that is not limited to untied ranks. If no ties exist in either $x_1, ..., x_g$ or $y_1, ..., y_g$, then

$$\mu = \frac{1}{g^2} \sum_{i=1}^{g} \sum_{j=1}^{g} |i - j|$$

$$= \frac{2}{g^2} \sum_{i=1}^{g-1} \sum_{j=i+1}^{g} (j - i)$$

$$= \frac{1}{g^2} \sum_{i=1}^{g-1} \left[g(g+1) + i^2 - i(2g+1) \right]$$

$$= \frac{g(g-1)}{6g^2} \left[6(g+1) + (2g-1) - 3(2g+1) \right]$$

$$= \frac{g^2 - 1}{3g},$$

and Spearman's footrule is given by

$$R = 1 - \frac{3g\delta}{g^2 - 1}.$$

TABLE 4.14. Example data set for ordinal data
with $g = 6$ objects, $b = 2$ observers, and $r = 1$
dimension.

Object	Observer A	Observer B
1	1	2
2	2.5	2
3	2.5	2
4	4	6
5	5	4
6	6	5

Thus, the footrule is generalized to include tied ranks on x and y, and R is shown to be a special case of $\Re$ when no ties are present (Berry and Mielke, 1997c).[5] $\Re$, like R, is a chance-corrected measure of agreement since the expected disagreement is $E[\delta] = \mu$.

To illustrate the measurement of agreement with tied ranks, consider the data listed in Table 4.14, where each of two observers is asked to rank six objects in terms of quality, with 6 indicating highest quality and 1 indicating lowest quality. For these data, $g = 6$, $b = 2$, $r = 1$, $\delta = 1.0000$, $\mu = 1.8889$, and $\Re = 0.4706$, indicating 47 percent agreement between the two observers above and beyond what is expected by chance.

If δ and μ are redefined as

$$\delta = \frac{1}{g} \sum_{i=1}^{g} \Delta(x_i, y_i)$$

and

$$\mu = \frac{1}{g^2} \sum_{i=1}^{g} \sum_{j=1}^{2} \Delta(x_i, y_i),$$

respectively, where

$$\Delta(x_i, y_i) = \left[\sum_{k=1}^{r} (x_{ik} - y_{ik})^2 \right]^{1/2},$$

then

$$\Re = 1 - \frac{\delta}{\mu}$$

and Spearman's footrule is expanded to incorporate multiple dimensions. Again, the footrule R is a special case of $\Re$ for a single response variable

---

[5]Adapted and reprinted with permission of Psychological Reports from K.J. Berry and P.W. Mielke, Jr. Spearman's footrule as a measure of agreement. *Psychological Reports*, 1997, 80, 839–846. Copyright © 1997 by Psychological Reports.

TABLE 4.15. Example data set for multiple dimensions with ranked data, $g = 6$ objects, $b = 2$ observers, and $r = 3$ dimensions.

	Observer					
	A			B		
Object	Color	Shape	Label	Color	Shape	Label
1	1	1	2	1	2	3
2	5	2	3	6	1	2
3	2	5	6	3	4	5
4	6	3	5	5	3	6
5	3	6	4	4	6	1
6	4	4	1	2	5	4

TABLE 4.16. Example layout of proportions p and $1 - p$ with $p = 0.6$ and $1 - p = 0.4$.

	Proportions									
Variable	0.2			0.6					0.2	
x	1	2	3	4	5	6	7	8	9	10
y	10	9	3	4	5	6	7	8	2	1

when no ties are present. To illustrate the measurement of agreement for more than one dimension, consider the data listed in Table 4.15, where two observers are asked to rank order six new product packaging combinations in terms of three attributes: color, shape, and label. For these data, $g = 6$, $b = 2$, $r = 3$, $\delta = 2.1994$, $\mu = 3.9233$, and $\Re = 0.4394$, indicating 44 percent agreement among the two observers above and beyond what is expected by chance.

It is not generally recognized that under special conditions Spearman's rank-order correlation coefficient, ρ, is also a chance-corrected measure of agreement. When x and y consist of ranks from 1 to g with no ties, or x includes tied ranks and y is a permutation of x, then Spearman's ρ is both a measure of correlation and a chance-corrected measure of agreement since any deviation from perfect agreement also counts as a deviation from perfect correlation (Krippendorff, 1970a, p. 144).

To compare the large sample properties of $\Re$ and ρ, consider a worst-case scenario with large g, no ties on either x or y, $\Re = R$, and where some proportion, p, of the x and y values is in perfect agreement and the remaining proportion, $1 - p$, is in maximum disagreement. If the x values are arranged sequentially, then p represents the middle proportion of the x and y values and there are $(1 - p)/2$ values at either extreme. Table 4.16 contains an example based on $g = 10$ ranked observations that illustrates the proportions of interest. In this example, the middle six of ten scores are in perfect agreement and $p = 0.6$. The two sets of two

TABLE 4.17. Large sample $\Re$ and ρ values for various proportions of maximum disagreement, $1 - p$, from 0.0 to 1.0.

$1 - p$	$\Re$	ρ
0.0	1.000	1.000
0.1	0.715	0.458
0.2	0.460	0.024
0.3	0.235	−0.314
0.4	0.040	−0.568
0.5	−0.125	−0.750
0.6	−0.260	−0.872
0.7	−0.365	−0.946
0.8	−0.440	−0.984
0.9	−0.485	−0.998
1.0	−0.500	−1.000

scores at either end are arranged to provide the proportion of maximum disagreement $1 - p = 0.4$. If g is large, then $\Re$ and ρ are given by

$$\Re = 1 - \frac{3\left(1 - p^2\right)}{2}$$

and

$$\rho = 1 - 2\left(1 - p^3\right),$$

respectively. Table 4.17 contains large sample comparisons of $\Re$ and ρ for values of the proportion of maximum disagreement, $1 - p$, from 0.0 to 1.0. When the proportion of extreme disagreement is only 0.2, ρ is essentially zero; the exact value when $\rho = 0$ is $1 - p = 0.2063$. On the other hand, $\Re$ does not attain zero until $1 - p = 0.4227$. The ρ measure of agreement is heavily influenced by a small proportion of cases that are in disagreement because ρ is based on squared Euclidean differences between x and y. In contrast, $\Re$ focuses on agreement rather than disagreement and is less affected by extreme disagreement values since it is based on ordinary Euclidean differences between x and y. The results given in Table 4.17 demonstrate that $\Re$ provides a significant advantage over ρ for assessing agreement in paired ranks when g is large and no ties exist on either x or y. The values of $\Re$ and ρ listed in Table 4.17 for all proportions of maximum disagreement from 0.0 to 1.0 indicate that ρ is a relatively uninformative measure of chance-corrected agreement because the squared disagreement differences contribute a disproportionate influence on the agreement coefficient. In contrast, $\Re$ provides an informative indicator of chance-corrected agreement for all values of $1 - p$, even under maximum disagreement (Berry and Mielke, 1997c).

TABLE 4.18. Example data set for interval data with $g = 12$ objects, $b = 2$ observers, and $r = 2$ dimensions.

| | Observer | | | |
| | A | | B | |
Object	Distance	Elevation	Distance	Elevation
1	120	10	125	10
2	80	15	85	20
3	100	5	95	10
4	150	20	140	15
5	75	10	60	5
6	50	5	60	10
7	50	20	50	25
8	20	20	25	15
9	90	15	90	15
10	95	25	90	20
11	100	25	90	20
12	70	5	70	5

Interval Measurement

The construction of $\Delta(x_{i1}, x_{i2})$ makes an extension of $\Re$ to interval measurement straightforward. For interval data, x is simply a vector of $r \geq 1$ measurements. Here, an observer assigns a vector of $r \geq 1$ scores to each observation. In this case, $\Re$ measures the degree to which the two observers agree on their scoring, above and beyond what is expected by chance. If x_{i1k} and x_{i2k} $(k = 1, ..., r)$ agree, $\Delta(x_{i1}, x_{i2})$ is zero; if x_{i1k} and x_{i2k} $(k = 1, ..., r)$ disagree, $\Delta(x_{i1}, x_{i2})$ is the Euclidean distance between the points in an r-dimensional space, measured in score units (Berry and Mielke, 1988b). If $r \geq 2$, the previously described Euclidean commensuration may be applied.

To illustrate the measurement of agreement for interval level variables, consider the data listed in Table 4.18, where each of two observers is asked to estimate distance and elevation, in meters, of 12 distant objects. For these data, $g = 12$, $b = 2$, $r = 2$, $\delta = 7.1305$, $\mu = 37.6931$, and $\Re = 0.8108$, indicating 81 percent agreement between the two observers above and beyond what is expected by chance.

4.5.2 Multiple Observers

A simple modification to the computation of δ and μ generalizes $\Re$ to measure agreement among multiple observers (Berry and Mielke, 1988b,

TABLE 4.19. Example data set for multiple observers with ranked data, $g = 8$ objects, $b = 4$ observers, and $r = 1$ dimension.

Object	Observer			
	A	B	C	D
1	6	7	8	8
2	8	5	4	7
3	1	3	6	4
4	2	1	2	2
5	3	2	1	1
6	5	6	7	5
7	4	4	3	3
8	7	8	5	6

1998a). Thus, δ may be redefined as

$$\delta = \left[g \binom{b}{2} \right]^{-1} \sum_{i=1}^{g} \sum_{s<t} \Delta\left(x_{is},\, x_{it}\right),$$

where

$$\Delta\left(x_{is},\, x_{it}\right) = \left[\sum_{k=1}^{r} \left(x_{isk} - x_{itk}\right)^2 \right]^{1/2},$$

b is the number of observers (i.e., blocks), and $\sum_{s<t}$ is the sum over all s and t such that $1 \leq s < t \leq b$. The reformulation of μ is given by

$$\mu = \left[g^2 \binom{b}{2} \right]^{-1} \sum_{i=1}^{g} \sum_{j=1}^{g} \sum_{s<t} \Delta\left(x_{is},\, x_{jt}\right),$$

where

$$\Delta\left(x_{is},\, x_{jt}\right) = \left[\sum_{k=1}^{r} \left(x_{isk} - x_{jtk}\right)^2 \right]^{1/2}.$$

To illustrate the measurement of agreement for multiple observers, consider the data listed in Table 4.19, where each of four observers is asked to rank order eight objects in terms of preference, with 1 indicating most preferred and 8 indicating least preferred. For these data, $g = 8$, $b = 4$, $r = 1$, $\delta = 1.4167$, $\mu = 2.6250$, and $\Re = 0.4603$, indicating 46 percent agreement among the four observers above and beyond what is expected by chance.

The coefficient of agreement $\Re$ is a generalization of Cohen's (1960) κ to ordinal and interval data and to multiple observers. It preserves the desired qualities of κ in that it is chance-corrected, Euclidean-based, and applicable to the measurement of reliability. If $b > 2$ and the level of measurement is nominal, $\Re = 1 - \delta/\mu$ is equivalent to Conger's (1980) reformulation of a statistic proposed by Fleiss (1971) for multiple observers. It should be mentioned that among the three general concepts of agreement suggested by Hubert (1977), $\Re$ employs the pairwise definition of agreement.

The generalization of Cohen's (1960) κ to multiple observers for nominal data is the special case of $\Re$ when the distance space is restricted to an r-dimensional simplex. An r-dimensional simplex consists of r distinct points where the distance between any pair of distinct points is unity and where the distance between any two coincident points at any one of the r positions is zero. In this context, Cohen's (1960) κ is the special case of $\Re$ when $b = 2$, and the measure of agreement corresponding to Cochran's (1950) Q test is the special case of $\Re$ when $r = 2$. That is, Cochran's (1950) Q test involves b observers, g observations, and a two-dimensional simplex (Mielke, 1986). Incidentally, the measure of agreement corresponding to McNemar's (1947) test for change is the special case of both Cohen's κ and the measure of agreement corresponding to Cochran's (1950) Q test because $b = r = 2$ in these cases (Berry and Mielke, 1988b).

When the distance space is not limited to an r-dimensional simplex (e.g., it could instead be an r-dimensional Euclidean space), then other agreement measures may be considered. If the distance space is a one-dimensional Euclidean space and the observations are rank-order statistics of the g observations associated with each of the b observers, then the measure of agreement corresponding to Spearman's (1904, 1906) footrule is, as previously noted, a special case of $\Re$ when $b = 2$.

If the distance space is redefined as a nonmetric space of squared Euclidean distances (Mielke, 1986, 1987) where

$$\Delta\left(x_{is},\, x_{jt}\right) = \sum_{k=1}^{r}\left(x_{isk} - x_{jtk}\right)^{2},$$

then a variety of classical measures of association become special cases of $\Re$. If $r = 1$ and if the g observations are rank-order statistics associated with each of the b observers, then Spearman's (1904, 1906) rank correlation coefficient, ρ, is identical to $\Re$ when $b = 2$. Similarly, the extension to b observers of Spearman's (1904, 1906) ρ is the measure of association corresponding to Friedman's (1937) two-way analysis of variance for ranks and Kendall's (1948) coefficient of concordance (Mielke, 1984). If the restriction of rank-order statistics is removed and interval-level measurements are used with $r = 1$, then the permutation version of the Pearson product-moment correlation coefficient is a special case of $\Re$ when $b = 2$ (Mielke, 1984). In addition, the b observer extension of the permutation version of Pearson's product-moment correlation coefficient is the measure of association corresponding to a randomized block analysis of variance (Mielke, 1984).

4.5.3 Test of Significance

Since, for any problem and any level of measurement, $\Re$ is simply a linear transformation of δ, a test of significance for δ is a test of significance for $\Re$. Thus, the P-value for an observed value of δ (δ_o) is the probability, under the null hypothesis, given by $P(\delta \leq \delta_o \,|\, H_0)$. As the b blocks are specified, the randomization associated with a randomized block experiment is confined to all permutations of the g observations within each block. Under the null hypothesis, each of the

$$M = (g!)^b$$

possible permutations occurs with equal probability $(1/M)$. Thus, the exact probability of the observed $\Re$ ($\Re_o$) is the proportion of the M possible values of $\Re$ equal to or greater than $\Re_o$ or, equivalently, the proportion of δ values equal to or less than δ_o. When the number of permutations becomes large, the Pearson type III probability distribution may be employed to attain an approximate P-value where the exact mean, variance, and skewness of δ are given by

$$\mu = \frac{1}{M} \sum_{j=1}^{M} \delta_j,$$

$$\sigma^2 = \frac{1}{M} \sum_{j=1}^{M} \delta_j^2 - \mu^2,$$

and

$$\gamma = \left(\frac{1}{M} \sum_{j=1}^{M} \delta_j^3 - 3\mu\sigma^2 - \mu^3 \right) \Big/ \sigma^3,$$

respectively (Berry and Mielke, 1988b, 1990).

To illustrate the test of significance for $\Re$, consider the data listed in Table 4.20, where each of three referees is asked to evaluate eight submitted journal manuscripts on a 10-point scale, with 10 indicating the highest rating. For these data, $g = 8$, $b = 3$, $r = 1$, $\delta_o = 1.0833$, $\mu = 2.9479$, and $\Re_o = 0.6325$, indicating 63 percent agreement among the three referees above and beyond what is expected by chance. In addition, $\sigma^2 = 0.1658$, $\gamma = -0.5000$, and the Pearson type III P-value is 0.1765×10^{-3}. Also, a resampling approximation with $L = 1,000,000$ yields a P-value of 0.4600×10^{-4}.

In the case of $b = 2$, when both x and y consist entirely of untied ranks from 1 to g and y is a permutation of x, then methods exist to determine the probability of an observed value of Spearman's footrule R under the null hypothesis that any of the $g!$ orderings of either the x or y values is

TABLE 4.20. Example data set for a test of significance with $g = 8$ objects, $b = 3$ observers, and $r = 1$ dimension.

Object	Observer		
	A	B	C
1	8	8	7
2	6	5	4
3	1	1	3
4	9	9	8
5	5	7	4
6	3	2	3
7	4	3	5
8	2	2	1

equally likely to occur. If

$$G = \sum_{i=1}^{g} |x_i - y_i| = g\delta,$$

then, since R is a linear transformation of G, the probability of an observed G is the probability of an observed R. Tables of the exact cumulative distribution function (cdf) of G are given by Ury and Kleinecke (1979) for $2 \le g \le 10$ and approximate results based on Monte Carlo methods are given for $11 \le g \le 15$. Franklin (1988) reported the exact cdf of G for $11 \le g \le 18$, and both Franklin (1988) and Ury and Kleinecke (1979) discussed the rate of convergence to an approximating normal distribution and the use of a continuity correction to be applied to the cdf of G. Salama and Quade (1990) used Markov chain properties to obtain the exact cdf of G for $4 \le g \le 40$, corrected some tabled values in Franklin (1988), and further investigated the adequacy of approximations to the distribution of G.

If either x or y contains tied values, then the calculation of probabilities is more complex. Because $\Re$ is merely a linear transformation of δ, the probability of an observed δ is the probability of an observed $\Re$. Thus, the probability value for δ_o is the probability under the null hypothesis given by $P(\delta \le \delta_o \mid H_0)$. In the case of no tied values for either x or y, the exact mean, variance, and skewness of δ, under the null hypothesis, are given by

$$\mu = \frac{g^2 - 1}{3g},$$

$$\sigma^2 = \frac{(g + 1)(2g^2 + 7)}{45g^2},$$

and

$$\gamma = -\frac{(g-2)(2g^2+31)}{[49(g+1)(2g^2+7)^3/20]^{1/2}},$$

respectively (Berry and Mielke, 1997c; Mielke, 1984).

4.5.4   Two Independent Groups of Observers

It is often of interest to evaluate the difference between measures of agreement obtained from two independent groups of observers. For example, if written essays are scored by a group of professional educators on a set of criteria (e.g., punctuation and grammar) and are scored independently by a group of graduate students on the same set of criteria, it may be interesting to know (1) the amount of agreement among the professional educators, (2) the amount of agreement among the graduate students, and (3) the difference in agreement between the two groups.

For convenience, let $\Re_1$ ($\Re_2$) indicate the measure of agreement for group 1 (group 2), and let μ_1 (μ_2), σ_1^2 (σ_2^2), and γ_1 (γ_2) denote the mean, variance, and skewness, respectively, for the δ statistic corresponding to group 1 (group 2). Under the null hypothesis, H_0, $\Re_1 = \Re_2$, and groups 1 and 2 are independent. If $D = \Re_1 - \Re_2$, then the exact mean, variance, and skewness of D under H_0 are given by

$$\mu_D = 0,$$

$$\sigma_D^2 = \frac{\mu_1^2\sigma_2^2 + \mu_2^2\sigma_1^2}{\mu_1^2\mu_2^2},$$

and

$$\gamma_D = \frac{\mu_1^3\sigma_2^3\gamma_2 - \mu_2^3\sigma_1^3\gamma_1}{\mu_1^3\mu_2^3\sigma_D^3},$$

respectively (Berry and Mielke, 1997a).[6] Then, the Pearson type III P-value is based on the standardized statistic $T = D/\sigma_D$ and on γ_D.

Cicchetti and Heavens (1981) provided a Z statistic that evaluates the difference between two independent values of Cohen's (1960) κ agreement measure. Although the $\Re$ measure of agreement reduces to κ when there are only two observers, a single subject response, and a nominal level of measurement, $\Re$ is a much more general measure of agreement that allows for multiple observers, multiple subject responses, and any level of measurement. In addition, because the Z statistic of Cicchetti and Heavens (1981) uses the standard error of κ derived by Fleiss and Cicchetti

---

[6]Adapted and reprinted with permission of Sage Publications, Inc. from K.J. Berry and P.W. Mielke, Jr. Agreement measure comparisons between two sets of independent raters. *Educational and Psychological Measurement*, 1997, 57, 360–364. Copyright © 1997 by Sage Publications, Inc.

(1978) and Fleiss et al., (1969), its inferential asymptotic solution requires large sample sizes before normality is achieved; otherwise, the Z statistic overestimates the true probability value. Cicchetti and Heavens (1981) recommended a minimum of $3k^2$ subjects, where k is the number of categories. Thus, for example, $k = 7$ categories would require a minimum of 147 subjects. By contrast, the probability of differences between two $\Re$ values is based on an inferential nonasymptotic solution, and a sample size of only $g = 10$ is sufficient for all analyses of differences between two $\Re$ measures.

To illustrate the analysis of the difference between two independent values of $\Re$, consider a set of $g = 40$ undergraduate essays evaluated by two independent sets of graders on six canons of writing excellence: clarity, organization, accuracy, spelling, grammar, and punctuation. One set of graders is composed of $b = 3$ faculty members in English composition, and the second set of graders consists of $b = 8$ advanced graduate students in English composition. Each of the $r = 6$ attributes is scored on a scale of 1 to 10 by each of the graders. For the $b = 3$ faculty members in group 1, $\Re_1 = 0.1158$, $\mu_1 = 1.2705$, $\sigma_1^2 = 0.4678 \times 10^{-3}$, and $\gamma_1 = -0.3415$. For the $b = 8$ graduate students in group 2, $\Re_2 = 0.1978$, $\mu_2 = 1.6024$, $\sigma_2^2 = 0.1010 \times 10^{-2}$, and $\gamma_2 = -0.2843$. The analysis yields $D = -0.0820$, $\sigma_D^2 = 0.6832 \times 10^{-3}$, $T = -3.1380$, $\gamma_D = -0.2985 \times 10^{-1}$, and the probability of a D this large or larger under H_0: $\mu_D = 0$, is 0.1966×10^{-2} (Berry and Mielke, 1997a).

4.5.5   Agreement With a Standard

A number of research problems require the measurement of agreement between multiple observers and a standard, or "correct," set of responses. Several investigators have considered this requirement. Guetzkow (1950) introduced procedures to measure agreement among multiple observers coding objects when each object belongs to a known category. Tukey (1950) criticized this approach because of the assumption that each object is either coded correctly with 100% certainty or it is coded at random. Light (1971) provided a test for the joint agreement of multiple observers with a correct set of responses, and Hubert (1977) offered a "target rater" measure of agreement that is identical to the measure proposed by Light (1971) but uses a much simpler formula for the variance.

The measures of agreement proposed by Guetzkow (1950), Light (1971), and Hubert (1977) are limited to nominal level data and a single response. The measure of agreement $\Re$ can easily be adapted to measure the agreement of multiple observers with a standard set of responses (Berry and Mielke, 1997b).[7] In addition, $\Re$ can be used with any level of measurement

---

[7]Adapted and reprinted with permission of Sage Publications, Inc. from K.J. Berry and P.W. Mielke, Jr. Measuring the joint agreement between multiple raters and a standard. *Educational and Psychological Measurement*, 1997, 57, 527–530. Copyright © 1997 by Sage Publications, Inc.

and with multivariate responses. If r is the number of responses for each of g objects scored by m raters, and the index of the standard set is denoted by s, then the measure of agreement, $\Re$, between the m raters and the standard set is defined by

$$\Re = 1 - \frac{\delta}{\mu}$$

with δ, the index of disagreement, given by

$$\delta = \sum_{i=1}^{m} \delta_i,$$

where

$$\delta_i = \frac{1}{g} \sum_{j=1}^{g} \left[\sum_{k=1}^{r} (x_{jsk} - x_{jik})^2 \right]^{1/2}$$

for $i = 1, ..., m$ and μ is the expected value of δ under H_0, namely,

$$\mu = \sum_{i=1}^{m} \mu_i,$$

where

$$\mu_i = \frac{1}{g^2} \sum_{j=1}^{g} \sum_{l=1}^{g} \left[\sum_{k=1}^{r} (x_{jsk} - x_{lik})^2 \right]^{1/2}.$$

If $m = 1$, $r = 1$, and the responses are categorical, then $\Re$ reduces to Cohen's κ statistic. Because $\Re$ is a linear function of δ, the probability (P) of an observed $\Re$ $(\Re_o)$, under H_0, is the probability of an observed δ (δ_o), under H_0, given by

$$P\left(\Re \geq \Re_o \,|\, H_0 \right) = P\left(\delta \leq \delta_o \,|\, H_0 \right).$$

Under H_0, each of the

$$M = (g!)^m$$

possible permutations of the m observers has an equal probability $(1/M)$ of occurrence. Because the calculation of exact probability values is necessarily limited to small values of M, approximate probability values based on the Pearson type III probability distribution can be obtained. Because the m observers yield independent ratings, the exact mean, variance, and skewness of δ are given by

$$\mu = \sum_{i=1}^{m} \mu_i,$$

$$\sigma^2 = \sum_{i=1}^{m} \sigma_i^2,$$

TABLE 4.21. Example data set for agreement with a standard where each of $b = 3$ observers (A, B, and C) estimates the height (H), width (W), and depth (D) of $g = 5$ objects.

Object	Observer								
	A			B			C		
	H	W	D	H	W	D	H	W	D
1	8.0	9.2	6.0	8.2	9.0	6.5	8.2	9.0	6.5
2	10.5	2.5	11.0	11.2	3.0	11.5	9.5	2.8	12.5
3	17.6	4.5	13.0	20.0	4.5	15.0	21.4	4.5	17.0
4	9.0	12.0	14.2	9.0	12.5	14.0	9.5	13.5	14.4
5	14.6	6.0	7.5	14.2	6.0	8.0	14.5	5.5	9.2

and

$$\gamma = \frac{\sum_{i=1}^{m} \kappa_{3i}}{\sigma^3},$$

respectively, where μ_i, σ_i^2, and κ_{3i} denote the first three exact cumulants of δ_i for $i = 1, ..., m$.

As an example, consider an application where each of three observers estimates the height, width, and depth of five objects, in centimeters. The data are given in Table 4.21, where Observer A estimates the height, width, and depth of object 1 as 8.0, 9.2, and 6.0, respectively; Observer B estimates the height, width, and depth of object 1 as 8.2, 9.0, and 6.5, respectively; and so on. Observer A is considered the standard, or correct, set of responses against which Observers B and C are compared. Analysis of these data with $m = 3$, $r = 3$, and $g = 5$ yields $\delta = 1.4167$, $\mu = 16.6913$, $\sigma = 6.3936$, $\gamma = -0.4699$, $\Re = 0.7504$, and the approximate Pearson type III P-value is 0.6130×10^{-4}.

5
Regression Analysis, Prediction, and Agreement

Evaluations of the regression, prediction, and agreement methods described in this chapter are based on the permutation approach. In addition, emphasis is again placed on statistical procedures that closely correspond to the geometrical structure of the data in question. Following some preliminary historical comments regarding linear regression, general descriptions of permutation-based multiple linear regression analyses are presented. MRPP analyses of least (sum of) absolute deviations (LAD) for multiple regression and, more generally, least sum (of) Euclidean distances (LSED) for multivariate multiple regression residuals are described for various experimental designs. MRPP regression analyses, Cade–Richards regression analyses, and classical ordinary least (sum of) squared deviations (OLS) regression analyses are compared. Next, MRPP confidence intervals for regression parameters are described. Since the validation of prediction models is a major concern for many fields, the results of recent studies involving drop-one cross-validation and the use of either LAD or OLS regression are discussed. In addition, effects on agreement by various conditions such as sample size, population agreement value, inclusion of redundant predictors, and varying severity of data contamination are examined. Finally, linear and nonlinear multivariate multiple regression models and their applications are discussed.

5.1   Historical Perspective

As described by Sheynin (1973), the initial known use of regression by D. Bernoulli (circa 1734) for astronomical prediction problems involved least (sum of) absolute deviations (LAD) regression. The distance function associated with LAD regression is the common Euclidean distance between observed and predicted response values. Further work in developing LAD regression was accomplished by R.J. Boscovich (circa 1755), P.S. Laplace (circa 1789), and C.F. Gauss (circa 1809). Sheynin (1973) points out that Gauss developed linear programming for the sole purpose of estimating the parameters associated with LAD regression; Gauss consequently had to utilize his previously developed ordinary least (sum of) squared deviations (OLS) regression (which was independently developed by A.M. Legendre) simply because calculus provided an efficient way to estimate the parameters associated with OLS regression. Thus, OLS regression is a default procedure that was introduced only because Gauss lacked appropriate computational equipment to solve linear programming problems. The American mathematician and astronomer N. Bowditch (circa 1809) immediately attacked OLS regression because squared residuals unduly overemphasize questionable observations in comparison to the absolute residuals associated with LAD regression (Sheynin, 1973). There are many important topics involving permutation methods for multiple regression such as quantile estimates and rank score tests that have not been considered here (Cade and Richards, 2006; Cade et al., 2006).

5.2   OLS and LAD Regressions

OLS linear regression has long been recognized as a useful tool in many kinds of research. The optimal properties of estimators of OLS regression parameters are well known when the errors are normally distributed. In practice, however, the assumption of normality is rarely justified. LAD linear regression is often superior to OLS regression when the errors are not normally distributed (Blattberg and Sargent, 1971; Dielman, 1986, 1989; Mathew and Nordström, 1993; Pfaffenberger and Dinkel, 1978; Wilson, 1978). Estimators of OLS regression parameters can be severely affected by unusual values in either the criterion variable or in one or more of the predictor variables. This is due to the weight given to each data point when minimizing the sum of squared errors. In contrast, LAD regression is less sensitive to the effects of unusual values because the errors are not squared. This is analogous to the effect of extreme values on the mean and median as measures of location (Dielman, 1986). In this section, the robust nature of LAD regression is illustrated with a simple example and the effects of distance, leverage, and influence are examined (Berry and Mielke, 1998b).[1]

For clarity and efficiency, the illustration and ensuing discussion are limited to simple linear regression with one predictor variable (x) and one criterion variable (y). Consider N paired x_I and y_I observed values for $I = 1, ..., N$. For the OLS regression equation given by

$$\hat{y}_I = \hat{\alpha} + \hat{\beta} x_I,$$

where $\hat{y}_I$ is the Ith of N predicted criterion values and x_I is the Ith of N predictor values, and $\hat{\alpha}$ and $\hat{\beta}$ are the least squared parameter estimates of the intercept and slope, respectively, and are given by

$$\hat{\beta} = \frac{\sum_{I=1}^{N} (y_I - \bar{y})(x_I - \bar{x})}{\sum_{I=1}^{N} (x_I - \bar{x})^2}$$

and

$$\hat{\alpha} = \bar{y} - \hat{\beta}\bar{x},$$

where $\bar{x}$ and $\bar{y}$ are the sample means of variables x and y, respectively. Estimates of OLS regression parameters are computed by minimizing the sum of the squared differences between the observed and predicted criterion values, namely,

$$\sum_{I=1}^{N} (y_I - \hat{y}_I)^2 .$$

For the LAD regression equation given by

$$\tilde{y}_I = \tilde{\alpha} + \tilde{\beta} x_I,$$

where $\tilde{y}_I$ is the Ith of N predicted values, x_I is the Ith of N predictor values, and $\tilde{\alpha}$ and $\tilde{\beta}$ are the least absolute parameter estimates of the intercept and slope, respectively. Unlike OLS regression, no simple expressions can be given for $\tilde{\alpha}$ and $\tilde{\beta}$. However, values for $\tilde{\alpha}$ and $\tilde{\beta}$ may be found by linear programming (Barrodale and Roberts, 1973, 1974). Estimates of LAD regression parameters are computed by minimizing the sum of the absolute differences between the observed and predicted criterion values, namely,

$$\sum_{I=1}^{N} |y_I - \tilde{y}_I|.$$

---

[1]Adapted and reprinted with permission of Perceptual and Motor Skills from K.J. Berry and P.W. Mielke, Jr. Least sum of absolute deviations regression: distance, leverage, and influence. *Perceptual and Motor Skills*, 1998, 86, 1063–1070. Copyright © 1998 by Perceptual and Motor Skills.

TABLE 5.1. Data for a perfect linear regression with one predictor variable.

Variable	Value								
x	1	2	3	4	5	6	7	8	9
y	9	8	7	6	5	4	3	2	1

Portnoy and Koenker (1997) discuss algorithms for fitting LAD regression models based on large data sets, which may be more efficient than algorithms for fitting OLS regression models.

5.2.1 Some OLS and LAD Comparisons

Three useful diagnostics for assessing the potential effects of extreme values on regression estimators are distance, leverage, and influence (Berry and Mielke, 1998b). In general terms, distance refers to the possible presence of unusual values in the criterion variable (y) and is typically measured as the deviation of a value from the center of the criterion variable. Leverage refers to the possible presence of unusual values in a predictor variable. In the case of a single predictor, leverage is typically measured as the deviation of a value from the center of the predictor variable (x). Influence incorporates both distance and leverage and refers to the possible presence of unusual values in some combination of the criterion variable and predictor variable, i.e., both y and x.

Since OLS regression is based on squared residuals and LAD regression is based on absolute residuals, OLS regression is intuitively far more sensitive to extreme residual values while LAD regression is more robust. To illustrate the effects of extreme residual values on the estimates of OLS and LAD regression parameters, consider an example of linear regression with one predictor and a single extreme data point. This simplified example permits the isolation and assessment of distance, leverage, and influence and allows comparison of the effects of an atypical value on estimates of OLS and LAD regression parameters. The data for a linear regression with one predictor variable are listed in Table 5.1.

The data in Table 5.1 consist of nine data points with $x_I = I$ and $y_I = 10-I$ for $I = 1, ..., 9$ and describe a perfect negative linear relationship between x and y. Figure 5.1 displays the data in Table 5.1 and indicates the directions of unusual values implicit in direction, leverage, and influence.

5.2.2 Distance

If a tenth bivariate value is added to the nine bivariate values given in Table 5.1, where $x_{10} = y_{10} = 5$, the new data point is located at the common mean and median of both x and y and does not affect the perfect linear relationship. If x_{10} is held constant at 5, but y_{10} takes on additional

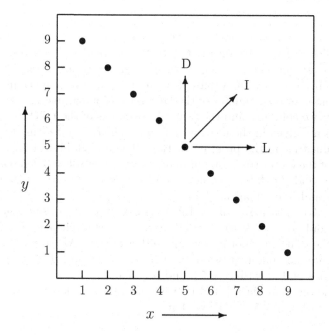

FIGURE 5.1. Scatterplot of the data in Table 5.1 with directions of distance (D), influence (I), and leverage (L) indicated.

values of 6, 7, ..., 30, 40, 60, 80, 100, then the effects of distance on the two regression models can be observed. The vertical movement of y_{10} with x_{10} held constant is displayed in Figure 5.1. In Table 5.2, the values of x_{10} and y_{10} are given in the first two columns, the $\hat{\alpha}$ and $\hat{\beta}$ estimates of the OLS regression parameters are given in the next two columns, and the $\tilde{\alpha}$ and $\tilde{\beta}$ estimates of the LAD regression parameters are given in the last two columns. The $\tilde{\alpha}$ and $\tilde{\beta}$ LAD regression parameter estimates were obtained using the program of Barrodale and Roberts (1974). The estimates of the OLS regression parameters listed in Table 5.2 demonstrate that $\hat{\alpha}$ systematically changes with increases in distance, but $\hat{\beta}$ remains constant at -1.0. In contrast, estimates of the LAD regression parameters are unaffected by changes in distance, remaining constant at $\tilde{\alpha} = 10.0$ and $\tilde{\beta} = -1.0$ for $x_{10} = 5$ and any value of y_{10}. Given the bivariate data listed in Table 5.1 and an additional bivariate data point with $x_{10} = 5$, it follows that

$$\sum_{I=1}^{10} |y_I - \tilde{y}_I| = |y_{10} - 5|.$$

5.2.3 Leverage

If a tenth bivariate value is added to the nine bivariate values given in Table 5.1, where y_{10} is 5 and x_{10} takes on the values 5, 6, ..., 30, 40, 60, 80, 100, then the effects of leverage on the two regression models can be observed. The horizontal movement of x_{10} with y_{10} held constant is displayed in Figure 5.1. In Table 5.3, the values of x_{10} and y_{10} are given in the first two columns, the $\hat{\alpha}$ and $\hat{\beta}$ estimates of the OLS regression parameters are given in the next two columns, and the $\tilde{\alpha}$ and $\tilde{\beta}$ estimates of the LAD regression parameters are given in the last two columns. The $\tilde{\alpha}$ and $\tilde{\beta}$ estimates were again obtained using the program of Barrodale and Roberts (1974). The estimates of the OLS regression parameters listed in Table 5.3 demonstrate that both $\hat{\alpha}$ and $\hat{\beta}$ exhibit complex changes with increases in leverage. In contrast, $\tilde{\alpha}$ and $\tilde{\beta}$ are unaffected for $y_{10} = 5$ and $5 \leq x_{10} \leq 24$. For $y_{10} = 5$ and $x_{10} \geq 26$, the estimates of the LAD regression parameters change from $\tilde{\alpha} = 10.0$ and $\tilde{\beta} = -1.0$ to $\tilde{\alpha} = 5.0$ and $\tilde{\beta} = 0.0$. When $y_{10} = 5$ and $x_{10} = 25$, the solution is not unique and either of two LAD regression lines is appropriate, i.e., one regression line with $\tilde{\alpha} = 10.0$ and $\tilde{\beta} = -1.0$ and a second regression line with $\tilde{\alpha} = 5.0$ and $\tilde{\beta} = 0.0$.

Given the bivariate data listed in Table 5.1 and an additional bivariate data point with $y_{10} = 5$, it follows that

$$\sum_{I=1}^{10} |y_I - \tilde{y}_I| \leq 20.0$$

for $x_{10} \leq 25$ and

$$\sum_{I=1}^{10} |y_I - \tilde{y}_I| = 20.0$$

for $x_{10} \geq 25$. When $x_{10} \leq 25$, the LAD regression line defined by $\tilde{\alpha} = 10.0$ and $\tilde{\beta} = -1.0$ yields the minimum sum of absolute differences. However, when $x_{10} \geq 25$, the LAD regression line defined by $\tilde{\alpha} = 5.0$ and $\tilde{\beta} = 0.0$ that passes through point (x_{10}, y_{10}) yields the minimum sum of absolute differences. For $x_{10} = 25$, the LAD regression line is not unique. Although this is an interesting property of LAD regression and can easily be illustrated with one predictor and a small number of data points, in practice any extreme value would have to be so far removed from the center of the x distribution to be considered a "grossly aberrant" value (Rousseeuw, 1984).

5.2.4 Influence

If a tenth bivariate value is added to the nine bivariate values given in Table 5.1, where $x_{10} = y_{10}$ take on the values 5, 6, ..., 30, 40, 60, 80, 100, then the effects of influence on the two regression models can be observed. The diagonal movement of (x_{10}, y_{10}) is displayed in Figure 5.1. In Table 5.4,

TABLE 5.2. Effects of distance on intercepts and slopes of least squared and least absolute regression models.

x_{10}	y_{10}	Least squared $\hat{\alpha}$	$\hat{\beta}$	Least absolute $\tilde{\alpha}$	$\tilde{\beta}$
5	5	10.0000	-1.0000	10.0000	-1.0000
5	6	10.1000	-1.0000	10.0000	-1.0000
5	7	10.2000	-1.0000	10.0000	-1.0000
5	8	10.3000	-1.0000	10.0000	-1.0000
5	9	10.4000	-1.0000	10.0000	-1.0000
5	10	10.5000	-1.0000	10.0000	-1.0000
5	11	10.6000	-1.0000	10.0000	-1.0000
5	12	10.7000	-1.0000	10.0000	-1.0000
5	13	10.8000	-1.0000	10.0000	-1.0000
5	14	10.9000	-1.0000	10.0000	-1.0000
5	15	11.0000	-1.0000	10.0000	-1.0000
5	16	11.1000	-1.0000	10.0000	-1.0000
5	17	11.2000	-1.0000	10.0000	-1.0000
5	18	11.3000	-1.0000	10.0000	-1.0000
5	19	11.4000	-1.0000	10.0000	-1.0000
5	20	11.5000	-1.0000	10.0000	-1.0000
5	21	11.6000	-1.0000	10.0000	-1.0000
5	22	11.7000	-1.0000	10.0000	-1.0000
5	23	11.8000	-1.0000	10.0000	-1.0000
5	24	11.9000	-1.0000	10.0000	-1.0000
5	25	12.0000	-1.0000	10.0000	-1.0000
5	26	12.1000	-1.0000	10.0000	-1.0000
5	27	12.2000	-1.0000	10.0000	-1.0000
5	28	12.3000	-1.0000	10.0000	-1.0000
5	29	12.4000	-1.0000	10.0000	-1.0000
5	30	12.5000	-1.0000	10.0000	-1.0000
5	40	13.5000	-1.0000	10.0000	-1.0000
5	60	15.5000	-1.0000	10.0000	-1.0000
5	80	17.5000	-1.0000	10.0000	-1.0000
5	100	19.5000	-1.0000	10.0000	-1.0000

the values of x_{10} and y_{10} are given in the first two columns, the $\hat{\alpha}$ and $\hat{\beta}$ estimates of the OLS regression parameters are given in the next two columns, and the $\tilde{\alpha}$ and $\tilde{\beta}$ estimates of the LAD regression parameters are given in the last two columns. The estimates of the OLS regression parameters listed in Table 5.4 demonstrate that both $\hat{\alpha}$ and $\hat{\beta}$ exhibit complex changes with increases in influence. In contrast, $\tilde{\alpha}$ and $\tilde{\beta}$ do not change for $5 \leq x_{10} = y_{10} \leq 24$. For $x_{10} = y_{10} \geq 26$, the estimates of the LAD regression parameters change from $\tilde{\alpha} = 10.0$ and $\tilde{\beta} = -1.0$ to $\tilde{\alpha} = 0.0$ and

TABLE 5.3. Effects of leverage on intercepts and slopes of least squared and least absolute regression models.

x_{10}	y_{10}	Least squared		Least absolute	
		$\hat{\alpha}$	$\hat{\beta}$	$\tilde{\alpha}$	$\tilde{\beta}$
5	5	10.0000	−1.0000	10.0000	−1.0000
6	5	10.0246	−0.9852	10.0000	−1.0000
7	5	9.9057	−0.9434	10.0000	−1.0000
8	5	9.6696	−0.8811	10.0000	−1.0000
9	5	9.3548	−0.8065	10.0000	−1.0000
10	5	9.0000	−0.7273	10.0000	−1.0000
11	5	8.6364	−0.6494	10.0000	−1.0000
12	5	8.2853	−0.5764	10.0000	−1.0000
13	5	7.9592	−0.5102	10.0000	−1.0000
14	5	7.6637	−0.4515	10.0000	−1.0000
15	5	7.4000	−0.4000	10.0000	−1.0000
16	5	7.1670	−0.3552	10.0000	−1.0000
17	5	6.9620	−0.3165	10.0000	−1.0000
18	5	6.7822	−0.2829	10.0000	−1.0000
19	5	6.6244	−0.2538	10.0000	−1.0000
20	5	6.4857	−0.2286	10.0000	−1.0000
21	5	6.3636	−0.2066	10.0000	−1.0000
22	5	6.2559	−0.1874	10.0000	−1.0000
23	5	6.1604	−0.1706	10.0000	−1.0000
24	5	6.0756	−0.1559	10.0000	−1.0000
25	5	6.0000	−0.1429	10.0000	−1.0000
26	5	5.9324	−0.1313	5.0000	0.0000
27	5	5.8717	−0.1211	5.0000	0.0000
28	5	5.8170	−0.1119	5.0000	0.0000
29	5	5.7676	−0.1037	5.0000	0.0000
30	5	5.7229	−0.0964	5.0000	0.0000
40	5	5.4387	−0.0516	5.0000	0.0000
60	5	5.2264	−0.0216	5.0000	0.0000
80	5	5.1464	−0.0117	5.0000	0.0000
100	5	5.1063	−0.0073	5.0000	0.0000

$\tilde{\beta} = 1.0$. When $x_{10} = y_{10} = 25$, either of two LAD regression lines holds since the solution is not unique, i.e., one regression line with $\tilde{\alpha} = 10.0$ and $\tilde{\beta} = -1.0$ and a second regression line with $\tilde{\alpha} = 0.0$ and $\tilde{\beta} = 1.0$.

Given the bivariate data listed in Table 5.1 and an additional bivariate data point $x_{10} = y_{10}$ (which is allowed to vary), it follows that

$$\sum_{I=1}^{10} |y_I - \tilde{y}_I| \leq 40$$

for $5 \leq x_{10} = y_{10} \leq 25$ and

$$\sum_{I=1}^{10} |y_I - \tilde{y}_I| = 40$$

for $x_{10} = y_{10} \geq 25$. When $(x_{10} = y_{10} \leq 25)$ or $(x_{10} = y_{10} \geq 25)$, the LAD regression line defined by ($\tilde{\alpha} = 10.0$ and $\tilde{\beta} = 1.0$) or ($\tilde{\alpha} = 0.0$ and $\tilde{\beta} = 1.0$), respectively, yields the minimum sum of absolute differences, i.e., the line is not unique when $x_{10} = y_{10} = 25$.

It should be noted that the shift in the LAD regression line is a consequence of only the leverage component of influence. For these data, the LAD regression line is defined by $\tilde{\alpha} = 10.0$ and $\tilde{\beta} = -1.0$ if $|x_{10} - 5| \leq 20.0$, and the regression line is unique if $|x_{10} - 5| < 20.0$ or $y_{10} = 10 - x_{10}$.

LAD regression is a robust alternative to OLS regression, especially when errors are generated by fat-tailed distributions (Dielman and Pfaffenberger, 1988; Dielman and Rose, 1994; Taylor, 1974). Fat-tailed distributions involve an abundance of extreme values, and OLS regression gives disproportionate weight to such values. In practice, LAD regression is virtually unaffected by the presence of a few extreme values. Although the effects of distance, leverage, and influence are illustrated by only a simplified example of perfect linear regression with one predictor, the results extend to more general regression models. If a less than perfect regression model with m predictors is considered, then the estimators of the LAD regression parameters are unaffected by unusual y_I values when the leverage effect is absent. In addition, only exceedingly extreme values of the predictors $(x_1, ..., x_m)$ have an impact on the estimation of the LAD regression parameters.

5.3 MRPP Regression Analyses of Linear Models

Permutation multiple regression analyses of experimental designs with univariate dependent values are given by Mielke and Berry (1997a, 2002a).[2] In comparison with other permutation methods for this purpose (Cade and Richards, 1996; Freedman and Lane, 1983; Manly, 1997, pp. 154–170; also see Section 5.4), the method of Mielke and Berry (1997a) is based strictly on coupled combinations of the observed dependent and independent values (Mielke and Berry, 2002b). Considered here are the natural extensions of permutation multiple regression analyses described by Mielke and Berry (1997a) to applications involving multivariate dependent values

---

[2]Adapted and reprinted with permission of Psychological Reports from P.W. Mielke, Jr. and K.J. Berry, Multivariate multiple regression analyses: A permutation method for linear models. *Psychological Reports*, 2002, 91, 3–9. Copyright © 2002 by Psychological Reports.

TABLE 5.4. Effects of influence on intercepts and slopes of least squared and least absolute regression models.

x_{10}	y_{10}	Least squared		Least absolute	
		$\hat{\alpha}$	$\hat{\beta}$	$\tilde{\alpha}$	$\tilde{\beta}$
5	5	10.0000	−1.0000	10.0000	−1.0000
6	6	10.0493	−0.9704	10.0000	−1.0000
7	7	9.8113	−0.8868	10.0000	−1.0000
8	8	9.3392	−0.7621	10.0000	−1.0000
9	9	8.7097	−0.6129	10.0000	−1.0000
10	10	8.0000	−0.4545	10.0000	−1.0000
11	11	7.2727	−0.2987	10.0000	−1.0000
12	12	6.5706	−0.1527	10.0000	−1.0000
13	13	5.9184	−0.0204	10.0000	−1.0000
14	14	5.3273	0.0971	10.0000	−1.0000
15	15	4.8000	0.2000	10.0000	−1.0000
16	16	4.3339	0.2895	10.0000	−1.0000
17	17	3.9241	0.3671	10.0000	−1.0000
18	18	3.5644	0.4342	10.0000	−1.0000
19	19	3.2487	0.4924	10.0000	−1.0000
20	20	2.9714	0.5429	10.0000	−1.0000
21	21	2.7273	0.5868	10.0000	−1.0000
22	22	2.5117	0.6251	10.0000	−1.0000
23	23	2.3208	0.6587	10.0000	−1.0000
24	24	2.1512	0.6882	10.0000	−1.0000
25	25	2.0000	0.7143	10.0000	−1.0000
26	26	1.8647	0.7374	0.0000	1.0000
27	27	1.7433	0.7579	0.0000	1.0000
28	28	1.6340	0.7762	0.0000	1.0000
29	29	1.5353	0.7925	0.0000	1.0000
30	30	1.4458	0.8072	0.0000	1.0000
40	40	0.8774	0.8968	0.0000	1.0000
60	60	0.4528	0.9569	0.0000	1.0000
80	80	0.2928	0.9766	0.0000	1.0000
100	100	0.2126	0.9853	0.0000	1.0000

(Mielke and Berry, 2002a). The extensions were prompted by a recently developed multivariate least sum (of) Euclidean distances (LSED) multiple regression algorithm (Kaufman et al., 2002). Like the permutation multiple regression analyses based on univariate dependent values, the extensions to multivariate dependent values are highly resistant to extreme values.

Consider the multivariate multiple regression model given by

$$y_{Ik} = \sum_{j=1}^{m} x_{Ij} \beta_{jk} + e_{Ik} \tag{5.1}$$

for $I = 1, ..., N$ and $k = 1, ..., r$, where y_{Ik} represents the Ith of N measurements for the kth of r response variables, possibly affected by a treatment; x_{Ij} is the jth of m covariates associated with the Ith response, where $x_{I1} = 1$ if the model includes an intercept; β_{jk} denotes the jth of m regression parameters for the kth of r response variables; and e_{Ik} designates the error associated with the Ith of N measurements for the kth of r response variables. If the estimates of β_{jk} that minimize

$$\sum_{I=1}^{N} \left(\sum_{k=1}^{r} e_{Ik}^2 \right)^{1/2}$$

are denoted by $\tilde{\beta}_{jk}$ for $j = 1, ..., m$ and $k = 1, ..., r$, then the N r-dimensional residuals of the LSED multivariate multiple regression model are given by

$$\tilde{e}_{Ik} = y_{Ik} - \sum_{j=1}^{m} x_{Ij} \tilde{\beta}_{jk}$$

for $I = 1, ..., N$ and $k = 1, ..., r$. Note that the univariate LAD multiple regression model is a special case when $r = 1$. An algorithm to obtain the $\tilde{\beta}_{jk}$ values is given by Kaufman et al. (2002). In comparison to multivariate multiple regression models that minimize

$$\sum_{I=1}^{N} \sum_{k=1}^{r} |e_{Ik}|,$$

$$\sum_{I=1}^{N} \left(\sum_{k=1}^{r} |e_{Ik}| \right)^2,$$

or

$$\sum_{I=1}^{N} \sum_{k=1}^{r} e_{Ik}^2,$$

only the LSED multivariate multiple regression model does not vary with coordinate rotation and possesses the desired geometrical attributes of satisfying the triangle inequality of a metric (Mielke, 1987; Kaufman et al., 2002).

Incidentally, if $L0$ and $L1$ denote the minimum values of

$$\sum_{I=1}^{N} \left(\sum_{k=1}^{r} e_{Ik}^2 \right)^{1/2}$$

under the reduced model (H_0) and the full model (H_1), respectively, then an alternative effect size measure is given by

$$1 - \frac{L1}{L0}$$

(Berry and Mielke, 2002; McKean and Sievers, 1987).

5.3.1 Permutation Test

Mielke and Berry (1997a) used MRPP to analyze univariate residuals from a LAD multiple regression. Extension of the univariate procedure to multivariate residuals is straightforward. Let the N r-dimensional residuals, $(\tilde{e}_{I1}, ..., \tilde{e}_{Ir})$ for $I = 1, ..., N$ obtained from a LSED multivariate multiple regression model algorithm (Kaufman et al., 2002), be partitioned into g treatment groups of sizes $n_1, ..., n_g$ where $n_i \geq 2$ for $i = 1, ..., g$ and

$$\sum_{i=1}^{g} n_i = N.$$

The MRPP analysis of the multivariate residuals depends on the statistic given by

$$\delta = \sum_{i=1}^{g} C_i \xi_i$$

where $C_i = n_i/N$ is a positive weight for the ith of g treatment groups that minimizes the variability of δ,

$$\sum_{i=1}^{g} C_i = 1,$$

and ξ_i, the average pairwise Euclidean distance among the n_i r-dimensional residuals in the ith of g treatment groups, is defined by

$$\xi_i = \binom{n_i}{2}^{-1} \sum_{K=1}^{N-1} \sum_{L=K+1}^{N} \left[\sum_{j=1}^{r} (\tilde{e}_{Kj} - \tilde{e}_{Lj})^2 \right]^{1/2} \Psi_{Ki} \Psi_{Li},$$

where

$$\Psi_{Ii} = \begin{cases} 1 & \text{if } (\tilde{e}_{I1}, ..., \tilde{e}_{Ir}) \text{ is in the } i\text{th treatment group,} \\ 0 & \text{otherwise.} \end{cases}$$

The null hypothesis (H_0) specifies that each of the

$$M = \frac{N!}{\prod_{i=1}^{g} n_i!}$$

possible allocations of the N r-dimensional residuals to the g treatment groups is equally likely. Under H_0, the permutation distribution of δ assigns equal probabilities to the resulting M values of δ. Since small values of δ imply a concentration of similar residuals within the g treatment groups, H_0 is rejected when the observed value of δ, δ_0, is small. Thus, the exact MRPP P-value associated with δ_0 is given by

$$P\text{-value} = P\left(\delta \leq \delta_0 | H_0\right) = \frac{\text{number of } \delta \text{ values} \leq \delta_0}{M}.$$

To obtain MRPP P-values, either exact and/or approximate (resampling and Pearson type III moment) algorithms may be used (see Section 2.3). These exact and approximate methods for obtaining P-values either eliminate or substantially reduce any parametric assumptions regarding the r-dimensional residuals.

Since the multivariate multiple regression technique couples the dependent and independent values (Mielke and Berry, 2002b), a single set of observed multivariate residuals is obtained. Consequently, an exact MRPP analysis of the multivariate residuals guarantees that the type I statistical error is controlled. The univariate and multivariate regression methods are termed "MRPP regression analyses." The initial applications of MRPP regression analyses involved weather modification studies (Mielke et al., 1982; Smith et al., 1997; Wong et al., 1983).

5.3.2 Example

To illustrate the residual permutation analyses, consider an unbalanced randomized block experimental design. The Harter Self-perception Profile for Children is an inventory composed of 36 self-reporting items used to assess self-concept in children aged 8 years and older (Harter, 1985). Six subscales are associated with the Harter Self-perception Profile: Scholastic Competence, Social Acceptance, Athletic Competence, Physical Appearance, Behavioral Conduct, and Global Self-Worth. Suppose that the inventory is given to a sample of fifth-grade students in three neighborhood schools. Within each school (A, B, C) the inventory is administered in both the Fall and Spring semesters. The results for two of the subscales (Social Acceptance and Physical Appearance) are summarized in Table 5.5 with a small sample of $N = 16$ subjects for purposes of illustration. Although the residual permutation analyses can easily accommodate many dimensions, larger numbers of subjects, and more complicated designs, the example is intentionally kept simple to illustrate the procedures.

Analysis of Schools

The model under H_0 for the analysis of Schools is given by

$$y_{Ik} = x_{I1}\beta_{1k} + x_{I2}\beta_{2k} + e_{Ik}$$

TABLE 5.5. Bivariate data on social acceptance and physical appearance (y_1, y_2) for an unbalanced randomized block design.

Semester	School		
	A	B	C
Fall	49, 102	63, 84	45, 107
		60, 89	50, 100
			42, 111
			46, 104
Spring	48, 103	66, 83	
	58, 94	74, 79	
	51, 100	69, 88	
	55, 97	27, 114	
		71, 82	

where $I = 1, ..., 16$ and $k = 1, 2$ correspond to Expression (5.1). The values of the $\mathbf{X}$ and $\mathbf{Y}$ matrices (x_{Ij} and y_{Ik}) are given in Table 5.6 where $x_{I1} = 1$ for the intercept, $x_{I2} = 1$ (0) for the Fall (Spring) semester, and y_{Ik} denotes the kth response of the Ith student. If δ_o denotes the observed value of δ, then the exact permutation analysis based on $M = 1,441,440$ permutations yields $\delta_o = 12.8587$ with an exact P-value of $6,676/1,441,440 \doteq 0.4631 \times 10^{-2}$, the resampling permutation procedure based on $L = 1,000,000$ yields $\delta_o = 12.8587$ with an approximate P-value of 0.4689×10^{-2}, and the Pearson type III moment approximation permutation analysis yields $\delta_o = 12.8587$ with an approximate P-value of 0.4701×10^{-2}. Since the exact P-value is obviously preferred for this example, the resampling and moment approximation P-values are included to demonstrate that they closely approximate the exact P-value.

Analysis of Semesters

The model under H_0 for the analysis of Semesters is given by

$$y_{Ik} = x_{I1}\beta_{1k} + x_{I2}\beta_{2k} + x_{I3}\beta_{3k} + e_{Ik}$$

where $I = 1, ..., 16$ and $k = 1, 2$ correspond to Expression (5.1). The values of the $\mathbf{X}$ and $\mathbf{Y}$ matrices (x_{Ij} and y_{Ik}) are given in Table 5.7 where $x_{I1} = 1$ for the intercept, (x_{I2}, x_{I3}) is $(1, 0)$, $(0, 1)$ and $(0, 0)$ for School A, B, and C, respectively, and y_{Ik} denotes the kth response of the Ith student. The exact permutation analysis based on $M = 11,440$ permutations yields $\delta_o = 12.0535$ with an exact P-value of $2,090/11,440 \doteq 0.1827$, the resampling permutation procedure based on $L = 1,000,000$ yields $\delta_o = 12.0535$ with an approximate P-value of 0.1826, and the Pearson type III moment approximation permutation analysis yields $\delta_o = 12.0535$ with an approximate P-value of 0.1901. Again, the resampling and moment approximation P-values closely estimate the exact P-value.

TABLE 5.6. Data file containing the **X** and **Y** matrices for the analysis of schools.

School	**X** Matrix		**Y** Matrix	
A	1	1	49	102
	1	0	48	103
	1	0	58	94
	1	0	51	100
	1	0	55	97
B	1	1	63	84
	1	1	60	89
	1	0	66	83
	1	0	74	79
	1	0	69	88
	1	0	27	114
	1	0	71	82
C	1	1	45	107
	1	1	50	100
	1	1	42	111
	1	1	46	104

TABLE 5.7. Data file containing the **X** and **Y** matrices for the analysis of semesters.

Semester	**X** Matrix			**Y** Matrix	
Fall	1	1	0	49	102
	1	0	1	63	84
	1	0	1	60	89
	1	0	0	45	107
	1	0	0	50	100
	1	0	0	42	111
	1	0	0	46	104
Spring	1	1	0	48	103
	1	1	0	58	94
	1	1	0	51	100
	1	1	0	55	97
	1	0	1	66	83
	1	0	1	74	79
	1	0	1	69	88
	1	0	1	27	114
	1	0	1	71	82

5.3.3 Discussion

Experimental designs involving univariate dependent values, e.g., one-way, Latin square, factorial, nested, split-plot, etc., with and without covariates, and amenable to MRPP regression analyses (Berry and Mielke, 1998c, 1999a, 1999b; Mielke and Berry, 1997a) may also be analyzed with MRPP regression when multivariate dependent values are encountered. MRPP regression analyses are based on coupled dependent and independent values. Simulated decoupled univariate multiple regression analyses suggested by Freedman and Lane (1983) motivated the LSED univariate multiple regression analysis by Cade and Richards (1996). As a consequence of decoupling the dependent and independent values, these decoupled analyses are based on unobservable residuals (Mielke and Berry, 2002b) and, therefore, raise questions of validity. Moreover, an extension of the Cade and Richards (1996) LSED univariate regression analysis to the multivariate dependent value case requires time-consuming repeated simulations of multivariate multiple regression fits for the decoupled dependent and independent values (Mielke and Berry, 2002b). In contrast, MRPP regression analyses require a single multivariate multiple regression fit for the coupled dependent and independent values.

Compared with classical parametric approaches, this Euclidean-distance multivariate multiple regression method is exceedingly robust to extreme values and, being a permutation test, does not depend on artificial assumptions such as normality, homogeneity, and independence. Further, the permutation approach allows for the choice of calculating exact or approximate P-values.

An MRPP regression analysis is an exact permutation method under H_0. Because the N observed pairings between the "coupled" response and covariate values ($y_{I1}, ..., y_{Ir}$ and $x_{I1}, ..., x_{Im}$ for $I = 1, ..., N$) are preserved in this analysis, the resulting N residuals are unchanged for any of the $N!$ exchangeable sequences of the N coupled values. Thus, the N residuals are exchangeable random variables under H_0 and, since MRPP is an exact permutation test, the resulting MRPP regression analysis of the fixed collection of N residuals is also exact. An immediate consequence of this last statement is that any variation of the MRPP regression analysis is also exact, e.g., the choice of either LAD or OLS regression and the choice of distance function. Besides yielding exact permutation tests, coupling also avoids the obvious feature of "decoupling" in which a multitude of unobserved pairings of the response and covariate values occur. The decoupled pairings then yield analyses based on unobserved residuals, which are not compatible with the notion of data-dependent analyses. The differences between the coupled and decoupled methods account for the P-value discrepancies associated with the regression analyses discussed in Section 5.5.

TABLE 5.8. Example data for a one-way randomized design with $g = 3$ treatments and $N = 26$ subjects.

A_1	A_2	A_3
15	17	6
18	22	9
12	15	12
12	12	11
9	20	11
10	14	8
12	15	13
20	20	30
	21	7

5.3.4 Examples of MRPP Regression Analyses

MRPP regression analysis will be illustrated with a series of examples. Each example is based on a published data set. Although, for the most part, the examples illustrate analyses of balanced designs, the permutation approach as already shown is applicable to unbalanced experimental designs. The following examples demonstrate the use of MRPP regression analyses with a one-way randomized design, a one-way randomized design with a covariate, a two-way factorial design, a one-way block design, a balanced two-way block design, an unbalanced two-way block design, a Latin square design, and a split-plot design. While these examples are confined to $r = 1$ for brevity, the MRPP regression analyses hold for $r \geq 2$. Complex color pattern analyses with $r > 1$ are both described and termed LSED–MRPP analyses by Endler and Mielke (2005). In addition, Endler and Mielke (2005) use effect size to illustrate a variety of alternative multivariate residual paterns that MRPP with $v = 1$ can detect (see Section 2.3.5).

5.3.5 One-Way Randomized Design

Consider a one-way randomized design with fixed effects in which $N = 26$ subjects are randomly assigned to one of $g = 3$ treatments (Berry and Mielke, 1999a).[3] The design and data are from Stevens (1990, p. 70) and are given in Table 5.8.

A design matrix for the LAD regression is given in Table 5.9, where the first column of 1 values provides for the intercept and the second column

---

[3] Adapted and reprinted with permission of Psychological Reports from K.J. Berry and P.W. Mielke, Jr. Least absolute regression residuals: analyses of randomized designs. *Psychological Reports*, 1999, 84, 947–954. Copyright © 1999 by Psychological Reports.

contains the scores ordered by the three treatments. Thus, the $N = 26$ scores in Table 5.9 are listed according to the original random assignment of the subjects to the $g = 3$ treatments with the first $n_1 = 8$ subjects, the next $n_2 = 9$ subjects, and the last $n_3 = 9$ subjects associated with treatments A_1, A_2, and A_3, respectively. Because the purpose of the analysis is to examine differences among treatments, a reduced LAD regression model is constructed without a variate for treatments. The full regression model is

$$y_{ij} = \Theta + \tau_i + e_{ij},$$

where Θ is an unknown population centering constant, τ_i denotes the ith treatment effect $(i = 1, ..., g)$, and e_{ij} is the error associated with the jth subject $(j = 1, ..., n_i)$. Then, the reduced regression model is given by

$$y_{ij} = \Theta + e_{ij}.$$

Consequently, for this single-factor experiment, the design matrix for the reduced model is composed solely of a code for the intercept. The MRPP regression analysis examines the regression residuals for differences in treatments.

The MRPP regression analysis yields $\delta_o = 5.2308$, $\mu = 6.1262$, $\sigma^2 = 0.7809 \times 10^{-1}$, $\gamma = -1.5124$, $T_o = -3.2041$, and a Pearson type III P-value of 0.1171×10^{-1}, where δ_o and T_o are the observed values of δ and T, respectively. A resampling approximation with $L = 1{,}000{,}000$ yields $\delta_o = 5.2308$ and a P-value of 0.1209×10^{-1}. In contrast, a conventional one-way analysis of variance yields $F(2, 24) = 2.6141$ and a P-value of 0.9485×10^{-1}, based on Snedecor's F distribution. Clearly, the permutation approach with a Euclidean distance function can produce results that differ substantially from the classical one-way analysis of variance.

5.3.6 One-Way Randomized Design with a Covariate

Consider a one-way randomized design with a covariate in which $N = 47$ rats are randomly assigned to one of $g = 5$ treatments (Berry and Mielke, 1999a). Conti and Musty (1984) bilaterally injected either a placebo, or 0.1, 0.5, 1, or 2 micrograms (μg) of tetrahydrocannibinol, the major active ingredient in marijuana, into the nucleus accumbens of each rat. The dependent variable was locomotor activity measured 10 minutes after the injection, and the covariate was a baseline measurement taken 10 minutes before the injection. The covariate design permits testing of differences among the treatments after the effect of the covariate has been partialled out of the analysis. The data are from Howell (1997, p. 589) and are given in Table 5.10.

A design matrix for the LAD regression is given in Table 5.11, where the 47 rats were randomly assigned to the $g = 5$ treatments with the first $n_1 = 10$ rats, the next $n_2 = 10$ rats, the next $n_3 = 9$ rats, the

TABLE 5.9. Design matrix and data for a one-
way randomized design.

Matrix	Score
1	15
1	18
1	12
1	12
1	9
1	10
1	12
1	20
1	17
1	22
1	15
1	12
1	20
1	14
1	15
1	20
1	21
1	6
1	9
1	12
1	11
1	11
1	8
1	13
1	30
1	7

next $n_4 = 8$ rats, and the last $n_5 = 10$ rats associated with the control,
0.1 μg, 0.5 μg, 1 μg, and 2 μg treatments, respectively. In Table 5.11, the
first column (all 1 values) provides for the intercept, the second column
lists the corresponding covariate values (prescores), and the third column
lists the responses, possibly affected by the treatments (postscores). The
MRPP regression analysis examines the LAD regression residuals for different treatment levels; consequently, no dummy codes for treatment levels
are included in Table 5.11 because this information is implicit in the ordering of the $g = 5$ treatment levels. The MRPP regression analysis yields
$\delta_o = 0.7962$, $\mu = 0.9178$, $\sigma^2 = 0.1100 \times 10^{-2}$, $\gamma = -1.0579$, $T_o = -3.6689$,
and a Pearson type III P-value of 0.4132×10^{-2}, where δ_o and T_o are the
observed values of δ and T, respectively. A resampling approximation with

TABLE 5.10. Example data for a one-way randomized design with a covariate
with $g = 5$ treatments and $N = 47$ subjects.

Control		0.1 μg		0.5 μg		1 μg		2 μg	
Pre	Post	Pre	Post	Pre	Post	Pre	Post	Pre	Post
4.34	1.30	1.55	0.93	7.18	5.10	6.94	2.29	4.00	1.44
3.50	0.94	10.56	4.44	8.33	4.16	6.10	4.75	4.10	1.11
4.33	2.25	8.39	4.03	4.05	1.54	4.90	3.48	3.62	2.17
2.76	1.05	3.70	1.92	10.78	6.36	3.69	2.76	3.92	2.00
4.62	0.92	2.40	0.67	6.09	3.96	4.76	1.67	2.90	0.84
5.40	1.90	1.83	1.70	7.78	4.51	4.30	1.51	2.90	0.99
3.95	0.32	2.40	0.77	5.08	3.76	2.32	1.07	1.82	0.44
1.55	0.64	7.67	3.53	2.86	1.92	7.35	2.35	4.94	0.84
1.42	0.69	5.79	3.65	6.30	3.84			5.69	2.84
1.90	0.93	9.58	4.22					5.54	2.93

$L = 1,000,000$ yields $\delta_o = 0.7962$ and a P-value of 0.4128×10^{-2}. In contrast, a conventional OLS regression analysis yields $F(4, 41) = 4.6978$ and a P-value of 0.3257×10^{-2}.

5.3.7   Factorial Design

Consider a 2×3 factorial design with four subjects in each treatment combination where the purpose is to investigate the role of drive level and size of reward on the learning of a discrimination problem by monkeys (Berry and Mielke, 1999a). In this experiment, two like objects and one different object are presented to the subjects, and the task is to select the nonduplicated object. The dependent variable is the number of correct selections in 20 trials. Factor A, with $a = 2$ treatment levels, is the drive level of the subject, either 1 or 24 hours of food deprivation, and Factor B, with $b = 3$ treatment levels, is the size of reward, either 1, 3, or 5 grapes. The design and data are from Keppel (1982, p. 197) and are given in Table 5.12.

Although design matrices of either dummy or effect codes are appropriate for one-way randomized designs and for block designs, the main effects of factorial designs should not be analyzed with design matrices constructed with dummy codes whenever Method 1 of Overall and Spiegel (1969) is utilized (Berry et al., 1998). Method 1 of Overall and Spiegel (1969) is also known as the "regression method" and involves estimation of the independent effects of each factor adjusted for all other factors in the model. Method 1 of Overall and Spiegel (1969) tests the interaction and main effects by comparing the full regression model with appropriate reduced regression models. To illustrate, consider a two-way fixed-effects factorial

TABLE 5.11. Design matrix, consisting of the intercept and pretest measurements, and posttest measurements (scores) for a one-way randomized design with a covariate.

Matrix		Score	Matrix		Score
1	4.34	1.30	1	6.09	3.96
1	3.50	0.94	1	7.78	4.51
1	4.33	2.25	1	5.08	3.76
1	2.76	1.05	1	2.86	1.92
1	4.62	0.92	1	6.30	3.84
1	5.40	1.90			
1	3.95	0.32	1	6.94	2.29
1	1.55	0.64	1	6.10	4.75
1	1.42	0.69	1	4.90	3.48
1	1.90	0.93	1	3.69	2.76
			1	4.76	1.67
1	1.55	0.93	1	4.30	1.51
1	10.56	4.44	1	2.32	1.07
1	8.39	4.03	1	7.35	2.35
1	3.70	1.92			
1	2.40	0.67	1	4.00	1.44
1	1.83	1.70	1	4.10	1.11
1	2.40	0.77	1	3.62	2.17
1	7.67	3.53	1	3.92	2.00
1	5.79	3.65	1	2.90	0.84
1	9.58	4.22	1	2.90	0.99
			1	1.82	0.44
1	7.18	5.10	1	4.94	0.84
1	8.33	4.16	1	5.69	2.84
1	4.05	1.54	1	5.54	2.93
1	10.78	6.36			

TABLE 5.12. Data on correct responses of four subjects for two levels of deprivation (A) and three levels of reward (B).

A_1			A_2		
B_1	B_2	B_3	B_1	B_2	B_3
1	13	9	15	6	14
4	5	16	6	18	7
0	7	18	10	9	6
7	15	13	13	15	13

design with factors A and B (as in Table 5.12). The full model is given by

$$\mu_{ij} = \mu + \alpha_i + \beta_j + \gamma_{ij},$$

where μ_{ij} is the population mean of scores at factors A_i and B_j, μ is the population grand mean, α_i is the main effect of factor A, β_j is the main effect of factor B, and γ_{ij} is the interaction effect of factors A_i and B_j. The reduced model for testing the interaction is given by

$$\mu_{ij} = \mu + \alpha_i + \beta_j,$$

and the reduced models for testing the effects of factors A and B are given by

$$\mu_{ij} = \mu + \beta_j + \gamma_{ij}$$

and

$$\mu_{ij} = \mu + \alpha_i + \gamma_{ij},$$

respectively. In each case, the appropriate reduced regression model is compared with the full regression model.

Method 1 tests hypotheses about unweighted factor means and is commonly used whenever unequal cell frequencies can be attributed to chance. Method 1 is preferred by most researchers for both balanced and unbalanced designs; see, for example, Carlson and Timm (1974), Howell and McConaughy (1982), Lewis and Keren (1977), and Overall et al. (1975). For an alternative point of view and related discussions, see Appelbaum and Cramer (1974), Cramer and Appelbaum (1980), O'Brien (1976), Overall et al. (1981), and Rawlings (1972, 1973).

A design matrix of effect codes to analyze factor A is given on the left-hand side of Table 5.13, where the first column of 1 values provides for the intercept, the second and third columns contain the codes for factor B, the fourth and fifth columns contain the codes for the $A \times B$ interaction, and the last column lists the $N = 24$ scores listed according to the original random assignment of the subjects to the $a = 2$ levels of factor A with the first $n_1 = 12$ subjects and the last $n_2 = 12$ subjects associated with treatment levels A_1 and A_2, respectively. No effect codes for factor A are given in Table 5.13 because this information is implicit in the ordering of the $a = 2$ levels. The right-hand side of Table 5.13 contains a design matrix of effect codes to analyze factor B, where the first column of 1 values provides for the intercept, the second column contains the codes for factor A, the third and fourth columns contain the codes for the $A \times B$ interaction, and the last column lists the $N = 24$ scores listed according to the original random assignment of the subjects to the $b = 3$ levels of factor B with the first $n_1 = 8$ subjects, the next $n_2 = 8$ subjects, and the last $n_3 = 8$ subjects associated with treatment levels B_1, B_2, and B_3, respectively. No effect codes for factor B are given in Table 5.13 because this information is implicit in the ordering of the $b = 3$ levels.

TABLE 5.13. Design matrices and data for the main effects of factors A and B in a two-way factorial design.

Deprivation (A)						Reward (B)				
Matrix					Score	Matrix				Score
1	1	0	1	0	1	1	1	1	0	1
1	1	0	1	0	4	1	1	1	0	4
1	1	0	1	0	0	1	1	1	0	0
1	1	0	1	0	7	1	1	1	0	7
1	0	1	0	1	13	1	−1	−1	0	15
1	0	1	0	1	5	1	−1	−1	0	6
1	0	1	0	1	7	1	−1	−1	0	10
1	0	1	0	1	15	1	−1	−1	0	13
1	−1	−1	−1	−1	9					
1	−1	−1	−1	−1	16	1	1	0	1	13
1	−1	−1	−1	−1	18	1	1	0	1	5
1	−1	−1	−1	−1	13	1	1	0	1	7
						1	1	0	1	15
1	1	0	−1	0	15	1	−1	0	−1	6
1	1	0	−1	0	6	1	−1	0	−1	18
1	1	0	−1	0	10	1	−1	0	−1	9
1	1	0	−1	0	13	1	−1	0	−1	15
1	0	1	0	−1	6					
1	0	1	0	−1	18	1	1	−1	−1	9
1	0	1	0	−1	9	1	1	−1	−1	16
1	0	1	0	−1	15	1	1	−1	−1	18
1	−1	−1	1	1	14	1	1	−1	−1	13
1	−1	−1	1	1	7	1	−1	1	1	14
1	−1	−1	1	1	6	1	−1	1	1	7
1	−1	−1	1	1	13	1	−1	1	1	6
						1	−1	1	1	13

The MRPP regression analysis for factor A yields $\delta_o = 5.0758$, $\mu = 5.0725$, $\sigma^2 = 0.3309 \times 10^{-1}$, $\gamma = -2.1270$, $T_o = 0.1811 \times 10^{-1}$, and a Pearson type III P-value of 0.3665, where δ_o and T_o are the observed values of δ and T, respectively. A resampling approximation with $L = 1{,}000{,}000$ yields $\delta_o = 5.0758$ and a P-value of 0.3841. In contrast, a conventional OLS regression analysis yields $F(1, 18) = 1.3091$ and a P-value of 0.2675. The MRPP regression analysis for factor B yields $\delta_o = 5.0000$, $\mu = 5.3333$, $\sigma^2 = 0.8069 \times 10^{-1}$, $\gamma = -1.4639$, $T_o = -1.1735$, and a Pearson type III P-value of 0.1195. A resampling approximation with $L = 1{,}000{,}000$ yields $\delta_o = 5.0000$ and a P-value of 0.1255. In contrast, a conventional OLS regression analysis yields $F(2, 18) = 3.0545$ and a P-value of 0.7208×10^{-1}.

TABLE 5.14. Design matrix and data for the $A \times$ B interaction in a two-way factorial design.

Matrix				Score
1	1	1	0	1
1	1	1	0	4
1	1	1	0	0
1	1	1	0	7
1	−1	1	0	15
1	−1	1	0	6
1	−1	1	0	10
1	−1	1	0	13
1	1	0	1	13
1	1	0	1	5
1	1	0	1	7
1	1	0	1	15
1	−1	0	1	6
1	−1	0	1	18
1	−1	0	1	9
1	−1	0	1	15
1	1	−1	−1	9
1	1	−1	−1	16
1	1	−1	−1	18
1	1	−1	−1	13
1	−1	−1	−1	14
1	−1	−1	−1	7
1	−1	−1	−1	6
1	−1	−1	−1	13

A design matrix of effect codes to analyze the $A \times B$ interaction is given in Table 5.14, where the first column of 1 values provides for the intercept, the second column contains the codes for factor A, the third and fourth columns contain the codes for factor B, and the last column lists the $N = 24$ scores listed according to the original random assignment of the subjects to the $ab = 6$ levels of the $A \times B$ interaction. No effect codes for factors A and B are given in Table 5.14 because this information is implicit in the ordering of the treatments. The MRPP regression analysis for the $A \times B$ interaction yields $\delta_o = 5.3333$, $\mu = 5.5000$, $\sigma^2 = 0.2650$, $\gamma = -0.7571$, $T_o = -0.3237$, and a Pearson type III P-value of 0.3311. A resampling approximation with $L = 1,000,000$ yields $\delta_o = 5.3333$ and a P-value of 0.3483. In contrast, a conventional OLS regression analysis yields $F(2, 18) = 3.9273$ and a P-value of 0.3843×10^{-1}.

TABLE 5.15. Stress data for three work station systems on six controllers.

Controller	System		
	A_1	A_2	A_3
1	15	15	18
2	14	14	14
3	10	11	15
4	13	12	17
5	16	13	16
6	13	13	13

5.3.8 One-Way Block Design

One-way randomized block designs are common in experimental research. When the same subjects are used in each treatment, the design is sometimes termed a "repeated-measures" or "within-subjects" design. Consider a complete randomized block design where $b = 6$ air traffic controllers (blocks) are tested on $a = 3$ work station systems (treatments). The dependent variable is controller stress. This is a randomized block design in which each controller is tested on all three systems and the order in which the systems are assigned to the controllers is chosen randomly (Berry and Mielke, 1998d).[4] The design and data are from Anderson et al. (1994, p. 471) and are given in Table 5.15.

A design matrix for the LAD regression is given in Table 5.16, where the first column of 1 values provides for the intercept, the next five columns contain dummy codes for the blocks, and the last column lists the stress scores listed according to the original random assignment of the subjects to the $a = 3$ treatment levels with the first $n_1 = 6$ subjects, the next $n_2 = 6$ subjects, and the last $n_3 = 6$ subjects associated with treatment levels A_1, A_2, and A_3, respectively. The test examines the regression residuals for differences in treatment levels. Consequently, there are no dummy codes for treatments in Table 5.16 because this information is implicit in the ordering of the $a = 3$ treatments. The MRPP regression analysis yields $\delta_o = 1.2889$, $\mu = 1.6078$, $\sigma^2 = 0.1353 \times 10^{-1}$, $\gamma = -1.1459$, $T_o = -2.7417$, and a Pearson type III P-value of 0.1663×10^{-1}, where δ_o and T_o are the observed values of δ and T, respectively. A resampling approximation with $L = 1,000,000$ yields $\delta_o = 1.2889$ and a P-value of 0.5607×10^{-1}. In contrast, a conventional OLS regression analysis yields $F(2, 10) = 5.5263$ and a P-value of 0.2418×10^{-1}.

---

[4]Adapted and reprinted with permission of Psychological Reports from K.J. Berry and P.W. Mielke, Jr. Least absolute regression residuals: analyses of block designs. *Psychological Reports*, 1998, 83, 923–929. Copyright © 1998 by Psychological Reports.

TABLE 5.16. Design matrix and data for a one-way block design.

Matrix						Score
1	0	0	0	0	0	15
1	1	0	0	0	0	14
1	0	1	0	0	0	10
1	0	0	1	0	0	13
1	0	0	0	1	0	16
1	0	0	0	0	1	13
1	0	0	0	0	0	15
1	1	0	0	0	0	14
1	0	1	0	0	0	11
1	0	0	1	0	0	12
1	0	0	0	1	0	13
1	0	0	0	0	1	13
1	0	0	0	0	0	18
1	1	0	0	0	0	14
1	0	1	0	0	0	15
1	0	0	1	0	0	17
1	0	0	0	1	0	16
1	0	0	0	0	1	13

TABLE 5.17. Data on reaction times of three subjects (S) for three target shapes (A) on three experimental days (B).

Subject	B_1			B_2			B_3		
	A_1	A_2	A_3	A_1	A_2	A_3	A_1	A_2	A_3
S_1	3.1	2.9	2.4	1.9	2.0	1.7	1.6	1.9	1.5
S_2	5.7	6.8	5.3	4.5	5.7	4.4	4.4	5.3	3.9
S_3	9.7	10.9	8.0	7.4	10.5	6.6	6.9	8.9	6.0

5.3.9   Balanced Two-Way Block Design

Consider a two-way randomized block design, also called a two-way within-subjects design, in which three subjects (S) are asked to detect targets in a visual array (Berry and Mielke, 1998d). The targets are of three shapes (A) and are presented a specified number of times in a random order to each subject. An average response time is recorded for each subject for each target shape. Repeating the experiment on three successive days (B) permits an evaluation of practice effects and the interaction between practice effects and target shape. The design and data are from Myers and Well (1991, p. 260) and are given in Table 5.17.

A design matrix to analyze factor A is given on the left-hand side of Table 5.18 where the first column of 1 values provides for the intercept, the next two columns contain the dummy codes for factor B, and the last column lists the scores summed over the $b = 3$ levels of factor B (e.g., $3.1 + 1.9 + 1.6 = 6.6$) and ordered by the $a = 3$ treatment levels with the first $n_1 = 3$ sums, the next $n_2 = 3$ sums, and the last $n_3 = 3$ sums associated with treatment levels A_1, A_2, and A_3, respectively. There are no dummy codes for factor A on the left-hand side of Table 5.18 because this information is implicit in the ordering of the $a = 3$ treatments. A design matrix to analyze factor B is given on the right-hand side of Table 5.18, where the first column of 1 values provides for the intercept, the next two columns contain the dummy codes for factor A, and the last column lists the scores summed over the $a = 3$ levels of factor A (e.g., $3.1 + 2.9 + 2.4 = 8.4$) and ordered by the $b = 3$ treatment levels with the first $n_1 = 3$ sums, the next $n_2 = 3$ sums, and the last $n_3 = 3$ sums associated with treatment levels B_1, B_2, and B_3, respectively. There are no dummy codes for factor B on the right-hand side of Table 5.18 because this information is implicit in the ordering of the $b = 3$ treatments.

The MRPP regression analysis for factor A yields $\delta_o = 1.8889$, $\mu = 2.9889$, $\sigma^2 = 0.1214$, $\gamma = -0.9981$, $T_o = -3.1567$, and a Pearson type III P-value of 0.8191×10^{-2}, where δ_o and T_o are the observed values of δ and T, respectively. A resampling approximation with $L = 1,000,000$ yields $\delta_o = 1.8889$ and a P-value of 0.3568×10^{-2}. In comparison, a conventional OLS regression analysis yields $F(2,4) = 3.9282$ and a P-value of 0.1138. The corresponding residual analysis for factor B yields $\delta_o = 0.7556$, $\mu = 2.5889$, $\sigma^2 = 0.2007$, $\gamma = -1.0522$, $T_o = -4.0921$, and a Pearson type III P-value of 0.2181×10^{-2}. A resampling approximation with $L = 1,000,000$ yields $\delta_o = 0.7556$ and a P-value of 0.3504×10^{-2}. In comparison, a conventional OLS regression analysis yields $F(2,4) = 22.5488$ and a P-value of 0.6637×10^{-2}.

A design matrix to analyze the $A \times B$ interaction is given in Table 5.19, where the first column of 1 values provides for the intercept, the second and third columns contain the dummy codes for subjects, the fourth and fifth columns contain the dummy codes for factor A, the sixth and seventh columns contain the dummy codes for factor B, and the next eight columns contain the $S \times A$ and $S \times B$ dummy codes. The last column in Table 5.19 lists the scores ordered by the $ab = 9$ levels of the $A \times B$ interaction. There are no dummy codes for the $A \times B$ interaction in Table 5.19 because this information is implicit in the ordering of the $ab = 9$ interactions. The MRPP regression analysis for the $A \times B$ interaction yields $\delta_o = 0.1926$, $\mu = 0.2063$, $\sigma^2 = 0.4252 \times 10^{-3}$, $\gamma = -1.5766$, $T_o = -0.6632$, and a Pearson type III P-value of 0.2033. A resampling approximation with $L = 1,000,000$ yields $\delta_o = 0.1926$ and a P-value of 0.2367. In comparison, a conventional OLS regression analysis yields $F(4,8) = 1.5591$ and a P-value of 0.2744.

TABLE 5.18. Design matrices and data for target shape (A) and experimental days (B) in a two-way block design.

Target shape (A)				Experimental days (B)			
Matrix			Score	Matrix			Score
1	0	0	6.6	1	0	0	8.4
1	1	0	14.6	1	1	0	17.8
1	0	1	24.0	1	0	1	28.6
1	0	0	6.8	1	0	0	5.6
1	1	0	17.8	1	1	0	14.6
1	0	1	30.3	1	0	1	24.5
1	0	0	5.6	1	0	0	5.0
1	1	0	13.6	1	1	0	13.6
1	0	1	20.6	1	0	1	21.8

Reanalysis of Between-Subjects Factors A and B

The previously-discussed classical analyses by Myers and Well (1991) based on summations are often employed. In order to account for the individual responses in the analyses of factor A and factor B, an alternative approach is described. A design matrix to analyze factor A is given in Table 5.20, where the first column of 1 values provides for the intercept, the second and third columns contain the dummy codes for factor B, the fourth and fifth columns contain the dummy codes for subjects, the sixth through ninth columns contain the dummy codes for the $B \times S$ interactions, and the last column lists the response scores ordered by the $a = 3$ treatment levels of factor A with the first $n_1 = 9$ scores, the next $n_2 = 9$ scores, and the last $n_3 = 9$ scores associated with treatment levels A_1, A_2, and A_3, respectively. There are no dummy codes for factor A in Table 5.20 because this information is implicit in the ordering of the $a = 3$ treatments. The MRPP regression analysis for factor A yields $\delta_o = 0.5759$, $\mu = 0.9533$, $\sigma^2 = 0.1341 \times 10^{-2}$, $\gamma = -1.3364$, $T_o = -10.3052$, and a Pearson type III P-value of 0.7139×10^{-6}. A resampling approximation with $L = 1{,}000{,}000$ yields $\delta_o = 0.5759$ and a P-value of 0.0000. In comparison, a conventional OLS regression analysis yields $F(2, 16) = 13.3711$ and a P-value of 0.3856×10^{-3}.

A design matrix to analyze factor B is given in Table 5.21, where the first column of 1 values provides for the intercept, the second and third columns contain the dummy codes for factor A, the fourth and fifth columns contain the dummy codes for subjects, the sixth through ninth columns contain the dummy codes for the $A \times S$ interactions, and the last column lists the response scores ordered by the $b = 3$ treatment levels with the first $n_1 = 9$ scores, the next $n_2 = 9$ scores, and the last $n_3 = 9$ scores associated with treatment levels B_1, B_2, and B_3, respectively. There are no dummy codes for factor B in Table 5.21 because this information is implicit

TABLE 5.19. Design matrix and data for target shape (A) and experimental days (B) interaction.

Matrix															Score
1	0	0	0	0	0	0	0	0	0	0	0	0	0	0	3.1
1	1	0	0	0	0	0	0	0	0	0	0	0	0	0	5.7
1	0	1	0	0	0	0	0	0	0	0	0	0	0	0	9.7
1	0	0	1	0	0	0	0	0	0	0	0	0	0	0	2.9
1	1	0	1	0	0	0	1	0	0	0	0	0	0	0	6.8
1	0	1	1	0	0	0	0	0	1	0	0	0	0	0	10.9
1	0	0	0	1	0	0	0	0	0	0	0	0	0	0	2.4
1	1	0	0	1	0	0	0	1	0	0	0	0	0	0	5.3
1	0	1	0	1	0	0	0	0	0	1	0	0	0	0	8.0
1	0	0	0	0	1	0	0	0	0	0	0	0	0	0	1.9
1	1	0	0	0	1	0	0	0	0	0	1	0	0	0	4.5
1	0	1	0	0	1	0	0	0	0	0	0	0	1	0	7.4
1	0	0	1	0	1	0	0	0	0	0	0	0	0	0	2.0
1	1	0	1	0	1	0	1	0	0	0	1	0	0	0	5.7
1	0	1	1	0	1	0	0	0	1	0	0	0	1	0	10.5
1	0	0	0	1	1	0	0	0	0	0	0	0	0	0	1.7
1	1	0	0	1	1	0	0	1	0	0	1	0	0	0	4.4
1	0	1	0	1	1	0	0	0	0	1	0	0	1	0	6.6
1	0	0	0	0	0	1	0	0	0	0	0	0	0	0	1.6
1	1	0	0	0	0	1	0	0	0	0	0	1	0	0	4.4
1	0	1	0	0	0	1	0	0	0	0	0	0	0	1	6.9
1	0	0	1	0	0	1	0	0	0	0	0	0	0	0	1.9
1	1	0	1	0	0	1	1	0	0	0	0	1	0	0	5.3
1	0	1	1	0	0	1	0	0	1	0	0	0	0	1	8.9
1	0	0	0	1	0	1	0	0	0	0	0	0	0	0	1.5
1	1	0	0	1	0	1	0	1	0	0	0	1	0	0	3.9
1	0	1	0	1	0	1	0	0	0	1	0	0	0	1	6.0

in the ordering of the $b = 3$ treatments. The MRPP regression analysis for factor B yields $\delta_o = 0.3500$, $\mu = 0.8462$, $\sigma^2 = 0.1359 \times 10^{-2}$, $\gamma = -1.5402$, $T_o = -13.4574$, and a Pearson type III P-value of 0.4133×10^{-7}. A resampling approximation with $L = 1,000,000$ yields $\delta_o = 0.3500$ and a P-value of 0.0000. In comparison, a conventional OLS regression analysis yields $F(2, 16) = 43.4252$ and a P-value of 0.3430×10^{-6}.

The three factor A reanalysis P-values (0.7139×10^{-6}, 0.0000, 0.3856×10^{-3}) correspond to the three factor A classical analysis P-values ($0.8191 \times$

TABLE 5.20. Design matrix and data for target shape (A).

Matrix									Score
1	0	0	0	0	0	0	0	0	3.1
1	1	0	0	0	0	0	0	0	1.9
1	0	1	0	0	0	0	0	0	1.6
1	0	0	1	0	0	0	0	0	5.7
1	1	0	1	0	1	0	0	0	4.5
1	0	1	1	0	0	1	0	0	4.4
1	0	0	0	1	0	0	0	0	9.7
1	1	0	0	1	0	0	1	0	7.4
1	0	1	0	1	0	0	0	1	6.9
1	0	0	0	0	0	0	0	0	2.9
1	1	0	0	0	0	0	0	0	2.0
1	0	1	0	0	0	0	0	0	1.9
1	0	0	1	0	0	0	0	0	6.8
1	1	0	1	0	1	0	0	0	5.7
1	0	1	1	0	0	1	0	0	5.3
1	0	0	0	1	0	0	0	0	10.9
1	1	0	0	1	0	0	1	0	10.5
1	0	1	0	1	0	0	0	1	8.9
1	0	0	0	0	0	0	0	0	2.4
1	1	0	0	0	0	0	0	0	1.7
1	0	1	0	0	0	0	0	0	1.5
1	0	0	1	0	0	0	0	0	5.3
1	1	0	1	0	1	0	0	0	4.4
1	0	1	1	0	0	1	0	0	3.9
1	0	0	0	1	0	0	0	0	8.0
1	1	0	0	1	0	0	1	0	6.6
1	0	1	0	1	0	0	0	1	6.0

10^{-2}, 0.3568×10^{-2}, 0.1138), respectively. Also, the three factor B reanalysis P-values (0.4133×10^{-7}, 0.0000, 0.3430×10^{-6}) correspond to the three factor B classical analysis P-values (0.2181×10^{-2}, 0.3504×10^{-2}, 0.6637×10^{-2}), respectively. Thus, the summation approach used in many classical analyses can suppress substantial information contained in the individual responses.

TABLE 5.21. Design matrix and data for experimental days
(B).

Matrix									Score
1	0	0	0	0	0	0	0	0	3.1
1	1	0	0	0	0	0	0	0	2.9
1	0	1	0	0	0	0	0	0	2.4
1	0	0	1	0	0	0	0	0	5.7
1	1	0	1	0	1	0	0	0	6.8
1	0	1	1	0	0	1	0	0	5.3
1	0	0	0	1	0	0	0	0	9.7
1	1	0	0	1	0	0	1	0	10.9
1	0	1	0	1	0	0	0	1	8.0
1	0	0	0	0	0	0	0	0	1.9
1	1	0	0	0	0	0	0	0	2.0
1	0	1	0	0	0	0	0	0	1.7
1	0	0	1	0	0	0	0	0	4.5
1	1	0	1	0	1	0	0	0	5.7
1	0	1	1	0	0	1	0	0	4.4
1	0	0	0	1	0	0	0	0	7.4
1	1	0	0	1	0	0	1	0	10.5
1	0	1	0	1	0	0	0	1	6.6
1	0	0	0	0	0	0	0	0	1.6
1	1	0	0	0	0	0	0	0	1.9
1	0	1	0	0	0	0	0	0	1.5
1	0	0	1	0	0	0	0	0	4.4
1	1	0	1	0	1	0	0	0	5.3
1	0	1	1	0	0	1	0	0	3.9
1	0	0	0	1	0	0	0	0	6.9
1	1	0	0	1	0	0	1	0	8.9
1	0	1	0	1	0	0	0	1	6.0

5.3.10   Unbalanced Two-Way Block Design

Consider the analysis of an unbalanced randomized block experimental design (Mielke and Berry, 1997a).[5] Analyses of unbalanced designs proceed in the same manner as analyses of balanced designs. However, some added detail is provided in this example analysis of an unbalanced two-way block design. The Piers–Harris Children's Self-Concept Scale is an inventory

---

[5] Adapted and reprinted with permission of Psychological Reports from P.W. Mielke, Jr. and K. J. Berry. Permutation covariate analyses of residuals based on Euclidean distance. *Psychological Reports*, 1997, 81, 795–802. Copyright © 1997 by Psychological Reports.

TABLE 5.22. Data set for an unbalanced randomized block design.

Semester	School		
	A	B	C
Fall	49	63	45
		60	50
			42
			46
Spring	48	66	
	58	74	
	51	69	
	55	27	
		71	

composed of 80 descriptive statements in which children select a "yes" or "no" response (Piers, 1984). Suppose that the inventory is given to a sample of fifth-grade children in three neighborhood schools. Within each school (A, B, and C) the inventory is administered in both Fall and Spring semesters. The results are summarized in Table 5.22 with a small sample of $N = 16$ subjects for purposes of illustration. The only restriction in MRPP regression analyses is that the number of residuals in each treatment group must be at least two.

The full regression model is given by

$$y_{ijk} = \Theta + \tau_i + \lambda_j + e_{ijk},$$

where Θ is an unknown population centering constant; τ_i denotes the semester treatment effect with $i = 1, 2$; λ_j denotes the school block effect with $j = 1, 2, 3$; and e_{ijk} is the error associated with the kth subject, $k = 1, ..., n_{ij}$. Two reduced models are considered. Reduced model 1 examines differences among schools; thus, blocking factor school is removed from the full model by setting $\lambda_j = 0$ for $j = 1, 2, 3$. Reduced model 2 examines differences between semesters; thus, treatment factor semester is removed from the full model by setting $\tau_i = 0$ for $i = 1, 2$.

To test reduced model 1, an appropriate design matrix is incorporated into the regression model. A dummy coded design matrix is given on the left-hand side of Table 5.23, together with the scale scores. The first column of 1 values provides for the intercept, and the second column contains the dummy codes for semesters. The data are arranged according to school, with the first $n_1 = 5$ scores, the next $n_2 = 7$ scores, and the last $n_3 = 4$ scores associated with schools A, B, and C, respectively. There are no dummy codes for schools on the left-hand side of Table 5.23 because this information is implicit in the ordering of the scores by school. A LAD regression yields $\tilde{\beta}_1 = \tilde{\Theta} + \tilde{\tau}_1 = 49$ and $\tilde{\beta}_2 = \tilde{\tau}_2 - \tilde{\tau}_1 = 9$. The use of

TABLE 5.23. Design matrices, scores, and residuals for the unbalanced randomized block design.

School analysis				Semester analysis				
Matrix		Score	Residual	Matrix			Score	Residual
1	0	49	0	1	0	0	49	−2
1	1	48	−10	1	1	0	63	−3
1	1	58	0	1	1	0	60	−6
1	1	51	−7	1	0	1	45	−1
1	1	55	−3	1	0	1	50	4
				1	0	1	42	−4
1	0	63	14	1	0	1	46	0
1	0	60	11					
1	1	66	8	1	0	0	48	−3
1	1	74	16	1	0	0	58	7
1	1	69	11	1	0	0	51	0
1	1	27	−31	1	0	0	55	4
1	1	71	13	1	1	0	66	0
				1	1	0	74	8
1	0	45	−4	1	1	0	69	3
1	0	50	1	1	1	0	27	−39
1	0	42	−7	1	1	0	71	5
1	0	46	−3					

dummy coding places emphasis on treatment differences. Thus, $\tilde{\beta}_1 = 49$ is the sample median of the treatment assigned a value of zero — in this case, Fall semester. The difference between treatments is given by $\tilde{\beta}_2 = 9$. Thus, the median of Spring semester is $\tilde{\beta}_1 + \tilde{\beta}_2 = 49 + 9 = 58$. These values can be verified from the data in Table 5.22.

The residuals obtained from the LAD regression are listed on the left-hand side of Table 5.23. The residuals contain information on the block effect controlled for treatment differences, i.e., schools controlled for semesters. The MRPP regression analysis on the residuals yields $\delta_o = 9.1875$, $\mu = 13.0917$, $\sigma^2 = 0.9870$, $\gamma = -1.3618$, $T_o = -3.9297$, and a Pearson type III P-value of 0.4218×10^{-2}, where δ_o and T_o are the observed values of δ and T, respectively. A resampling approximation with $L = 1{,}000{,}000$ yields a P-value of 0.4287×10^{-2}. The exact P-value is $6{,}232/1{,}441{,}440 = 0.4323 \times 10^{-2}$. In contrast, a conventional OLS regression analysis yields $F(2,10) = 1.7897$ and a P-value of 0.2088. The marked difference in the P-values obtained from the MRPP regression analyses based on absolute residuals (0.4218×10^{-2} and 0.4287×10^{-2}) and the conventional OLS regression analysis based on squared residuals (0.2088) is due to the extreme value 27 in the Spring semester in school B, which has a residual of -31.

A dummy coded design matrix to test reduced model 2 with semesters removed is given on the right-hand side of Table 5.23, together with the scale scores. The first column of 1 values provides for the intercept, and the second and third columns contain the dummy codes for schools. The data are arranged according to semester, with the first $n_1 = 7$ scores and the next $n_2 = 9$ scores associated with the Fall and Spring semesters, respectively. There are no dummy codes for semester on the right-hand side of Table 5.23 because this information is implicit in the ordering of the scores by semester (Fall and Spring). The LAD regression yields three estimated regression parameters. The sample median of school A is given by $\tilde{\beta}_1 = \Theta + \tilde{\lambda}_1 = 51$. The block difference between schools A and B is given by $\tilde{\beta}_2 = \tilde{\lambda}_2 - \tilde{\lambda}_1 = 15$, yielding a sample median for school B of $\tilde{\beta}_1 + \tilde{\beta}_2 = 51 + 15 = 66$. The block difference between schools A and C is given by $\tilde{\beta}_3 = \tilde{\lambda}_3 - \tilde{\lambda}_1 = -5$, yielding a sample median for school C of $\tilde{\beta}_1 + \tilde{\beta}_3 = 51 - 5 = 46$. Nonunique solutions are not unusual in LAD regression. The sample median for school C is, in fact, any value from 45 to 46. The residuals obtained from the LAD regression are listed in Table 5.23. The residuals contain information on the treatment effect, which was controlled for blocks, i.e., semesters controlled for schools. The MRPP regression analysis yields $\delta_0 = 8.9167$, $\mu = 9.2750$, $\sigma^2 = 0.8836 \times 10^{-1}$, $\gamma = -2.0713$, $T_0 = -1.2055$, and a Pearson type III P-value of 0.1094. A resampling approximation with $L = 1,000,000$ yields a P-value of 0.1026. The exact P-value is $1,173/11,440 = 0.1025$. The corresponding P-value for a conventional OLS regression analysis yields $F(1, 12) = 4.1938$ and a P-value of 0.8629. The considerable difference in the P-values obtained from the MRPP regression analyses based on absolute residuals (0.1094 and 0.1026) and the conventional OLS regression analysis based on squared residuals (0.8629) is again due to the extreme value 27 in the Spring semester in school B with a residual of -39.

5.3.11   Latin Square Design

Consider a Latin square experiment involving repeated measurements in which four subjects (S) are tested four times on treatment A (Berry and Mielke, 1998d). The design and data are from Ferguson (1981, p. 349) and are given in Table 5.24, where B refers to the ordinal position in which the levels of A are administered. Thus, the first subject receives the four treatments in the order A_2, A_4, A_1, A_3, etc.

A design matrix to analyze A is given in Table 5.25, where the first column of 1 values provides for the intercept, the second through fourth columns contain the dummy codes for S, the fifth through seventh columns contain the dummy codes for B, and the last column lists the scores ordered by the $a = 4$ levels of A, with the first $n_1 = 4$ scores, the next $n_2 = 4$ scores, the next $n_3 = 4$ scores, and the last $n_4 = 4$ scores associated with treatment levels A_1, A_2, A_3, and A_4, respectively. There are no dummy codes for A in Table 5.25 because this information is contained in the

TABLE 5.24. Design and data for a Latin square design with four subjects (S), four treatments (A), and four orders (B).

	Design					Observations			
Subject	B_1	B_2	B_3	B_4	Subject	B_1	B_2	B_3	B_4
S_1	A_2	A_4	A_1	A_3	S_1	10	21	5	14
S_2	A_3	A_1	A_2	A_4	S_2	12	7	11	19
S_3	A_1	A_3	A_4	A_2	S_3	6	16	24	12
S_4	A_4	A_2	A_3	A_1	S_4	22	8	17	9

TABLE 5.25. Design matrix and data for treatment (A) in a Latin square design.

Matrix							Score
1	0	0	0	0	1	0	5
1	1	0	0	1	0	0	7
1	0	1	0	0	0	0	6
1	0	0	1	0	0	1	9
1	0	0	0	0	0	0	10
1	1	0	0	0	1	0	11
1	0	1	0	0	0	1	12
1	0	0	1	1	0	0	8
1	0	0	0	0	0	1	14
1	1	0	0	0	0	0	12
1	0	1	0	1	0	0	16
1	0	0	1	0	1	0	17
1	0	0	0	1	0	0	21
1	1	0	0	0	0	1	19
1	0	1	0	0	1	0	24
1	0	0	1	0	0	0	22

ordering of the $a = 4$ treatment levels in the last column. The MRPP regression analysis of the LAD residuals for A yields $\delta_o = 6.2083$, $\mu = 8.2750$, $\sigma^2 = 0.5603$, $\gamma = -1.0750$, $T_o = -2.7609$, and a Pearson type III P-value of 0.1545×10^{-1}, where δ_o and T_o are the observed values of δ and T, respectively. A resampling approximation with $L = 1{,}000{,}000$ yields $\delta_o = 6.2083$ and a P-value of 0.2073×10^{-1}. In contrast, a conventional OLS regression analysis yields $F(3, 6) = 40.7277$ and a P-value of 0.2204×10^{-3}.

A design matrix to analyze B is given in Table 5.26, where the first column of 1 values provides for the intercept, the second through fourth columns contain the dummy codes for S, the fifth through seventh columns contain the dummy codes for A, and the last column lists the scores ordered by the $b = 4$ treatment levels of B, with the first $n_1 = 4$ scores, the next

TABLE 5.26. Design matrix and data for order (B) in a Latin square design.

Matrix							Score
1	0	0	0	1	0	0	10
1	1	0	0	0	1	0	12
1	0	1	0	0	0	0	6
1	0	0	1	0	0	1	22
1	0	0	0	0	0	1	21
1	1	0	0	0	0	0	7
1	0	1	0	0	1	0	16
1	0	0	1	1	0	0	8
1	0	0	0	0	0	0	5
1	1	0	0	1	0	0	11
1	0	1	0	0	0	1	24
1	0	0	1	0	1	0	17
1	0	0	0	0	1	0	14
1	1	0	0	0	0	1	19
1	0	1	0	1	0	0	12
1	0	0	1	0	0	0	9

$n_2 = 4$ scores, the next $n_3 = 4$ scores, and the last $n_4 = 4$ scores associated with treatment levels B_1, B_2, B_3, and B_4, respectively. There are no dummy codes for B in Table 5.26 because this information is implicit in the ordering of the $b = 4$ treatments in the last column. The MRPP regression analysis of the LAD residuals for B yields $\delta_o = 1.7917$, $\mu = 1.8583$, $\sigma^2 = 0.3481 \times 10^{-1}$, $\gamma = -1.0149$, $T_o = -0.3573$, and a Pearson type III P-value of 0.3066. A resampling approximation with $L = 1,000,000$ yields $\delta_o = 1.7917$ and a P-value of 0.4961. In contrast, a conventional OLS regression analysis yields $F(3,6) = 0.5602$ and a P-value of 0.6606.

5.3.12   Split-Plot Design

Imagine an experiment that considers two treatment factors, A and B, with a and b levels, respectively, so that there are ab treatment combinations. If each testing session requires h hours of a subject's time and every subject is to be tested under all treatment combinations, each subject will require ab testing sessions and abh hours of testing time. If this is unreasonable, then with S subjects available, assign $n = S/a$ subjects to each level of factor A and test each subject under all levels of factor B. This experimental design is called a split-plot design. More specifically, it is a repeated measures split-plot design in which subjects are randomly assigned to the a levels of factor A (i.e., plots), and each subject is then tested under all b levels of

TABLE 5.27. Scores on a 60-point vocabulary test for $S = 12$ subjects on three types of lectures (A) over three replications (B).

Factor A	Subject	Factor B		
		B_1	B_2	B_3
A_1	S_1	53	51	35
	S_2	49	34	18
	S_3	47	44	32
	S_4	42	48	27
A_2	S_5	47	42	16
	S_6	42	33	10
	S_7	39	13	11
	S_8	37	16	6
A_3	S_9	45	35	29
	S_{10}	41	33	21
	S_{11}	38	46	30
	S_{12}	36	40	20

factor B (i.e., subplots). The design is also called a mixed factorial design with one between-subjects factor (A) and one within-subjects factor (B), or an $A \times (B \times S)$ design (Keppel, 1982).

Consider an experimental design in which factor A is type of lecture (physical science, social science, and history) and factor B is three 60-point vocabulary tests administered at different times following the lecture. Four of $S = 12$ subjects are randomly assigned to each of the three lectures, and each subject is tested immediately after the lecture, two weeks later, and two weeks following the second test (Berry and Mielke, 1999b).[6] The design and data are from Keppel and Zedeck (1989) and are given in Table 5.27.

Analysis of Factor B

A design matrix of effect codes for the MRPP regression analysis of factor B is given in Table 5.28, where the first column of 1 values provides for the intercept, the next 11 columns contain effect codes for the subjects with S nested within factor A, and the next four columns contain effect codes for the $A \times B$ interaction. The last column lists the 36 scores ordered by the $b = 3$ treatment levels of factor B, with the first $n_1 = 12$ scores, the next $n_2 = 12$ scores, and the last $n_3 = 12$ scores associated with treatment levels B_1, B_2, and B_3, respectively. The MRPP regression

---

[6]Adapted and reprinted with permission of Psychological Reports from K.J. Berry and P.W. Mielke, Jr. Least absolute regression residuals: analyses of split-plot designs. *Psychological Reports*, 1999, 85, 445–453. Copyright © 1999 by Psychological Reports.

analysis examines the regression residuals for differences in treatment levels of factor B; consequently, there are no effect codes for factor B in the reduced regression model because this information is implicit in the ordering of the $b = 3$ treatments in the last column of Table 5.28. The MRPP regression analysis for factor B yields $\delta_o = 7.8283$, $\mu = 12.5460$, $\sigma^2 = 0.1675$, $\gamma = -1.3580$, $T_o = -11.5275$, and a Pearson type III P-value of 0.1495×10^{-6}, where δ_o and T_o are the observed values of δ and T, respectively. A resampling approximation with $L = 1{,}000{,}000$ yields $\delta_o = 7.8283$ and a P-value of 0.0000. In contrast, a conventional OLS regression analysis yields $F(2, 18) = 52.1842$ and a P-value of 0.3224×10^{-7}. It should be noted that the MRPP regression analysis is not unique for these data; see Section 5.2.

Analysis of the $A \times B$ Interaction

A design matrix of effect codes for the MRPP regression analysis of the $A \times B$ interaction is given in Table 5.29, where the first column of 1 values provides for the intercept, the next 11 columns contain effect codes for the subjects with S nested within factor A, and the next two columns contain the effect codes for factor B. The last column lists the $N = 36$ scores ordered by the $ab = 9$ levels of the $A \times B$ interaction. The coding for the $A \times B$ interaction is deleted in the reduced regression model because this information is implicit in the ordering of the scores in the last column of Table 5.29. The MRPP regression analysis for the $A \times B$ interaction yields $\delta_o = 5.2593$, $\mu = 5.6825$, $\sigma^2 = 0.1425$, $\gamma = -0.6865$, $T_o = -1.1212$, and a Pearson type III P-value of 0.1325. A resampling approximation with $L = 1{,}000{,}000$ yields $\delta_o = 5.2593$ and a P-value of 0.1403. In comparison, a conventional OLS regression analysis yields $F(4, 18) = 2.8114$ and a P-value of 0.5653×10^{-1}. It should be noted that the MRPP regression analysis is not unique for these data; see Section 5.2.

Analysis of Factor A

A design matrix of effect codes for the MRPP regression analysis of factor A is given in Table 5.30, where the first column of 1 values provides for the intercept and the second column lists the totals of scores summed over the b levels of factor B, e.g., $53 + 51 + 35 = 139$. These sums are ordered by the $a = 3$ treatment levels of factor A with the first four sums, the next four sums, and the last four sums associated with treatment levels A_1, A_2, and A_3, respectively. Because the purpose of the analysis is to examine differences among the levels of the between-subjects variable (i.e., plots), the design matrix for the reduced regression model is composed solely of a code for the intercept. The MRPP regression analysis for factor A yields $\delta_o = 19.4444$, $\mu = 27.0000$, $\sigma^2 = 7.4691$, $\gamma = -1.0598$, $T_o = -2.7646$, and a Pearson type III P-value of 0.1521×10^{-1}. A resampling approximation with $L = 1{,}000{,}000$ yields $\delta_o = 19.4444$ and a P-value of 0.1927×10^{-1}. In

TABLE 5.28. Design matrix and data for the main effects of factor B.

Matrix																Score
1	1	0	0	0	0	0	0	0	0	0	0	1	0	0	0	53
1	0	1	0	0	0	0	0	0	0	0	0	1	0	0	0	49
1	0	0	1	0	0	0	0	0	0	0	0	1	0	0	0	47
1	0	0	0	1	0	0	0	0	0	0	0	1	0	0	0	42
1	0	0	0	0	1	0	0	0	0	0	0	0	1	0	0	47
1	0	0	0	0	0	1	0	0	0	0	0	0	1	0	0	42
1	0	0	0	0	0	0	1	0	0	0	0	0	1	0	0	39
1	0	0	0	0	0	0	0	1	0	0	0	0	1	0	0	37
1	0	0	0	0	0	0	0	0	1	0	0	-1	-1	0	0	45
1	0	0	0	0	0	0	0	0	0	1	0	-1	-1	0	0	41
1	0	0	0	0	0	0	0	0	0	0	1	-1	-1	0	0	38
1	-1	-1	-1	-1	-1	-1	-1	-1	-1	-1	-1	-1	-1	0	0	36
1	1	0	0	0	0	0	0	0	0	0	0	0	0	1	0	51
1	0	1	0	0	0	0	0	0	0	0	0	0	0	1	0	34
1	0	0	1	0	0	0	0	0	0	0	0	0	0	1	0	44
1	0	0	0	1	0	0	0	0	0	0	0	0	0	1	0	48
1	0	0	0	0	1	0	0	0	0	0	0	0	0	0	1	42
1	0	0	0	0	0	1	0	0	0	0	0	0	0	0	1	33
1	0	0	0	0	0	0	1	0	0	0	0	0	0	0	1	13
1	0	0	0	0	0	0	0	1	0	0	0	0	0	0	1	16
1	0	0	0	0	0	0	0	0	1	0	0	0	0	-1	-1	35
1	0	0	0	0	0	0	0	0	0	1	0	0	0	-1	-1	33
1	0	0	0	0	0	0	0	0	0	0	1	0	0	-1	-1	46
1	-1	-1	-1	-1	-1	-1	-1	-1	-1	-1	-1	0	0	-1	-1	40
1	1	0	0	0	0	0	0	0	0	0	0	-1	0	-1	0	35
1	0	1	0	0	0	0	0	0	0	0	0	-1	0	-1	0	18
1	0	0	1	0	0	0	0	0	0	0	0	-1	0	-1	0	32
1	0	0	0	1	0	0	0	0	0	0	0	-1	0	-1	0	27
1	0	0	0	0	1	0	0	0	0	0	0	0	-1	0	-1	16
1	0	0	0	0	0	1	0	0	0	0	0	0	-1	0	-1	10
1	0	0	0	0	0	0	1	0	0	0	0	0	-1	0	-1	11
1	0	0	0	0	0	0	0	1	0	0	0	0	-1	0	-1	6
1	0	0	0	0	0	0	0	0	1	0	0	1	1	1	1	29
1	0	0	0	0	0	0	0	0	0	1	0	1	1	1	1	21
1	0	0	0	0	0	0	0	0	0	0	1	1	1	1	1	30
1	-1	-1	-1	-1	-1	-1	-1	-1	-1	-1	-1	1	1	1	1	20

TABLE 5.29. Design matrix and data for the interaction effects of factors A and B.

Matrix														Score
1	1	0	0	0	0	0	0	0	0	0	0	1	0	53
1	0	1	0	0	0	0	0	0	0	0	0	1	0	49
1	0	0	1	0	0	0	0	0	0	0	0	1	0	47
1	0	0	0	1	0	0	0	0	0	0	0	1	0	42
1	0	0	0	0	1	0	0	0	0	0	0	1	0	47
1	0	0	0	0	0	1	0	0	0	0	0	1	0	42
1	0	0	0	0	0	0	1	0	0	0	0	1	0	39
1	0	0	0	0	0	0	0	1	0	0	0	1	0	37
1	0	0	0	0	0	0	0	0	1	0	0	1	0	45
1	0	0	0	0	0	0	0	0	0	1	0	1	0	41
1	0	0	0	0	0	0	0	0	0	0	1	1	0	38
1	−1	−1	−1	−1	−1	−1	−1	−1	−1	−1	−1	1	0	36
1	1	0	0	0	0	0	0	0	0	0	0	0	1	51
1	0	1	0	0	0	0	0	0	0	0	0	0	1	34
1	0	0	1	0	0	0	0	0	0	0	0	0	1	44
1	0	0	0	1	0	0	0	0	0	0	0	0	1	48
1	0	0	0	0	1	0	0	0	0	0	0	0	1	42
1	0	0	0	0	0	1	0	0	0	0	0	0	1	33
1	0	0	0	0	0	0	1	0	0	0	0	0	1	13
1	0	0	0	0	0	0	0	1	0	0	0	0	1	16
1	0	0	0	0	0	0	0	0	1	0	0	0	1	35
1	0	0	0	0	0	0	0	0	0	1	0	0	1	33
1	0	0	0	0	0	0	0	0	0	0	1	0	1	46
1	−1	−1	−1	−1	−1	−1	−1	−1	−1	−1	−1	0	1	40
1	1	0	0	0	0	0	0	0	0	0	0	−1	−1	35
1	0	1	0	0	0	0	0	0	0	0	0	−1	−1	18
1	0	0	1	0	0	0	0	0	0	0	0	−1	−1	32
1	0	0	0	1	0	0	0	0	0	0	0	−1	−1	27
1	0	0	0	0	1	0	0	0	0	0	0	−1	−1	16
1	0	0	0	0	0	1	0	0	0	0	0	−1	−1	10
1	0	0	0	0	0	0	1	0	0	0	0	−1	−1	11
1	0	0	0	0	0	0	0	1	0	0	0	−1	−1	6
1	0	0	0	0	0	0	0	0	1	0	0	−1	−1	29
1	0	0	0	0	0	0	0	0	0	1	0	−1	−1	21
1	0	0	0	0	0	0	0	0	0	0	1	−1	−1	30
1	−1	−1	−1	−1	−1	−1	−1	−1	−1	−1	−1	−1	−1	20

TABLE 5.30. Design matrix and data for the main effects of factor A.

Matrix	Sum over B
1	139
1	101
1	123
1	117
1	105
1	85
1	63
1	59
1	109
1	95
1	114
1	96

comparison, a conventional OLS regression analysis yields $F(2, 9) = 6.7927$ and a P-value of 0.1592×10^{-1}.

Reanalysis of the Between-Subjects Factor

Consider a split-plot experiment with factor A as the between-subjects or plot variable and factor B as the within-subjects or subplot variable, such as described in the previous section (Berry and Mielke, 1999b). From the point of view of factor B alone, each subject is a block and the experiment is a randomized block design. On the other hand, because the S subjects are randomly assigned to the a levels of factor A, from the point of view of factor A, the experiment is a completely randomized design. In a split-plot experiment, comparisons among the levels of factor B at the same level of factor A are based on the same subject and therefore involve differences associated with only the levels of factor B. In contrast, comparisons among the levels of factor A involve differences associated with the levels of factor A commingled with differences among groups of subjects. The main effects of factor A are confounded with differences among groups of subjects, whereas the main effects of factor B are free of such confounding. This is illustrated by the comparison of the coding scheme for factor B in Table 5.28, in which the analysis is based on $N = 36$ scores, with the coding scheme for factor A in Table 5.30, in which the analysis is based on $S = 12$ sums of scores, totaled for each subject over the b levels of factor B.

A conventional split-plot analysis of variance is unable to decompose the confounding of factor A and subjects because the partitioning of the variance and the degrees-of-freedom into independent additive components would be violated. On the other hand, the MRPP regression analysis is a distribution-free test and is therefore able to analyze the main effects of factor A unencumbered by the restrictions imposed by variance and degrees-of-freedom considerations. An alternative design matrix of effect codes for the MRPP regression analysis of factor A is given in Table 5.31, where the first column of 1 values provides for the intercept, the next two columns contain effect codes for factor B, and the last column lists the $N = 36$ scores ordered by the $a = 3$ levels of factor A with the first $n_1 = 12$ scores, the next $n_2 = 12$ scores, and the last $n_3 = 12$ scores associated with treatment levels A_1, A_2, and A_3, respectively. The MRPP regression analysis for factor A yields $\delta_o = 8.1010$, $\mu = 10.1238$, $\sigma^2 = 0.1063$, $\gamma = -1.4949$, $T_o = -6.2056$, and a Pearson type III P-value of 0.2980×10^{-3}. A resampling approximation with $L = 1,000,000$ yields $\delta_o = 8.1010$ and a P-value of 0.2480×10^{-3}. An alternative OLS regression analysis in this context yields $F(2, 31) = 11.3924$ and a P-value of 0.1954×10^{-3}.

The MRPP regression analysis on the LAD residuals possesses several advantages over the conventional OLS regression analysis for split-plot designs. First, MRPP does not assume that the g treatment groups were drawn from a population with a specific distribution, such as a normal distribution. However, it is presumed that the unknown population distribution is common to each treatment group. If a location shift is of interest, then it is desirable that the shape of the unknown population distribution remain the same except for the shift (Mielke and Berry, 1994). This is analogous to the classical requirement of homogeneity of variance when normality is assumed. In fact, the only required assumption of MRPP is exchangeability. This is to say that, under the null hypothesis, all of the M possible allocations of the N residuals to the g treatment groups are equally likely. Second, MRPP analyzes the main effects of the between-subjects factor without utilizing sums over levels of the within-subjects factor (as would be done in a conventional OLS regression analysis). Third, since the use of sums is unnecessary, MRPP analyzes balanced and unbalanced designs equally well without any adjustments. If zero or more subjects are associated with the ith level of the between-subjects factor and the jth level of the within-subjects factor (i.e., in a potentially unbalanced design), MRPP is fully capable of analyzing the resulting split-plot experiment provided $n_i \geq 2$ for $i = 1, ..., g$. Regression analyses based on individual responses rather than sums of responses provide the basis to investigate unbalanced designs. Finally, MRPP is easily extended to more complex experimental designs, balanced or unbalanced, such as split-split-plot designs, where unbalanced conditions occur routinely.

TABLE 5.31. Design matrix and data for an alternative analysis of the main effects of factor A.

Matrix			Score
1	1	0	53
1	1	0	49
1	1	0	47
1	1	0	42
1	0	1	51
1	0	1	34
1	0	1	44
1	0	1	48
1	−1	−1	35
1	−1	−1	18
1	−1	−1	32
1	−1	−1	27
1	1	0	47
1	1	0	42
1	1	0	39
1	1	0	37
1	0	1	42
1	0	1	33
1	0	1	13
1	0	1	16
1	−1	−1	16
1	−1	−1	10
1	−1	−1	11
1	−1	−1	6
1	1	0	45
1	1	0	41
1	1	0	38
1	1	0	36
1	0	1	35
1	0	1	33
1	0	1	46
1	0	1	40
1	−1	−1	29
1	−1	−1	21
1	−1	−1	30
1	−1	−1	20

5.4   MRPP, Cade–Richards, and OLS Regression Analyses

Cade and Richards (1996) provide alternative permutation tests for regression analyses. To compare the MRPP regression analysis, the Cade–Richards regression analysis, and the classical OLS regression analysis, the Cade–Richards regression analysis is described. Consider the null hypothesis (H_0) that the regression model is

$$y_I = \mathbf{x}'_{0I}\,\beta_0 + e_{0I}$$

versus the alternative hypothesis (H_1) that the regression model is

$$y_I = \mathbf{x}'_{1I}\,\beta_1 + e_{1I},$$

where y_I, $\mathbf{x}_{0I}$, $\mathbf{x}_{1I}$, e_{0I}, and e_{1I} denote the response values, null predictor vector, alternative predictor vector, null error values, and alternative error values, respectively, for the Ith of N cases, and the vector of parameters β_0 is a strict subset of the vector of parameters β_1. If

$$\tilde{e}_{0I} = y_I - \mathbf{x}'_{0I}\,\tilde{\beta}_{0v}$$

and

$$\tilde{e}_{1I} = y_I - \mathbf{x}'_{1I}\,\tilde{\beta}_{1v}$$

denote the Ith of N residual pairs where

$$S_{ov} = \sum_{I=1}^{N} |\tilde{e}_{0I}|^{v}$$

and

$$T_{ov} = \sum_{I=1}^{N} |\tilde{e}_{1I}|^{v}$$

are minimized, then $\tilde{\beta}_{0v}$ and $\tilde{\beta}_{1v}$ are the associated parameter estimates, and $v = 1$ and $v = 2$ correspond to the LAD and OLS regression models, respectively. The observed Cade–Richards statistic is given by

$$R_{ov} = \frac{S_{ov}}{T_{ov}} - 1.$$

Let $z_I = \tilde{e}_{0I}$ $(I = 1, ..., N)$ denote the observed residuals under H_0, and let $z_{1(j)}, ..., z_{N(j)}$ denote the jth of L independent random orderings from the $N!$ possible orderings of $z_1, ..., z_N$. Also, let

$$R_{jv} = \frac{S_{jv}}{T_{jv}} - 1$$

be the jth of L Cade–Richards statistics obtained by replacing $y_1, ..., y_N$ with $z_{1(j)}, ..., z_{N(j)}$. Then, the resampling P-value approximation (P_v^*) of the Cade–Richards regression analysis is given by

$$P_v^* = \frac{1}{L} \sum_{j=1}^{L} \Psi\left(R_{jv}\right),$$

where

$$\Psi\left(R_{jv}\right) = \begin{cases} 1 & \text{if } R_{jv} \geq R_{ov}, \\ 0 & \text{if } R_{jv} < R_{ov}. \end{cases}$$

In addition, let P_m and P_c denote the P-values of the MRPP and classical OLS regression analyses, respectively. Two versions of statistic R_{ov} were introduced in an OLS context $(v = 2)$ by Freedman and Lane (1983) that involved $z_I = y_I$ and $z_I = \tilde{e}_{0I}$ for $I = 1, ..., N$. The choice of $z_I = \tilde{e}_{0I}$ is preferred to $z_I = y_I$ when the reduced model (H_0) nuisance parameters are non-zero (Anderson and Legendre, 1999; Kennedy and Cade, 1996).

Because the MRPP regression analysis is based on equally-likely allocations of the N observed residuals $(\tilde{e}_{01}, ..., \tilde{e}_{0N})$ to g distinct groups under H_0 with $v = 1$, the N observed response and null predictor vector pairs (y_I and x_{0I} for $I = 1, ..., N$) are coupled in this analysis since

$$\tilde{e}_{0I} = y_I - \mathbf{x}_{0I}' \tilde{\beta}_{01}$$

for $I = 1, ..., N$. In contrast, coupling of the N response and null predictor vector pairs is certain only for R_{o1}, the observed value of the Cade–Richards statistic.

Whereas the exact MRPP regression analysis under H_0 depends on the reference set of $N!$ equally-likely orderings of the observed N exchangeable coupled residuals, the exact Cade–Richards regression analysis under H_0 depends on the reference set of $N!$ equally-likely Cade–Richards test statistics that result when all $N!$ orderings of the observed N exchangeable coupled residuals are treated as the dependent variables. Except for the observed ordering of the N coupled residuals, the remaining $N! - 1$ Cade–Richards test statistics depend on decoupled residuals. Since the criteria of the MRPP and Cade–Richards regression analyses differ, their exact P-values will most likely be different. Since $N!$ is generally very large, the approximate Cade–Richards regression analysis is consequently based on a with-replacement random sample of L test statistics from the reference set of all $N!$ test satistics. Implicitly, coupling and decoupling are considered in recent work on exchangeability (Cade and Richards, 2006; Commenges, 2003; Good, 2002; Huh and Jhun, 2001). The residuals of a classical OLS regression are decoupled since the errors are assumed to be independent normal random variables. Thus, P-values obtained from the Cade–Richards regression analysis with $v = 2$ and the OLS regression analysis are expected to be similar (Mielke and Berry, 2002b).

TABLE 5.32. Comparative P-values for the MRPP (P_m), Cade–Richards with $v = 1$ (P_1^*) and $v = 2$ (P_2^*), and the classical (P_c) regression analyses.

Variable/Control	P_m	P_1^*	P_2^*	P_c
Schools/Semesters	0.0043	0.0019	0.2095	0.2088
Semester/Schools	0.1025	0.0513	0.8415	0.8629

An example based on the unbalanced two-way randomized block data in Table 5.22 demonstrates the differences between the MRPP, the Cade–Richards, and classical OLS regression analyses. The P-values obtained from the MRPP regression analysis (P_m), the Cade–Richards regression analysis for $v = 1$ and $v = 2$ $(P_1^*$ and $P_2^*)$, and the OLS regression analysis (P_c) are given in Table 5.32 with (1) schools controlled for semesters and (2) semesters controlled for schools. Each of the four Cade–Richards P-values are computed with $L = 100{,}000$ random reorderings of $z_1, ..., z_N$. The differences between the P_m and P_1^* values are due to the coupling and decoupling differences corresponding to exchangeable and independent random variables, respectively. The exchangeable and independent variable differences are supported by the fact that the P_2^* and P_c values are so similar. Due to the influence of a single value (see Section 2.8), the substantial difference between P_1^* and P_2^* of the Cade–Richards regression analyses with $v = 1$ and $v = 2$, respectively, is consistent with the analogous difference between MRPP P-values involving $v = 1$ and $v = 2$. Recent work pertaining to this example is given by Cade and Richards (2006).

As previously noted in Section 5.3, the MRPP regression analysis conveniently includes cases involving multivariate multiple regression. While conceptually feasible, the extension of the Cade–Richards regression analysis based on a with-replacement random sample of L test statistics to a multivariate multiple regression context is far more computationally intensive than the corresponding extension of MRPP regression analysis.

A further comment is that an MRPP regression analysis is limited to alternatives involving treatment group differences, whereas the Cade–Richards and OLS regression analyses can accommodate the previous alternatives and many more. For example, the MRPP regression analysis is unable to test H_0: $\mu_0(x) = \beta x$ versus H_1: $\mu_1(x) = \alpha + \beta x$, whereas tests of this type are routine for the Cade–Richards and OLS regression analyses. Kennedy and Cade (1996) and Anderson and Legendre (1999) compare randomization tests for use with multiple least squares regression.

5.4.1 Extension of MRPP Regression Analysis

Consider g multivariate populations with $m + 1$ variates $(y, x_1, ..., x_m)$ and cdfs $F_1, ..., F_g$. Assume that

$$F_i(y, x_1, ..., x_m) = F(y - \beta_{0i} - \beta_{1i}x_1 - \cdots - \beta_{mi}x_m)G(x_1, ..., x_m)$$

for $i = 1, ..., g$, i.e., the conditional *cdf* of y given $x_1, ..., x_m$ for the ith group is $F(y - \beta_{0i} - \cdots - \beta_{mi}x_m)$ and the marginal joint *cdf* of $(x_1, ..., x_m)$ is G for each group. Without loss of generality, assume that the median of F is 0. Consider testing H_0: $(\beta_{0i}, ..., \beta_{mi}) = (\beta_0, ..., \beta_m)$ for $i = 1, ..., g$ versus H_1: not all $(\beta_{0i}, ..., \beta_{mi})$ are equal. Under H_0, the F_i values are all equal, and the entire sample is identically and independently distributed. Hence, given the set of vectors $(y_j, x_{j1}, ..., x_{jm})$ for $j = 1, ..., n_1 + \cdots + n_g = N$, all possible ways of assigning the vectors to the g groups, respecting the sample sizes $n_1, ..., n_g$, are equally likely. Thus, the set of N coupled vectors are exchangeable under H_0. Consequently, the conditional null distribution of any function of the data can be computed exactly. In particular, the conditional null distribution of the MRPP δ statistic, based on the LAD residuals, can be computed. The proposed α-level decision rule is to reject H_0 if the observed value of δ is in the lower α-percentile of the permutation distribution of δ. Other methods, including least squares, could be used to fit the common regression model in place of LAD. For instance, any of the rank regression methods and other nonparametric methods could be used. The test is still exact under the given set of assumptions.

In normal theory linear models, an exact test (under normality) is available for testing H_0: $(\beta_{0i}, ..., \beta_{mi}) = (\beta_0, ..., \beta_m)$ for $i = 1, ..., g$ versus H_1: not all $(\beta_{0i}, ..., \beta_{mi})$ are equal under the following more general setting. Assume

$$F_i(y, x_1, ..., x_m) = F(y - \beta_{0i} - \beta_{1i}x_1 - \cdots - \beta_{mi}x_m)G_i(x_1, ..., x_m)$$

for $i = 1, ..., g$. Thus, the marginal joint *cdf*s for the g groups are allowed to be different. The hypothesis of interest is the same H_0 as before. While an exact test is available (F-test) for this hypothesis under traditional normal theory, an exact permutation test is not possible since, under H_0, the data vectors are no longer identically and independently distributed and, consequently, the residuals are not exchangeable.

To overcome this obstacle, one approach is to use a more restrictive null hypothesis, namely, H_0: $(\beta_{0i}, ..., \beta_{mi}) = (\beta_0, ..., \beta_m)$ and $G_i = G$ for $i = 1, ..., g$ versus H_1: the null hypothesis is false. Now, under H_0, the residuals are exchangeable and the MRPP regression test is exact. However, when H_0 is rejected, the reason for rejection may be because (1) $(\beta_{0i}, ..., \beta_{mi})$ are not equal for $i = 1, ..., g$, (2) G_i are not equal for $i = 1, ..., g$, or (3) both $(\beta_{0i}, ..., \beta_{mi})$ and G_i are not equal for $i = 1, ..., g$. It is therefore important to ensure that the test statistic chosen is sensitive to (1) and not to (2). On intuitive grounds, the proposed MRPP regression test statistic appears to meet this requirement, but no such theoretical results are available.

Another issue to be considered is: how sensitive is the type I error rate of the MRPP regression test to differences in the G_is under the null hypothesis H_0: $(\beta_{0i}, ..., \beta_{mi})$ are equal for $i = 1, ..., g$? If the actual type I error rates are close to the nominal rate, even when exact equality of the G_is does not hold, then the MRPP regression test can be used in practice to test this more general hypothesis.

5.4.2   Limitations of MRPP Regression Analysis

The following simple example serves to illustrate the consequence of the failure of the assumption that $G_i = G$ for $i = 1, ..., g$. Consider two groups consisting of a random sample of size $n_1 = 3$ drawn from population 1 and a second random sample of size $n_2 = 2$ drawn from population 2. Let x denote the covariate, y denote the response variable, $\{(x_{11}, y_{11}), (x_{12}, y_{12}), (x_{13}, y_{13})\}$ represent the sample data in Group 1, and $\{(x_{21}, y_{21}), (x_{22}, y_{22})\}$ represent the sample data in Group 2. Suppose the data arise according to one of two models specified under Case 1 and Case 2.

Case 1. For $i = 1, 2$ and $j = 1, ..., n_i$, the X_{ij} are independent and identically distributed random values 1 or 2 with probability 0.5. The regression equation is given by

$$Y_{ij} = X_{ij} + E_{ij},$$

where the E_{ij} are independent and identically distributed Bernoulli random values -1 and $+1$ with probability 0.5 and the E_{ij} are independent of X_{ij}.

Case 2. For $i = 1, 2$ and $j = 1, ..., n_i$, the X_{1j} are independent and identically distributed random values 1 or 2 with probability 0.5 and the X_{2j} are independent and identically distributed random values 2 or 3 with probability 0.5. The regression equation is given by

$$Y_{ij} = X_{ij} + E_{ij},$$

where the E_{ij} are independent and identically distributed Bernoulli random values -1 and $+1$ with probability 0.5 and the E_{ij} are independent of X_{ij}.

In Case 1, the marginal distribution of X and the conditional distribution of Y given X are the same for both groups. In Case 2, the marginal distribution of X for Group 1 is not the same as the marginal distribution of X for Group 2, but the conditional distribution of Y given X for Group 1 is the same as the conditional distribution of Y given X for Group 2. The null hypothesis under consideration is H_0: the conditional distribution of Y given X is the same for Groups 1 and 2. Simply put, the null hypothesis states that the Y values for the two groups have the same distribution after adjusting for the covariate X.

Analysis of Case 1

The totality of samples can be partitioned into six classes depending on the number of x values that are equal to 1. Label these classes as Class 0, Class 1, ..., Class 5. The label Class i refers to the class of samples in which there are exactly i points with $x = 1$. For this discussion, consider the class of

TABLE 5.33. Partial listing of the complete enumeration of 160 samples in class 1 based on $n_1 = 3$ data values in group 1 and $n_2 = 2$ data values in group 2.

Sample	Group 1	Group 2
1	(1,0), (2,1), (2,1)	(2,1), (2,1)
2	(1,0), (2,1), (2,1)	(2,1), (2,3)
⋮	⋮	⋮
159	(2,3), (2,3), (2,3)	(1,0), (2,1)
160	(2,3), (2,3), (2,3)	(2,1), (1,0)

TABLE 5.34. Partitions of the 160 samples in class 1 into 10 subclasses and associated frequencies.

	Subclass number									
Points	1	2	3	4	5	6	7	8	9	10
(1,0)	1	1	1	1	1	0	0	0	0	0
(1,2)	0	0	0	0	0	1	1	1	1	1
(2,1)	4	3	2	1	0	4	3	2	1	0
(2,3)	0	1	2	3	4	0	1	2	3	4
Frequency	5	20	30	20	5	5	20	30	20	5

samples where exactly one x value is equal to 1 and the four other x values are equal to 2, i.e., the samples in Class 1. Simple enumeration reveals that there are 160 samples that satisfy this condition, i.e., Class 1 contains 160 samples. The first two samples and the last two samples (using an arbitrary ordering) of the 160 possible samples in Class 1 are listed in Table 5.33. These 160 samples can be further partitioned according to the number of times each of the possible points (1,0), (1,2), (2,1), and (2,3) occurs in the sample, resulting in 10 subclasses with the frequencies given in Table 5.34. Note that the numbers in the last row of Table 5.34 sum to 160.

Given a particular sample realization with the point (1,0) occurring once, the point (2,1) occurring twice, and the point (2,3) occurring twice, but without knowledge of group membership, the conditional distribution of statistic δ is computed from the permutation distribution of δ based on random subdivisions of the observed set of the five data values into a group of $n_1 = 3$ data points and a second group of $n_2 = 2$ data points. This permutation distribution is the same as the conditional distribution of δ in which only samples that belong to the same subclass as the observed sample are considered.

The complete collection of 30 samples in subclass 3 of Table 5.34 are listed in Table 5.35. Table 5.35 also lists the 30 values of δ and the corresponding 30 P-values. The value of δ is the calculated MRPP statistic for

TABLE 5.35. Listing of the 30 samples in subclass 3 of Table 5.34 with associated δ values and corresponding P-values.

Group 1						Group 2					
x_{11}	y_{11}	x_{12}	y_{12}	x_{13}	y_{13}	x_{21}	y_{21}	x_{22}	y_{22}	δ	P-value
1	0	2	1	2	1	2	3	2	3	0.0	0.1
1	0	2	1	2	3	2	1	2	3	1.6	1.0
1	0	2	1	2	3	2	3	2	1	1.6	1.0
1	0	2	3	2	1	2	1	2	3	1.6	1.0
1	0	2	3	2	1	2	3	2	1	1.6	1.0
1	0	2	3	2	3	2	1	2	1	0.8	0.4
2	1	1	0	2	1	2	3	2	3	0.0	0.1
2	1	1	0	2	3	2	1	2	3	1.6	1.0
2	1	1	0	2	3	2	3	2	1	1.6	1.0
2	3	1	0	2	1	2	1	2	3	1.6	1.0
2	3	1	0	2	1	2	3	2	1	1.6	1.0
2	3	1	0	2	3	2	1	2	1	0.8	0.4
2	1	2	1	1	0	2	3	2	3	0.0	0.1
2	1	2	3	1	0	2	1	2	3	1.6	1.0
2	1	2	3	1	0	2	3	2	1	1.6	1.0
2	3	2	1	1	0	2	1	2	3	1.6	1.0
2	3	2	1	1	0	2	3	2	1	1.6	1.0
2	3	2	3	1	0	2	1	2	1	0.8	0.4
2	1	2	1	2	3	1	0	2	3	1.6	1.0
2	1	2	3	2	1	1	0	2	3	1.6	1.0
2	1	2	3	2	3	1	0	2	1	0.8	0.4
2	3	2	1	2	1	1	0	2	3	1.6	1.0
2	3	2	1	2	3	1	0	2	1	0.8	0.4
2	3	2	3	2	1	1	0	2	1	0.8	0.4
2	1	2	1	2	3	2	3	1	0	1.6	1.0
2	1	2	3	2	1	2	3	1	0	1.6	1.0
2	1	2	3	2	3	2	1	1	0	0.8	0.4
2	3	2	1	2	1	2	3	1	0	1.6	1.0
2	3	2	1	2	3	2	1	1	0	0.8	0.4
2	3	2	3	2	1	2	1	1	0	0.8	0.4

the analysis-of-covariance test of the null hypothesis of equality of groups after adjusting for the covariate, and the P-value is the probability of obtaining a δ value equal to or less than the observed δ, where the probability is calculated under the permutation distribution. When the distribution of the column of δ values is derived in Table 5.35, the conditional cumulative distribution function of δ, given the set of observed data values (without knowledge of group membership), takes the values 0.1, 0.4, and 1.0, corresponding to the δ values of 0.0, 0.8, and 1.6, respectively. Thus, it is verified,

TABLE 5.36. Listing of the 12 possible classes with $n_1 = 3$ data values in group 1 and $n_2 = 2$ data values in group 2.

| | Number of points with | | |
Class	$x = 1$	$x = 2$	$x = 3$
1	3	2	0
2	3	1	1
3	3	0	2
4	2	3	0
5	2	2	1
6	2	1	2
7	1	4	0
8	1	3	1
9	1	2	2
10	0	5	0
11	0	4	1
12	0	3	2

for this particular subclass of samples, that the conditional distribution of δ and the permutation distribution of δ are equal. This is well known and it is this fact that enables the use of the permutation distribution of δ to test the null hypothesis.

Analysis of Case 2

The situation is somewhat different in Case 2. The totality of all possible samples can now be divided into 12 classes, as given in Table 5.36. Note that there cannot be more than two points with $x = 3$ and there cannot be more than three points with $x = 1$ because of the chosen sample sizes for Group 1 and Group 2 (i.e., $n_1 = 3$ and $n_2 = 2$) and the corresponding marginal distributions of x.

Given a set of observed data with $n_1 = 3$ observations in Group 1 and $n_2 = 2$ observations in Group 2, the set must belong to exactly one of the 12 classes listed in Table 5.36. Suppose that it belongs to Class 5. Simple enumeration reveals that class 5 contains exactly 192 samples. Class 5 can be further partitioned into 18 subclasses based on the frequencies of occurrence of the possible sample points $(1,0)$, $(1,2)$, $(2,1)$, $(2,3)$, $(3,2)$, and $(3,4)$. The 18 subclasses are listed in Table 5.37. Note that the numbers in the last row sum to 192.

The complete collection of 24 samples in subclass 10 of Table 5.37 is listed in Table 5.38. Table 5.38 also lists the 24 values of δ and the corresponding 24 P-values. The value of δ is the calculated MRPP statistic for the analysis of covariance test of the null hypothesis of equality of groups after adjusting for the covariate, and the P-value is the probability of obtaining

TABLE 5.37. Partitions of the 192 samples in class 5 into 18 subclasses and associated frequencies.

Points	Subclass number																	
	1	2	3	4	5	6	7	8	9	10	11	12	13	14	15	16	17	18
(1,0)	2	2	2	2	2	2	1	1	1	1	1	1	0	0	0	0	0	0
(1,2)	0	0	0	0	0	0	1	1	1	1	1	1	2	2	2	2	2	2
(2,1)	2	2	1	1	0	0	2	2	1	1	0	0	2	2	1	1	0	0
(2,3)	0	0	1	1	2	2	0	0	1	1	2	2	0	0	1	1	2	2
(3,2)	1	0	1	0	1	0	1	0	1	0	1	0	1	0	1	0	1	0
(3,4)	0	1	0	1	0	1	0	1	0	1	0	1	0	1	0	1	0	1
Frequency	6	6	12	12	6	6	12	12	24	24	12	12	6	6	12	12	6	6

TABLE 5.38. Listing of the 24 samples in subclass 10 of Table 5.37 with associated δ values and corresponding P-values.

Group 1						Group 2				δ	P-value
x_{11}	y_{11}	x_{12}	y_{12}	x_{13}	y_{13}	x_{21}	y_{21}	x_{22}	y_{22}		
1	0	1	2	2	1	2	3	3	4	0.8	0.4
1	0	1	2	2	3	2	1	3	4	1.6	1.0
1	2	1	0	2	1	2	3	3	4	0.8	0.4
1	2	1	0	2	3	2	1	3	4	1.6	1.0
1	0	1	2	2	1	3	4	2	3	0.8	0.4
1	0	1	2	2	3	3	4	2	1	1.6	1.0
1	2	1	0	2	1	3	4	2	3	0.8	0.4
1	2	1	0	2	3	3	4	2	1	1.6	1.0
1	0	2	1	1	2	2	3	3	4	0.8	0.4
1	0	2	3	1	2	2	1	3	4	1.6	1.0
1	2	2	1	1	0	2	3	3	4	0.8	0.4
1	2	2	3	1	0	2	1	3	4	1.6	1.0
1	0	2	1	1	2	3	4	2	3	0.8	0.4
1	0	2	3	1	2	3	4	2	1	1.6	1.0
1	2	2	1	1	0	3	4	2	3	0.8	0.4
1	2	2	3	1	0	3	4	2	1	1.6	1.0
2	1	1	0	1	2	2	3	3	4	0.8	0.4
2	1	1	2	1	0	2	3	3	4	0.8	0.4
2	3	1	0	1	2	2	1	3	4	1.6	1.0
2	3	1	2	1	0	2	1	3	4	1.6	1.0
2	1	1	0	1	2	3	4	2	3	0.8	0.4
2	1	1	2	1	0	3	4	2	3	0.8	0.4
2	3	1	0	1	2	3	4	2	1	0.8	0.4
2	3	1	2	1	0	3	4	2	1	1.6	1.0

a δ equal to or less than the observed delta, where the P-value is calculated under the permutation distribution. When the distribution of the column of δ values is derived in Table 5.38, the conditional cumulative distribution function of δ, given the set of observed data values (without knowledge of group membership), takes the values 0.5 and 1.0, corresponding to the δ values of 0.8 and 1.6, respectively. However, for each of the 24 samples, the *cdf* of the permutation distribution of δ takes the values 0.4 and 1.0, corresponding to the δ values 0.8 and 1.6, respectively. Thus, for this subclass of samples, the conditional distribution of δ and the permutation distribution of δ are not equal. Therefore, the permutation test of H_0 is not exact, as expected. Nevertheless, note that the correspondence between the permutation distribution of δ and the conditional distribution of δ is quite close, even with such a small data set. This small example suggests that the permutation distribution of δ may provide a good approximation to the conditional distribution of δ under H_0.

5.5 MRPP Confidence Intervals for a Regression Parameter

Hail suppression generates considerable interest, on a worldwide basis, in the field of weather modification technology. Cloud seeding for hail suppression has been implemented in many parts of the world using a variety of techniques. Dennis (1980) discusses the processes by which seeding reduces damaging hail and, although some randomized experiments have provided significant evidence of seeding effects (e.g., Miller et al., 1975; Rudolph et al., 1994), others have not (e.g., Crow et al., 1979; Federer et al., 1986). In the face of conflicting experimental results, operational hail-suppression seeding projects continue, with evidence that some of the programs produce reductions in hail damage (e.g., Dessens, 1986; Markó et al., 1990; Mesinger and Mesinger, 1992; Simeonov, 1992).

Studies of hail damage to crops (Changnon, 1977, 1984) indicate that North Dakota experiences the highest insurance dollar loss of any state in the United States, while southwestern North Dakota has the highest ratio of damage claims paid to the insured's crop liability (Miller and Fuhs, 1987). Cloud seeding has been operational in western North Dakota since the 1950s, with regular hail-suppression operations taking place in some areas since 1961 (Rose and Jameson, 1986). Since 1976, seeding operations from aircraft in North Dakota have been organized as the North Dakota Cloud Modification Project (NDCMP). This ongoing project assumes that cloud seeding is effective in reducing hail damage to crops. It is important to examine available data for any evidence that may support or contradict this assumption.

Rose and Jameson (1986) and Miller and Fuhs (1987) conducted preliminary analyses of crop hail insurance data from western North Dakota and neighboring regions. They found indications of reduced hail damage in seeded areas. A further exploratory analysis of the same kind of data using more powerful statistical methods is desirable. In the following analysis, historical-period data and treatment-period data for both a target and a control area are examined (see Mielke et al., 1982). This approach combines features of both historical and target-control comparisons (Smith et al., 1997).[7]

5.5.1   The North Dakota Cloud Modification Project

Field operations of the NDCMP were initiated in 1976. The basic treatment strategy has remained the same over the succeeding years, although there have been some variations in seeding materials and delivery technology. The general approach is for aircraft to deliver glaciogenic seeding agents to summertime convective clouds. From 1976 to 1988, the target area included six continuously participating counties, comprising 26,278 km^2 in western North Dakota.

5.5.2   Crop Hail Insurance Data

Crop hail insurance data are available for western North Dakota and adjacent regions beginning in 1924. These data provide the yearly amount of insured crop liability and associated loss ratios (i.e., the ratio of damage claims paid, in dollars, to the insured's crop liabilities) for each county. The use of such data for evaluating seeding effects has limitations (Changnon, 1969, 1985). Among the limitations are (1) only a portion of the crop in any given area is insured, and the insured portion varies with time; (2) crop sensitivity to hail damage varies over the season; and (3) farming techniques, cropping patterns, crop yields, and crop values vary with time. Most importantly, insurance forms often include a "deductible" clause stipulating that no payment will be made for losses smaller than a specified fraction of the insured crop value. Consequently, loss payments cannot be directly equated to hail damage. However, insurance data have important advantages in that (1) they cover much larger areas than would be practical with hail-measurement instruments, (2) they are available for a long historical period, and (3) they are based on a relevant economic measure of the losses due to hail.

---

[7]Adapted and reprinted with permission of the American Meteorological Society from P.L. Smith, L.R. Johnson, D.L. Priegnitz, B.A. Boe, and P.W. Mielke, Jr. An exploratory analysis of crop-hail insurance data for evidence of cloud-seeding effects in North Dakota. *Journal of Applied Meteorology*, 1997, 36, 463–473. Copyright © 1997 by the American Meteorological Society.

The use of loss ratios, in the form of annual values based on areal totals of liabilities covered by insurance and calculated loss payments, mitigates the limitations of the hail insurance data. Seeding has been conducted in many of the counties of western North Dakota, but six counties were regularly seeded during the NDCMP treatment period of interest (1976 to 1988). Three southwestern counties (Bowman, Hettinger, and Slope) and three northern counties (McKenzie, Mountrail, and Ward) constitute the target area for these analyses, while 12 counties of eastern Montana (Carter, Custer, Daniels, Dawson, Fallon, McCone, Powder River, Prairie, Richland, Roosevelt, Sheridan, and Wibaux) provide an upwind control area. Although the control area is larger than the target area, the liabilities covered by insurance for the two areas are similar. The dollar liabilities, however, vary by a factor of about 10^3 over the period of record. Table 5.39 contains the annual values of the loss ratios for the 12 county control area in Montana and the NDCMP six county target area in North Dakota (CHIAA, 1978). Each of the NDCMP treatment years (1976 to 1988) is marked by an asterisk (∗). The year 1934 is omitted for the target area because the liability was extremely small.

5.5.3 Methodology

Described in this section is a method, based on the LAD regression approach, for deriving point and interval estimates of the difference between the target-area loss ratios for the historical years (1924 to 1975) and the NDCMP treatment years (1976 to 1988). The methodology is used to obtain permutation-based point and interval estimates. Let

$$y_I = \beta x_I + e_I$$

be the linear model for the n_h historical-period cases ($I = 1, ..., n_h$) and the n_t treatment-period cases ($I = n_h + 1, ..., n_h + n_t$). Here, y_I, x_I, and e_I denote the target, control, and error values of the Ith year, respectively, and β is an unknown scale parameter. A least sum of absolute deviations algorithm (Barrodale and Roberts, 1974) minimizes the sum given by

$$\sum_{I=1}^{n_h+n_t} |e_I|$$

and yields the LAD estimator of β ($\tilde{\beta}$) and the resulting LAD residuals given by

$$\tilde{e}_I = y_I - \tilde{\beta} x_I$$

for $I = 1, ..., n_h + n_t$.

The null hypothesis (H_0) states that the LAD residuals for the n_h historical-period cases and n_t treatment-period cases are from a common population. MRPP is used to compare the historical-period and treatment-period

LAD residuals under H_0. The MRPP statistic is given by

$$\delta = \frac{n_h \xi_h + n_t \xi_t}{n_h + n_t},$$

where

$$\xi_h = \binom{n_h}{2}^{-1} \sum_{I=2}^{n_h} \sum_{J=1}^{I-1} |\tilde{e}_I - \tilde{e}_J|$$

and

$$\xi_t = \binom{n_t}{2}^{-1} \sum_{I=n_h+2}^{n_h+n_t} \sum_{J=n_h+1}^{I-1} |\tilde{e}_I - \tilde{e}_J|.$$

The method may be implemented with either resampling or Pearson type III P-value approximations.

Consider adjusted historical dependent values given by $y_I^* = \Theta y_I$ for $I = 1, ..., n_h$, where Θ is a scale parameter chosen to make the median of the historical-period residuals the same as the median of the treatment-period residuals. Under H_0, $\Theta = 1$. The point estimator of Θ (Θ_M) is the value of Θ for which MRPP yields the largest P-value (P_{max}). Since the point estimator of Θ maximizes the P-value, the point estimator is analogous to a maximum likelihood estimator. Because MRPP detects both scale and location alternatives, P_{max} may be less than 1. Consequently, the lower and upper $1 - \alpha$ interval estimators of Θ (Θ_L and Θ_U, respectively) are obtained when the MRPP P-value is αP_{max}. While $\Theta = 1$ yields the P-value for the observed data, a search algorithm obtains the point and lower and upper $1 - \alpha$ interval estimators Θ_M, Θ_L, and Θ_U. Except for necessary modifications, a conceptually identical approach is applicable for obtaining either alternative confidence intervals for single parameters or confidence regions for multiple parameters. Smith et al. (1997) compared the present MRPP-based estimator results to corresponding results for double ratio and least squares regression estimators. The choice of estimators is far from exhaustive since alternative ratio estimators, such as those considered by Mielke and Medina (1983), have desirable properties.

5.5.4 Analysis Results

Utilizing Pearson type III P-values for the data in Table 5.39, the point estimate Θ_M is 0.547 (corresponding to a 45% reduction in the hail loss ratios during the NDCMP treatment-period years) and the lower and upper 90% interval estimates are $\Theta_L = 0.383$ (62% reduction) and $\Theta_U = 0.937$ (6% reduction), respectively. Thus, the entire 90% interval estimate during the NDCMP treatment-period years of 1976 to 1988 is comprised of reduced target-area loss ratios.

TABLE 5.39. Crop hail insurance loss ratios for the Montana control area and the NDCMP target area, 1924 to 1988.

Year	Control	Target	Year	Control	Target
1924	6.10	8.38	1957	6.17	4.04
1925	3.49	2.19	1958	4.89	2.95
1926	2.19	7.65	1959	4.02	6.23
1927	4.72	11.64			
1928	5.84	12.83	1960	6.27	8.79
1929	0.89	2.93	1961	9.05	31.4
			1962	10.07	18.04
1930	3.45	3.44	1963	12.25	19.75
1931	6.39	3.59	1964	7.60	13.35
1932	6.37	4.12	1965	4.64	4.36
1933	8.69	2.27	1966	5.21	4.97
1934	11.69	——	1967	0.91	1.48
1935	13.21	10.44	1968	3.16	7.58
1936	3.19	8.46	1969	6.50	3.74
1937	19.22	5.19			
1938	9.06	9.59	1970	4.86	3.20
1939	5.03	0.02	1971	11.56	8.79
			1972	4.09	5.15
1940	11.80	11.05	1973	0.79	0.96
1941	5.76	2.54	1974	2.17	1.11
1942	8.78	7.66	1975	7.32	6.39
1943	6.53	8.64	*1976	6.49	3.55
1944	13.74	4.70	*1977	3.29	2.97
1945	12.10	5.74	*1978	9.55	4.02
1946	10.74	6.12	*1979	3.87	2.22
1947	4.57	2.78			
1948	6.71	5.34	*1980	6.29	0.88
1949	2.26	10.90	*1981	11.94	5.26
			*1982	6.62	4.37
1950	0.48	2.06	*1983	7.60	3.73
1951	4.71	7.18	*1984	2.66	1.89
1952	3.31	9.99	*1985	1.39	1.23
1953	4.52	4.23	*1986	8.00	2.77
1954	7.32	8.81	*1987	1.97	9.06
1955	1.72	6.81	*1988	0.25	2.01
1956	6.28	15.25			

An asterisk (*) indicates a NDCMP treatment year.

5.6 LAD Regression Prediction Models

Consider the multiple linear regression model given by

$$y_I = \sum_{j=1}^{m} x_{Ij}\beta_j + e_I,$$

where y_I is the Ith of N observed values, x_{Ij} denotes the jth of m predictors associated with the Ith observed value, where $x_{I1} = 1$ if the model includes an intercept, β_j designates the jth of m regression parameters, and e_I represents the error associated with the Ith observed value. Since the desired fit consistent with Euclidean geometry between the N predicted values $(\tilde{y}_1, ..., \tilde{y}_N)$ and the N observed values $(y_1, ..., y_N)$ minimizes

$$\sum_{I=1}^{N} |\tilde{y}_I - y_I|,$$

the estimators of $\beta_1, ..., \beta_m$ that yield

$$\tilde{y}_I = \sum_{j=1}^{m} x_{Ij} \tilde{\beta}_j$$

for $I = 1, ..., N$ are the values $\tilde{\beta}_1, ..., \tilde{\beta}_m$. However, the permutation test in this situation is a special case of MRBP involving $b = 2$ (i.e., two blocks corresponding to the observed and predicted values) and $g = N$ (i.e., the number of observed values). Thus, the MRBP statistic is

$$\delta = \frac{1}{N} \sum_{I=1}^{N} |y_I - \tilde{y}_I|,$$

where the distribution of δ under H_0 assigns equal probabilities to each of the $M = (N!)^2$ possible allocations for the N positions associated with $y_1, ..., y_N$ and $\tilde{y}_1, ..., \tilde{y}_N$, i.e., $g = N$ and $b = 2$ in $M = (g!)^b$. Thus, the δ statistic compares the within-group clumping of response measurements with the model specified by random allocation under H_0. Since M is prohibitively large even for fairly small values of N, either the resampling or Pearson type III approximations for P-values described in Section 4.1 may be utilized.

Mielke et al. (1996a, 1997)[8] indicate substantial advantages for LAD regression over OLS regression in meteorological applications. These papers explore the effect of sample size, various types of contamination, and the inclusion of uninformative predictors on the shrinkage of the agreement measure $\Re$ in Expression (4.2), i.e., the reduction of the inflated agreement measure when data are fitted for a given sample to the anticipated agreement measure and when the estimated parameters are used with other random samples of the same size. It is shown in Mielke et al. (1997) that a drop-one cross-validation estimator is nearly an unbiased estimator of

---

[8]Adapted and reprinted with permission of the American Meteorological Society from P.W. Mielke, Jr., K.J. Berry, C.W. Landsea, and W.M. Gray. A single-sample estimate of shrinkage in meteorological forecasting. *Weather and Forecasting*, 1997, 12, 847–858. Copyright © 1997 by the American Meteorological Society.

shrinkage. This regression approach has been used to obtain forecast models of tropical cyclone activity (Mielke et al., 1996a, 1997). Berry and Mielke (1998b) compare LAD and OLS regression analyses, document the robustness of LAD regression, contrast the intuitive nature of LAD regression with the counterintuitive nature of OLS regression, and examine the effects of distance, leverage, and influence on LAD and OLS regression models.

5.6.1 Prediction and Cross-Validation

Meteorologists have long recognized the importance of quantifying forecasts. One of the primary tools of meteorological forecasting is multiple regression analysis (Murphy and Winkler, 1984) where, given sample data on a response variable y_i and associated predictor variables x_{ij} ($j = 1, ..., m$, $i = 1, ..., n$), m denotes the number of predictors, and n represents the number of events. The goal is to find some function of the x_{ij} values that is an accurate and precise predictor of y_i. It is generally recognized that any estimate of forecast skill grounded in a multiple regression model based on a sample of observations is characteristically higher than the forecast skill that would be obtained from a multiple regression model based on the entire population of observations (Barnston and van den Dool, 1993; Michaelsen, 1987; Mosteller and Tukey, 1977; Picard and Cook, 1984). It is also widely accepted that the fit of the multiple regression model to new sample data is nearly always less precise than the fit of the same multiple regression model to the original sample data on which the model was based. This is reflected in lower levels of forecast skill when sample-based multiple regression models are used to predict future events.

It is useful to have elementary terms to distinguish between the fit of a multiple regression model to the sample data on which the model has been determined and the fit of the same multiple regression model to an independent sample of data. The former is termed "retrospective" fit and the latter is termed "validation" fit (Copas, 1983). The term "shrinkage" denotes the drop in skill from retrospective fit to validation fit (Copas, 1983) and indicates how useful the sample-based regression coefficients will be for prediction on other data sets. For purposes of clarification, shrinkage involves the following four-step procedure. First, a multiple regression model is fit to a sample data set by optimizing the regression coefficients relative to a fitting criterion, e.g., least squares. Second, the goodness-of-fit of the multiple regression model is measured by an index, such as a squared multiple correlation coefficient. Third, the multiple regression model obtained is applied to an independent sample data set, and a second goodness-of-fit index is obtained for the independent data set. Fourth, a ratio of the two indices is constructed, where the goodness-of-fit index from the original data set is the denominator. This ratio is termed "shrinkage" since it is usually less than unity.

Mielke et al. (1996a) investigated the effects of sample size, type of regression model, and noise-to-signal ratio on the degree of shrinkage in five populations that differed in the amount and degree of contaminated data. Shrinkage was defined as the ratio of the validation fit of a sample regression equation to the retrospective fit of the same sample regression equation where the validation fit was assessed on five independent samples, averaged over 10,000 simulations for each sample, for a total of 50,000 values. Although this index of shrinkage is both rigorous and comprehensive, the use of six independent samples precludes its use in routine research situations. In this section, an estimate of shrinkage is developed that is based on a single sample and can easily be employed by researchers (Mielke et al., 1997). Comparisons with the index of shrinkage given by Mielke et al. (1996a) indicate that the single-sample estimate of shrinkage is very accurate under a wide variety of conditions. The single-sample estimate of shrinkage is related to cross-validation methods that have become standard for assessing the predictive validity of forecast skill.

Cross-Validation

Historically, users of multiple regression procedures have developed methods to assess how accurately sample regression coefficients estimate the corresponding population regression coefficients. The usual procedure is to test the sample regression coefficients on an independent set of sample data. This practice has come to be known as "cross-validation." A comprehensive historical background on cross-validation is provided by Geisser (1975), Mosteller and Tukey (1977), Snee (1977), and Stone (1974, 1978). Camstra and Boomsma (1992) present an extensive overview of the use of cross-validation in OLS regression, where the emphasis is on the prediction of individual observations, and in covariance structure analysis, where the emphasis is on future values of variances and covariances.

It is widely recognized that, to be useful, any sample regression equation must hold for data other than those on which the regression equation was developed. When sample data are used to determine the regression coefficients that best predict the response variable from the set of predictor variables, assuming that the variables to be used in the regression equation have already been selected, prediction performance is usually overestimated (Picard and Cook, 1984). Because the sample regression coefficients are determined by an optimizing process that is conditioned on the sample data, the regression equation generally provides better predictions for the sample data on which it is based than for any other data set. This is sometimes referred to as "testing on the training data" (Glick, 1978). It should be noted that the use of cross-validation precludes any manipulation of the data set prior to the development of the regression model and subsequent cross-validation.

In general, cross-validation involves determining the regression coefficients in one sample and applying the obtained coefficients to the predictor scores of another sample. The initial sample is termed the "calibration" or "training" sample, and the second sample is called the "validation" or "test" sample (Browne, 1975a, 1975b; Camstra and Boomsma, 1992; Huberty et al., 1987; MacCallum et al., 1994). The calibration sample is used to calculate the regression coefficients, and the predictive validity of the fitted equation is verified by the validation sample.

As defined, cross-validation requires two samples. Because a second sample is often not readily available, an alternative approach is sometimes used where a large sample is randomly split into two subsamples. One subsample is specified as the calibration sample, and the second sample is designated the validation sample. The many problems associated with this approach to cross-validation are summarized in Lachenbruch and Mickey (1968), Picard and Berk (1990), and Picard and Cook (1984). Setting aside the obvious loss of information in splitting samples (Browne and Cudeck, 1992), a significant problem is the difficulty in procuring large samples, which are not available in many research situations. In addition, when calibration sample sizes are small, the regression coefficients are less precise than those that would be obtained if the entire sample had been used (Horst, 1966). Mosier (1951) suggested a double cross-validation procedure where the regression coefficients are calculated for both the calibration and validation samples, and the two regression equations are cross-validated on the sample that was not used to establish the regression coefficients. Questions have been raised as to exactly what should be done when the results of the two cross-validations differ (Snee, 1977). It has been suggested that if the two sets of regression coefficients are not too different, then a new set of coefficients may be obtained from the combined calibration and validation samples (Mosier, 1951). Although no estimate of predictive validity is available for the combined sample, Mosier (1951) posited that it may be approximated by the average of the estimates of predictive validity obtained from the original calibration and validation samples.

Cross-validation is certainly not limited to just two samples. The data can be divided into more than two samples, and multiple cross-validations can be obtained. Multiple cross-validation involves partitioning an available sample of size N into a validation sample of size k and a calibration sample of size $N - k$. This approach is often termed "jackknifing." The cross-validation procedure is realized by withholding each validation sample of size k, calculating a regression model from the remaining calibration sample of size $N - k$, and validating each of the $\binom{N}{k}$ possible regression models on the remaining sample of size k held in reserve. Since $k = 1$ requires validating only N regression models on the remaining sample of size $k = 1$ held in reserve, this special case is both easily implemented and commonly used. In various literatures, the case where $k = 1$ is termed "drop-one cross-validation," "leave-one-out cross-validation," "hold-one-out cross-validation," or the "U method." Stone (1978) provides a thorough review of drop-one cross-validation. Drop-one cross-validation is an exhaustive method involving substantial redundancy in the participation of each data point (there is far more redundancy when $k > 1$). However, the exhaustive features of drop-one cross-validation may provide a comprehensive evaluation of predictive accuracy and a solid estimate of predictive skill (Barnston and van den Dool, 1993).

Drop-one cross-validation is usually credited to Lachenbruch (1967) or Lachenbruch and Mickey (1968). However, Toussaint (1974) has traced the drop-one method to earlier sources under different names (Glick, 1978). Currently, the drop-one method is the cross-validation procedure of choice, and it is not unusual to see the term "cross-validation" virtually equated with the drop-one method (Livezey et al., 1990; Nicholls, 1985).

For many researchers, the method of choice for cross-validation is to create a model based on one sample and test the model on a second sample that has been drawn from the same population. Alternatively, a model is created on a substantial portion of a sample and tested on the remaining portion of the sample. In either case, the selection of predictors can be based on information in the population or some other out-of-sample source, or the selection of predictors can involve subset selection based on in-sample information. In addition, the regression coefficients are nearly always based on information in the calibration sample. Much of the early work in cross-validation limited analyses to fixed models where the number and variety of predictors is determined a priori and not based on subset selection (Browne, 1975a, 1975b; Camstra and Boomsma, 1992; MacCallum et al., 1994). Thus, cross-validation in this context implies validation of the sample regression coefficients only. In those cases where subset selection is based on the sample information, cross-validation implies validation of both the subset selection process and the sample regression coefficients.

The advent of double cross-validation brought additional complications. Given fixed predictors, the regression coefficients from each sample are tested on the other sample, and any differences are consolidated by some form of weighted averaging of the regression coefficients (Subrahmanyam, 1972). However, given sample-based subset selection, there is the added complication that each sample will select a different number and/or a different set of predictors; in this situation, it may be much more difficult to resolve discrepancies between the two sample validation results. Browne (1970) provides results of random sampling experiments demonstrating the effects of failing to fix the predictors beforehand. With drop-one cross-validation, there may exist up to N different but overlapping sets of predictors and up to N different values for the regression coefficients for each predictor. The satisfactory and optimal combination of these differences appears very difficult; see, for example, Browne and Cudeck (1989) and MacCallum et al. (1994).

Statistical Measures

Let the population and sample sizes be denoted by $\mathcal{N}$ and N, respectively, let y_I denote the response variable, and let $x_{I1}, ..., x_{Im}$ denote the m predictor variables associated with the Ith of N events. Consider the linear regression model given by

$$y_I = \beta_0 + \sum_{j=1}^{m} \beta_j x_{Ij} + e_I,$$

where $\beta_0, ..., \beta_m$ are $m+1$ unknown parameters and e_I is the error term associated with the Ith of N events. Two types of regression models are of interest: least sum of absolute deviations (LAD) regression models and ordinary least sum of squared deviations (OLS) regression models. The LAD and OLS prediction equations are given by

$$\tilde{y}_I = \tilde{\beta}_0 + \sum_{j=1}^{m} \tilde{\beta}_j x_{Ij},$$

where $\tilde{y}_I$ is the predicted value of y_I and $\tilde{\beta}_0, ..., \tilde{\beta}_m$ minimize the expression

$$\sum_{I=1}^{N} |e_I|^v$$

with $v = 1$ and $v = 2$ associated with the LAD and OLS regression models, respectively.

A measure of agreement is employed to determine the correspondence between the y_I and $\tilde{y}_I$ values for $I = 1, ..., N$. Many researchers have utilized measures of agreement in assessing prediction accuracy (e.g., Badescu, 1993; Cotton et al., 1994; Elsner and Schmertmann, 1993; Gray et al., 1992; Hess and Elsner, 1994; Kelly et al., 1989; Lee et al., 1995; McCabe and Legates, 1992; Tucker et al., 1989; Willmott, 1982; and Willmott et al., 1985). Watterson (1996) provides a comprehensive comparison of various measures of agreement.

In this simulation study, the measure of agreement for both the LAD and OLS prediction equations is given by

$$\Re = 1 - \frac{\delta}{\mu_\delta},$$

where

$$\delta = \frac{1}{N} \sum_{I=1}^{N} |y_I - \tilde{y}_I|.$$

In this case, μ_δ is the average value over all $N!$ equally likely permutations of $y_1, ..., y_N$ relative to $\tilde{y}_1, ..., \tilde{y}_N$ under the null hypothesis that the N pairs

(y_I and $\tilde{y}_I$ for $I = 1, ..., N$) are merely the result of random assignment. This reduces to the simple computational form given by

$$\mu_\delta = \frac{1}{N^2} \sum_{I=1}^{N} \sum_{J=1}^{N} |y_I - \tilde{y}_J| \, .$$

Since $\Re$ is a chance-corrected measure of agreement (see Section 4.5), $\Re = 1.0$ implies that $\delta = 0$, $y_I = \tilde{y}_I$ for $I = 1, ..., N$, and, consequently, that all paired values of y_I and $\tilde{y}_I$ fall on a line with unit slope that passes through the origin, i.e., a perfect forecast. The choice of $\Re$ rather than the Pearson product-moment correlation coefficient (r) or the coefficient of determination (r^2) is based on the fact that the latter are measures of linearity and not measures of agreement. Also, the choice of the mean absolute error (MAE) for δ rather than the mean squared error (MSE) is because extreme values influence the squared Euclidean differences of the MSE far more than the Euclidean differences of the MAE. These choices are elaborated by Mielke et al. (1996a).

Data and Simulation Procedures

The present study investigates the accuracy and utility of a single-sample estimator of shrinkage. Also considered are the effects of sample size, type of regression model (LAD and OLS), and noise-to-signal ratio in five populations, which differ in the amount and the degree of contaminated data. Sample sizes (N) of 15, 25, 40, 65, 100, 160, 250, and 500 events are obtained from (1) a fixed population of $\mathcal{N} = 3,958$ events that, for the purpose of this study, is not contaminated with extreme cases; (2) a fixed population of $\mathcal{N} = 3,998$ events consisting of the initial population and 40 moderately extreme events (1% moderate contamination); (3) a fixed population of $\mathcal{N} = 3,998$ events consisting of the initial population and 40 very extreme events (1% severe contamination); (4) a fixed population of $\mathcal{N} = 4,158$ events consisting of the initial population and 200 moderately extreme events (5% moderate contamination); and (5) a fixed population of $\mathcal{N} = 4,158$ events consisting of the initial population and 200 very extreme events (5% severe contamination). The 3,958 available primary events used to construct each of the five populations used in this study consist of a response variable and $m = 10$ predictor variables.

The moderate 1% (5%) contamination consists of 40 (200) carefully designed additional events. The additional values of the independent variables were selected from the lowest and highest values of the specified independent variable in the initial population. Then, either the lowest or highest value was selected, based on a random binary choice. The associated values of the dependent variable were selected from the center of the distribution of the dependent variable in the initial population, near the median. The severe 1% (5%) contamination involves 40 (200) centered dependent-variable

values with the values of the independent variables placed at 2.5 times
the lower and upper values of the ranges associated with the corresponding independent variables in the initial population. The random sampling
of events from each population was implemented in the bootstrap context; that is, the random sampling was accomplished with replacement. It
should be noted that the contamination and examination of data sets containing extreme values is not new. Michaelsen (1987) analyzed data sets
containing naturally occurring extreme values. Barnston and van den Dool
(1993) contaminated Gaussian data sets with extreme values in a study of
cross-validated skill. As Barnston and van den Dool (1993) note, extreme
values are representative of many meteorological events and, in addition,
inclusion of very extreme values, up to ten standard deviations from the
mean (Barnston and van den Dool, 1993), may be important as "extreme
design experiments." Finally, it should be emphasized that the initial population was designed and constructed from real data. The added events
that contaminate the initial population create populations of data that are
contaminated relative to the initial population. Whatever contamination
preexists in the initial population of real data is unknown.

Two prediction models are considered for each of the five populations.
The first prediction model (Case 10) consists of $m = 10$ independent variables, and the second prediction model (Case 6) consists of $m = 6$ independent variables. In Case 10, four of the ten independent variables in the
initial population of $\mathcal{N} = 3{,}958$ events were found to contribute no information to the predictions. Case 6 is merely the prediction model with the four
noninformative independent variables of Case 10 deleted. The Case 10 and
Case 6 prediction models were both constructed from the initial fixed population of $\mathcal{N} = 3{,}958$ events. The reason for the choice of two prediction
models is to examine the effect of including noninformative independent
variables (i.e., noise) in a prediction model.

Findings and Discussion

The results of the study are summarized in Tables 5.40 through 5.49. In
these tables, each row is specified first by a sample size (N); second, by either $m = 10$ (Case 10) or $m = 6$ (Case 6) independent samples; and third,
by either a LAD or an OLS regression analysis. In Tables 5.40 through
5.44, the first column (C1) contains the true $\Re$ values for the designated
population calculated over all N events, and the second column (C2) contains the average of 10,000 randomly obtained sample estimates of $\Re$, $\hat{\Re}$,
where the $\tilde{y}$ values are based on the sample regression coefficients for each
of the 10,000 independent samples; that is, a measure of *retrospective fit*.
The third column (C3) measures the effectiveness of validating sample regression coefficients. In this column, the sample regression coefficients from
10,000 random samples were first obtained from column C2; then, for each
of these 10,000 sets of sample regression coefficients, an additional five

independent random samples of the same size ($N = 15, ..., 500$) were drawn from the population. The sample regression coefficients from C2 were then applied to each of the five new samples, and $\hat{\Re}$ values were computed for each of these five samples for a total of 50,000 values. The average of the 50,000 $\hat{\Re}$ values is reported in column C3, yielding a measure of *validation fit*. The fourth column (C4) contains the average of 10,000 randomly obtained drop-one sample $\hat{\Re}$ values, where each of the values is based on the same sample data, thus yielding one of the 10,000 sample $\hat{\Re}$ values comprising the averages in column C2. Thus, each value in column C4 represents the average of N times 10,000 $\hat{\Re}$ values. In Tables 5.45 through 5.49, the first column (C3/C2) contains the ratio of the average $\hat{\Re}$ value of C3 to the corresponding $\hat{\Re}$ value of C2; that is, the index of *shrinkage*. The second column (C4/C2) contains the ratio of the average $\hat{\Re}$ value of C4 to the average $\hat{\Re}$ value of C2; that is, the drop-one single-sample estimator of shrinkage, as measured by C3/C2. The third column (C4/C3) contains the ratio of the average $\hat{\Re}$ value of C4/C2 to the average $\hat{\Re}$ value of C3/C2; that is, the ratio of the drop-one single-sample estimator of shrinkage to the index of shrinkage. The fourth column (C3/C1) contains the ratio of the validation fit of C3 to the corresponding true fit, measured by the population $\Re$ value given in C1. The values of columns C1, C2, C3, C3/C2, and C3/C1 are contained in Mielke et al. (1996a).

It should be noted in this context that both C3 and C4 are free from any selection bias. Selection bias occurs when a subset of predictor variables is selected from the full set of predictor variables in the population based on information contained in the sample. In this study, selection bias has been controlled by selecting the two sets of predictor variables (i.e., Cases 10 and 6) from information contained in the population and not from information contained in any sample. Specifically, in the case of C3, the predictor variables were selected from information in the population, the regression coefficients were based on information contained in the sample for these (10 or 6) predetermined predictor variables, and then the regression coefficients were applied to five new independent samples of the same size and drawn from the same population. This process was repeated for 10,000 samples, producing 50,000 $\hat{\Re}$ values. Each C3 value is an average of these 50,000 values. Thus, although there is an optimizing bias due to retrospective fit, there is no selection bias. In the case of C4, the predictor variables were again selected from information contained in the population, and the regression coefficients were based on information contained in the sample, after dropping one observation. An $\hat{\Re}$ value was calculated from the set of $N - 1$ pairs of y and $\tilde{y}$ values and the procedure was repeated N times, dropping a different observation each time. The entire process was repeated for 10,000 samples, producing 10,000 $\hat{\Re}$ values where each value is based on N regression fits. Each C4 value is an average of these 50,000 $\hat{\Re}$ values. Thus, there is no selection bias. The advantage to this

TABLE 5.40. Population 1: initial population consisting of 3,958 noncontaminated events. Columns are (C1) true population $\Re$ values; (C2) retrospective fit based on the average of 10,000 sample $\hat{\Re}$ values using sample regression coefficients; (C3) validation fit based on the average of 50,000 sample $\hat{\Re}$ values; and (C4) drop-one single-sample estimate of shrinkage based on the average of 10,000 sample $\hat{\Re}$ values.

N	Case	Model	C1	C2	C3	C4
15	10	LAD	0.51495	0.83216	0.21959	0.19520
		OLS	0.51154	0.76579	0.24721	0.20980
	6	LAD	0.51130	0.69947	0.32214	0.29055
		OLS	0.50917	0.64059	0.34883	0.31267
25	10	LAD	0.51495	0.69659	0.34693	0.33158
		OLS	0.51154	0.63931	0.37427	0.35416
	6	LAD	0.51130	0.61963	0.39741	0.37757
		OLS	0.50917	0.57839	0.41795	0.39942
40	10	LAD	0.51495	0.62613	0.41279	0.40342
		OLS	0.51154	0.58533	0.43132	0.42250
	6	LAD	0.51130	0.57687	0.43965	0.42829
		OLS	0.50917	0.54955	0.45455	0.44493
65	10	LAD	0.51495	0.58265	0.45361	0.44876
		OLS	0.51154	0.55438	0.46425	0.45954
	6	LAD	0.51130	0.55102	0.46701	0.46115
		OLS	0.50917	0.53274	0.47611	0.47099
100	10	LAD	0.51495	0.55843	0.47627	0.47168
		OLS	0.51154	0.53790	0.48182	0.47803
	6	LAD	0.51130	0.53651	0.48269	0.47818
		OLS	0.50917	0.52353	0.48814	0.48429
160	10	LAD	0.51495	0.54290	0.49184	0.48998
		OLS	0.51154	0.52759	0.49302	0.49183
	6	LAD	0.51130	0.52727	0.49364	0.49187
		OLS	0.50917	0.51780	0.49598	0.49463
250	10	LAD	0.51495	0.53325	0.50076	0.50011
		OLS	0.51154	0.52141	0.49982	0.49965
	6	LAD	0.51130	0.52160	0.50012	0.50004
		OLS	0.50917	0.51454	0.50081	0.50080
500	10	LAD	0.51495	0.52527	0.50865	0.50660
		OLS	0.51154	0.51661	0.50562	0.50355
	6	LAD	0.51130	0.51685	0.50578	0.50422
		OLS	0.50917	0.51206	0.50500	0.50294

TABLE 5.41. Population 2: contaminated population of 3,998 events consisting of the initial population of 3,958 events and 40 moderately extreme events. Columns are (C1) true population $\Re$ values; (C2) retrospective fit based on the average of 10,000 sample $\hat{\Re}$ values using sample regression coefficients; (C3) validation fit based on the average of 50,000 sample $\hat{\Re}$ values; and (C4) drop-one single-sample estimate of shrinkage based on the average of 10,000 sample $\hat{\Re}$ values.

N	Case	Model	C1	C2	C3	C4
15	10	LAD	0.48886	0.83077	0.20662	0.18590
		OLS	0.45120	0.76387	0.23315	0.20030
	6	LAD	0.48220	0.69081	0.30215	0.28085
		OLS	0.44984	0.63008	0.32887	0.29919
25	10	LAD	0.48886	0.69099	0.32943	0.31682
		OLS	0.45120	0.63311	0.35703	0.33872
	6	LAD	0.48220	0.60467	0.37074	0.35322
		OLS	0.44984	0.56220	0.39249	0.37486
40	10	LAD	0.48886	0.61657	0.38947	0.38038
		OLS	0.45120	0.57548	0.40904	0.39914
	6	LAD	0.48220	0.55632	0.40805	0.39739
		OLS	0.44984	0.52658	0.42208	0.41204
65	10	LAD	0.48886	0.56622	0.42434	0.41918
		OLS	0.45120	0.53715	0.43587	0.43264
	6	LAD	0.48220	0.52586	0.43418	0.42843
		OLS	0.44984	0.50036	0.43615	0.43242
100	10	LAD	0.48886	0.53914	0.44413	0.43980
		OLS	0.45120	0.51555	0.44819	0.44515
	6	LAD	0.48220	0.51103	0.45081	0.44633
		OLS	0.44984	0.48556	0.44265	0.43940
160	10	LAD	0.48886	0.51867	0.45922	0.45747
		OLS	0.45120	0.49590	0.45266	0.45185
	6	LAD	0.48220	0.49982	0.46294	0.46082
		OLS	0.44984	0.47246	0.44554	0.44477
250	10	LAD	0.48886	0.50767	0.46914	0.46727
		OLS	0.45120	0.48257	0.45410	0.45271
	6	LAD	0.48220	0.49408	0.47041	0.46900
		OLS	0.44984	0.46486	0.44727	0.44579
500	10	LAD	0.48886	0.49896	0.47922	0.47885
		OLS	0.45120	0.46904	0.45367	0.45338
	6	LAD	0.48220	0.48999	0.47780	0.47740
		OLS	0.44984	0.45838	0.44897	0.44878

TABLE 5.42. Population 3: contaminated population of 3,998 events consisting of the initial population of 3,958 events and 40 very extreme events. Columns are (C1) true population $\Re$ values; (C2) retrospective fit based on the average of 10,000 sample $\hat{\Re}$ values using sample regression coefficients; (C3) validation fit based on the average of 50,000 sample $\hat{\Re}$ values; and (C4) drop-one single-sample estimate of shrinkage based on the average of 10,000 sample $\hat{\Re}$ values.

N	Case	Model	C1	C2	C3	C4
15	10	LAD	0.44873	0.83121	0.20082	0.18153
		OLS	0.29776	0.76468	0.22665	0.19527
	6	LAD	0.43722	0.69002	0.29357	0.27530
		OLS	0.27225	0.62930	0.31866	0.29310
25	10	LAD	0.44873	0.69172	0.31845	0.30758
		OLS	0.29776	0.63445	0.34486	0.32807
	6	LAD	0.43722	0.60065	0.35366	0.34098
		OLS	0.27225	0.55827	0.37435	0.36124
40	10	LAD	0.44873	0.61802	0.37532	0.36669
		OLS	0.29776	0.57769	0.39366	0.38507
	6	LAD	0.43722	0.54451	0.37879	0.37480
		OLS	0.27225	0.51698	0.39520	0.39098
65	10	LAD	0.44873	0.56667	0.40517	0.40388
		OLS	0.29776	0.53918	0.41701	0.41612
	6	LAD	0.43722	0.49965	0.38841	0.38981
		OLS	0.27225	0.47894	0.39580	0.39865
100	10	LAD	0.44873	0.53523	0.41757	0.41608
		OLS	0.29776	0.51541	0.42518	0.42465
	6	LAD	0.43722	0.47492	0.39691	0.39539
		OLS	0.27225	0.44794	0.38686	0.38850
160	10	LAD	0.44873	0.50458	0.42088	0.42080
		OLS	0.29776	0.48765	0.42113	0.42239
	6	LAD	0.43722	0.45708	0.40649	0.40508
		OLS	0.27225	0.41056	0.36825	0.37137
250	10	LAD	0.44873	0.48421	0.42473	0.42132
		OLS	0.29776	0.45964	0.40951	0.40740
	6	LAD	0.43722	0.44837	0.41433	0.41141
		OLS	0.27225	0.37856	0.34883	0.34694
500	10	LAD	0.44873	0.46656	0.43340	0.43378
		OLS	0.29776	0.40724	0.37716	0.37488
	6	LAD	0.43722	0.44242	0.42437	0.42319
		OLS	0.27225	0.33445	0.31859	0.31641

TABLE 5.43. Population 4: contaminated population of 4,158 events consisting of the initial population of 3,958 events and 200 moderately extreme events. Columns are (C1) true population $\mathfrak{R}$ values; (C2) retrospective fit based on the average of 10,000 sample $\hat{\mathfrak{R}}$ values using sample regression coefficients; (C3) validation fit based on the average of 50,000 sample $\hat{\mathfrak{R}}$ values; and (C4) drop-one single-sample estimate of shrinkage based on the average of 10,000 sample $\hat{\mathfrak{R}}$ values.

N	Case	Model	C1	C2	C3	C4
15	10	LAD	0.36924	0.82319	0.17630	0.16583
		OLS	0.31192	0.75362	0.19886	0.17653
	6	LAD	0.36698	0.66307	0.24413	0.23173
		OLS	0.30599	0.59807	0.26934	0.24821
25	10	LAD	0.36924	0.66658	0.26978	0.26159
		OLS	0.31192	0.60568	0.29496	0.28121
	6	LAD	0.36698	0.54840	0.28455	0.27086
		OLS	0.30599	0.50205	0.30704	0.29335
40	10	LAD	0.36924	0.57417	0.30939	0.30583
		OLS	0.31192	0.52983	0.33079	0.32601
	6	LAD	0.36698	0.48241	0.30925	0.29728
		OLS	0.30599	0.44501	0.32037	0.31236
65	10	LAD	0.36924	0.50310	0.33020	0.32513
		OLS	0.31192	0.46771	0.34046	0.33620
	6	LAD	0.36698	0.43752	0.32591	0.31565
		OLS	0.30599	0.39896	0.32084	0.31322
100	10	LAD	0.36924	0.45960	0.34149	0.33438
		OLS	0.31192	0.42314	0.33801	0.33372
	6	LAD	0.36698	0.41285	0.33750	0.32911
		OLS	0.30599	0.36963	0.31813	0.31226
160	10	LAD	0.36924	0.42656	0.34929	0.34577
		OLS	0.31192	0.38503	0.33172	0.32978
	6	LAD	0.36698	0.39421	0.34556	0.34131
		OLS	0.30599	0.34668	0.31471	0.31177
250	10	LAD	0.36924	0.40505	0.35441	0.35257
		OLS	0.31192	0.35909	0.32608	0.32541
	6	LAD	0.36698	0.38328	0.35161	0.34934
		OLS	0.30599	0.33194	0.31188	0.31066
500	10	LAD	0.36924	0.38708	0.36071	0.35695
		OLS	0.31192	0.33582	0.32013	0.31692
	6	LAD	0.36698	0.37622	0.36011	0.35656
		OLS	0.30599	0.31932	0.30961	0.30651

TABLE 5.44. Population 5: contaminated population of 4,158 events consisting of the initial population of 3,958 events and 200 very extreme events. Columns are (C1) true population $\Re$ values; (C2) retrospective fit based on the average of 10,000 sample $\hat{\Re}$ values using sample regression coefficients; (C3) validation fit based on the average of 50,000 sample $\hat{\Re}$ values; and (C4) drop-one single-sample estimate of shrinkage based on the average of 10,000 sample $\hat{\Re}$ values.

N	Case	Model	C1	C2	C3	C4
15	10	LAD	0.16541	0.82410	0.15671	0.14784
		OLS	0.13645	0.75637	0.17684	0.15684
	6	LAD	0.10284	0.65648	0.21212	0.21141
		OLS	0.08999	0.59195	0.23220	0.22483
25	10	LAD	0.16541	0.67046	0.23397	0.22978
		OLS	0.13645	0.61289	0.25467	0.24579
	6	LAD	0.10284	0.52745	0.22739	0.22995
		OLS	0.08999	0.48267	0.24628	0.24774
40	10	LAD	0.16541	0.57754	0.26244	0.26566
		OLS	0.13645	0.53669	0.27945	0.28149
	6	LAD	0.10284	0.42604	0.21735	0.22235
		OLS	0.08999	0.39821	0.23444	0.24104
65	10	LAD	0.16541	0.48744	0.26077	0.26526
		OLS	0.13645	0.46297	0.27581	0.27978
	6	LAD	0.10284	0.33718	0.19921	0.19730
		OLS	0.08999	0.30874	0.20295	0.20390
100	10	LAD	0.16541	0.40913	0.24710	0.24839
		OLS	0.13645	0.38873	0.25578	0.25838
	6	LAD	0.10284	0.27822	0.18593	0.18110
		OLS	0.08999	0.23511	0.17010	0.16837
160	10	LAD	0.16541	0.33696	0.23219	0.23301
		OLS	0.13645	0.30317	0.22288	0.22643
	6	LAD	0.10284	0.23075	0.17241	0.16991
		OLS	0.08999	0.17580	0.14063	0.13848
250	10	LAD	0.16541	0.28582	0.21974	0.22088
		OLS	0.13645	0.23539	0.19305	0.19305
	6	LAD	0.10284	0.19584	0.15837	0.15498
		OLS	0.08999	0.13849	0.11975	0.11718
500	10	LAD	0.16541	0.23315	0.20148	0.19745
		OLS	0.13645	0.17699	0.16198	0.15951
	6	LAD	0.10284	0.15889	0.14052	0.13570
		OLS	0.08999	0.11112	0.10326	0.09952

approach is that the optimizing bias can be isolated and examined while the selection bias is controlled. In addition, this approach is more conservative because validation fit is almost always better when subset selection is included (MacCallum et al., 1994). The disadvantage of this approach is that the results cannot be generalized to studies that selected both prediction variables and regression coefficients based on sample information. In addition, shrinkage may be increased.

The ratio values in column C3/C2 of Tables 5.45 through 5.49 provide a comprehensive index of shrinkage that serves as a benchmark against which the accuracy of the drop-one single-sample estimator of shrinkage given in column C4/C2 can be measured. The ratio values in column C4/C3 were obtained by dividing the ratio values in column C4/C2 by the corresponding ratio values in column C3/C2. They provide the comparison ratio values from which the drop-one single-sample estimator of shrinkage is evaluated.

For each of the five populations summarized in Tables 5.45 through 5.49, the ratio values in column C4/C3 are close to unity for samples with $N >$ 25. The few C4/C3 values that exceed 1.0 are probably due to sampling error. It should be noted that the C4/C3 ratios tend to be less than unity for the smaller sample sizes. When $N \leq 25$, reductions from unity of the C4/C3 values are 4.5%–11% for the LAD regression model and 4.5%–15% for the OLS regression model in Population 1. For Populations 2 through 5, the corresponding reductions are 4%–10% (LAD) and 4.5%–14% (OLS), 3.5%–9.5% (LAD) and 3.5%–14% (OLS), 3%–6% (LAD) and 4.5%–11% (OLS), and 0%–5.5% (LAD) and 0%–11% (OLS), respectively. Thus, the drop-one single-sample estimator (i.e., C4/C2) is an excellent estimator of shrinkage (i.e., C3/C2), although it is conservative for very small samples. This conclusion holds for all sample sizes greater than $N = 25$, both Cases (6 and 10), both regression models (LAD and OLS), and all five populations with differing degrees and amounts of data contamination.

Column C3/C1 in Tables 5.45 through 5.49 summarizes, in ratio format, the validation fit (C3) to the true population value (C1). This is sometimes designated as "expected skill" (Mielke et al., 1996a). In general, the C3/C1 values indicate the amount of skill that is expected relative to the true skill possible when an entire population is available. More specifically, the C3/C1 values indicate the expected reduction in fit of the y and $\tilde{y}$ values for future events (Mielke et al., 1996a). A C3/C1 value that is greater than 1.0 is cause for concern since this indicates that the sample regression coefficients provide a better validation fit, on the average, than would have been possible had the actual population been available.

Inspection of column C3/C1 in Table 5.45 reveals that the OLS regression model consistently performs better than the LAD regression model, Case 10 has lower values than Case 6, and the C3/C1 values increase with increasing sample size. Table 5.46, with 1% moderate contamination, yields a few C3/C1 values greater than 1.0, and they all appear with the OLS regression model. Table 5.47, with 1% severe contamination, shows the same pattern,

TABLE 5.45. Population 1: initial population consisting of 3,958 noncontaminated events. Columns are (C3/C2) index of shrinkage based on the ratio of validation fit to retrospective fit; (C4/C2) ratio of the drop-one single-sample estimator of shrinkage to retrospective fit; (C4/C3) ratio of the drop-one single-sample estimator of shrinkage to the index of shrinkage; and (C3/C1) expected skill based on the ratio of validation fit to the corresponding true fit.

N	Case	Model	C3/C2	C4/C2	C4/C3	C3/C1
15	10	LAD	0.264	0.235	0.889	0.426
		OLS	0.323	0.277	0.849	0.483
	6	LAD	0.461	0.415	0.902	0.630
		OLS	0.545	0.488	0.896	0.685
25	10	LAD	0.498	0.476	0.956	0.674
		OLS	0.585	0.554	0.946	0.732
	6	LAD	0.641	0.609	0.950	0.777
		OLS	0.723	0.691	0.956	0.821
40	10	LAD	0.659	0.644	0.977	0.802
		OLS	0.737	0.722	0.980	0.843
	6	LAD	0.762	0.742	0.974	0.860
		OLS	0.827	0.810	0.988	0.893
65	10	LAD	0.779	0.770	0.989	0.881
		OLS	0.837	0.829	0.990	0.908
	6	LAD	0.848	0.837	0.987	0.913
		OLS	0.894	0.884	0.989	0.935
100	10	LAD	0.853	0.845	0.990	0.925
		OLS	0.896	0.889	0.992	0.942
	6	LAD	0.900	0.891	0.991	0.944
		OLS	0.932	0.925	0.992	0.959
160	10	LAD	0.906	0.903	0.996	0.955
		OLS	0.934	0.932	0.998	0.965
	6	LAD	0.936	0.933	0.996	0.965
		OLS	0.958	0.955	0.997	0.974
250	10	LAD	0.939	0.938	0.999	0.972
		OLS	0.959	0.958	1.000	0.977
	6	LAD	0.959	0.959	1.000	0.978
		OLS	0.973	0.973	1.000	0.984
500	10	LAD	0.968	0.964	0.996	0.988
		OLS	0.985	0.975	0.996	0.988
	6	LAD	0.979	0.976	0.997	0.989
		OLS	0.986	0.982	0.991	0.992

TABLE 5.46. Population 2: contaminated population of 3,998 events consisting of the initial population of 3,958 events and 40 moderately extreme events. Columns are (C3/C2) index of shrinkage based on the ratio of validation fit to retrospective fit; (C4/C2) ratio of the drop-one single-sample estimator of shrinkage to retrospective fit; (C4/C3) ratio of the drop-one single-sample estimator of shrinkage to the index of shrinkage; and (C3/C1) expected skill based on the ratio of validation fit to the corresponding true fit.

N	Case	Model	C3/C2	C4/C2	C4/C3	C3/C1
15	10	LAD	0.249	0.224	0.900	0.423
		OLS	0.305	0.262	0.859	0.517
	6	LAD	0.437	0.407	0.930	0.627
		OLS	0.522	0.475	0.910	0.731
25	10	LAD	0.477	0.459	0.962	0.674
		OLS	0.564	0.535	0.949	0.791
	6	LAD	0.613	0.584	0.953	0.769
		OLS	0.698	0.667	0.955	0.873
40	10	LAD	0.632	0.617	0.977	0.797
		OLS	0.711	0.694	0.976	0.907
	6	LAD	0.733	0.714	0.974	0.846
		OLS	0.802	0.782	0.976	0.938
65	10	LAD	0.749	0.740	0.988	0.868
		OLS	0.811	0.805	0.993	0.966
	6	LAD	0.826	0.815	0.987	0.900
		OLS	0.872	0.864	0.991	0.970
100	10	LAD	0.824	0.816	0.990	0.909
		OLS	0.869	0.863	0.993	0.993
	6	LAD	0.882	0.873	0.990	0.935
		OLS	0.912	0.905	0.993	0.984
160	10	LAD	0.885	0.882	0.996	0.939
		OLS	0.913	0.911	0.998	1.003
	6	LAD	0.926	0.922	0.995	0.960
		OLS	0.943	0.941	0.998	0.990
250	10	LAD	0.924	0.920	0.996	0.960
		OLS	0.941	0.938	0.997	1.006
	6	LAD	0.952	0.949	0.997	0.964
		OLS	0.962	0.959	0.997	0.994
500	10	LAD	0.960	0.960	0.999	0.980
		OLS	0.967	0.967	0.999	1.005
	6	LAD	0.975	0.974	0.999	0.991
		OLS	0.979	0.979	1.000	0.998

TABLE 5.47. Population 3: contaminated population of 3,998 events consisting of the initial population of 3,958 events and 40 very extreme events. Columns are (C3/C2) index of shrinkage based on the ratio of validation fit to retrospective fit; (C4/C2) ratio of the drop-one single-sample estimator of shrinkage to retrospective fit; (C4/C3) ratio of the drop-one single-sample estimator of shrinkage to the index of shrinkage; and (C3/C1) expected skill based on the ratio of validation fit to the corresponding true fit.

N	Case	Model	C3/C2	C4/C2	C4/C3	C3/C1
15	10	LAD	0.242	0.218	0.904	0.448
		OLS	0.296	0.255	0.862	0.761
	6	LAD	0.425	0.399	0.938	0.671
		OLS	0.506	0.466	0.920	1.170
25	10	LAD	0.460	0.445	0.966	0.710
		OLS	0.544	0.517	0.951	1.158
	6	LAD	0.589	0.568	0.964	0.809
		OLS	0.671	0.647	0.965	1.375
40	10	LAD	0.607	0.593	0.977	0.836
		OLS	0.681	0.667	0.978	1.322
	6	LAD	0.696	0.688	0.989	0.866
		OLS	0.764	0.756	0.989	1.452
65	10	LAD	0.715	0.713	0.997	0.903
		OLS	0.773	0.772	0.998	1.400
	6	LAD	0.777	0.780	1.004	0.888
		OLS	0.826	0.832	1.007	1.454
100	10	LAD	0.780	0.777	0.996	0.931
		OLS	0.825	0.824	0.999	1.428
	6	LAD	0.836	0.833	0.996	0.908
		OLS	0.864	0.867	1.004	1.421
160	10	LAD	0.834	0.834	1.000	0.938
		OLS	0.864	0.866	1.003	1.414
	6	LAD	0.889	0.886	0.997	0.930
		OLS	0.897	0.905	1.008	1.353
250	10	LAD	0.877	0.870	0.992	0.947
		OLS	0.891	0.886	0.995	1.375
	6	LAD	0.924	0.918	0.993	0.948
		OLS	0.921	0.916	0.995	1.281
500	10	LAD	0.929	0.930	1.001	0.966
		OLS	0.926	0.921	0.994	1.267
	6	LAD	0.959	0.957	0.997	0.971
		OLS	0.953	0.946	0.993	1.170

TABLE 5.48. Population 4: contaminated population of 4,158 events consisting of the initial population of 3,958 events and 200 moderately extreme events. Columns are (C3/C2) index of shrinkage based on the ratio of validation fit to retrospective fit; (C4/C2) ratio of the drop-one single-sample estimator of shrinkage to retrospective fit; (C4/C3) ratio of the drop-one single-sample estimator of shrinkage to the index of shrinkage; and (C3/C1) expected skill based on the ratio of validation fit to the corresponding true fit.

N	Case	Model	C3/C2	C4/C2	C4/C3	C3/C1
15	10	LAD	0.214	0.201	0.941	0.477
		OLS	0.242	0.234	0.888	0.638
	6	LAD	0.368	0.349	0.949	0.665
		OLS	0.450	0.415	0.922	0.880
25	10	LAD	0.405	0.392	0.970	0.731
		OLS	0.487	0.464	0.953	0.946
	6	LAD	0.519	0.494	0.952	0.775
		OLS	0.612	0.584	0.955	1.003
40	10	LAD	0.539	0.533	0.988	0.838
		OLS	0.624	0.615	0.986	1.060
	6	LAD	0.641	0.616	0.961	0.843
		OLS	0.720	0.702	0.975	1.047
65	10	LAD	0.656	0.646	0.985	0.894
		OLS	0.728	0.719	0.987	1.091
	6	LAD	0.745	0.721	0.967	0.888
		OLS	0.804	0.785	0.976	1.049
100	10	LAD	0.743	0.728	0.979	0.925
		OLS	0.799	0.772	0.987	1.084
	6	LAD	0.817	0.797	0.975	0.920
		OLS	0.861	0.845	0.982	1.040
160	10	LAD	0.819	0.811	0.990	0.946
		OLS	0.862	0.857	0.994	1.063
	6	LAD	0.877	0.866	0.988	0.942
		OLS	0.908	0.899	0.991	1.028
250	10	LAD	0.875	0.870	0.995	0.960
		OLS	0.908	0.906	0.998	1.045
	6	LAD	0.917	0.911	0.994	0.958
		OLS	0.940	0.936	0.996	1.019
500	10	LAD	0.932	0.922	0.990	0.977
		OLS	0.953	0.944	0.990	1.026
	6	LAD	0.957	0.948	0.990	0.981
		OLS	0.970	0.960	0.990	1.012

TABLE 5.49. Population 5: contaminated population of 4,158 events consisting of the initial population of 3,958 events and 200 very extreme events. Columns are (C3/C2) index of shrinkage based on the ratio of validation fit to retrospective fit; (C4/C2) ratio of the drop-one single-sample estimator of shrinkage to retrospective fit; (C4/C3) ratio of the drop-one single-sample estimator of shrinkage to the index of shrinkage; and (C3/C1) expected skill based on the ratio of validation fit to the corresponding true fit.

N	Case	Model	C3/C2	C4/C2	C4/C3	C3/C1
15	10	LAD	0.190	0.179	0.943	0.947
		OLS	0.234	0.207	0.887	1.296
	6	LAD	0.323	0.322	0.997	2.063
		OLS	0.392	0.380	0.968	2.580
25	10	LAD	0.349	0.343	0.982	1.414
		OLS	0.416	0.401	0.965	1.866
	6	LAD	0.431	0.436	1.011	2.211
		OLS	0.467	0.513	1.006	2.737
40	10	LAD	0.454	0.460	1.012	1.587
		OLS	0.521	0.524	1.007	2.048
	6	LAD	0.510	0.522	1.023	2.113
		OLS	0.589	0.605	1.028	2.605
65	10	LAD	0.535	0.544	1.017	1.577
		OLS	0.596	0.604	1.014	2.021
	6	LAD	0.591	0.585	0.990	1.937
		OLS	0.657	0.660	1.005	2.255
100	10	LAD	0.604	0.607	1.005	1.494
		OLS	0.658	0.665	1.010	1.875
	6	LAD	0.668	0.651	0.974	1.808
		OLS	0.723	0.716	0.990	1.890
160	10	LAD	0.689	0.692	1.004	1.404
		OLS	0.735	0.747	1.016	1.633
	6	LAD	0.747	0.736	0.985	1.676
		OLS	0.800	0.788	0.985	1.563
250	10	LAD	0.769	0.773	1.005	1.328
		OLS	0.820	0.820	1.000	1.415
	6	LAD	0.809	0.791	0.979	1.540
		OLS	0.865	0.846	0.979	1.331
500	10	LAD	0.864	0.847	0.980	1.218
		OLS	0.915	0.901	0.985	1.187
	6	LAD	0.884	0.854	0.966	1.366
		OLS	0.929	0.896	0.964	1.147

but the C3/C1 ratio values are somewhat higher. Table 5.48, with 5% moderate contamination, continues the same motif, and Table 5.49, with 5% severe contamination, contains C3/C1 values considerably greater than 1.0 for nearly every case. It is abundantly evident that with only a small amount of moderate or severe contamination, the OLS regression model produces inflated estimates of expected skill. The LAD regression model, based on absolute deviations about the median, is relatively unaffected by even 1% severe contamination, but the OLS regression model, based on squared deviations about the mean, systematically overestimates the validation fit and yields inflated values of expected skill, i.e., C3/C1.

Since C3 (validation fit) values and C4 (drop-one single-sample validation fit) values are essentially the same for all five populations, both cases, both regression models, and all sample sizes, it is readily apparent that C4/C1 ratios would be nearly identical to the C3/C1 ratios in Tables 5.45 through 5.49. Consequently, caution should be exercised in using drop-one estimators with the OLS regression model because they will likely provide inflated estimates of validation fit when contaminated data are present. Because the drop-one estimate of shrinkage is equivalent to drop-one cross-validation, the same caution applies to drop-one cross-validation with an OLS regression model.

Although it is abundantly evident that OLS regression systematically overestimates validation fit, the reason for the optimistic C3/C1 values is not as manifest. It is obvious that the inflated estimates of expected skill for OLS regression in Tables 5.45 through 5.49 are systematically related to sample size, with larger sample sizes associated with C3/C1 values in excess of 1.0. This is probably due to a moderately or severely contaminated population event occurring in a single sample. Very small samples (e.g., $N = 15$) are not likely to include a contaminated event, whereas very large samples (e.g., $N = 500$) are much more likely to include one or more contaminated events. Table 5.50 provides the probability values that no contaminated population event belongs to a single sample for both 1% and 5% contamination. The probability that no contaminated event belongs to a single sample with 1% moderate or severe contamination in the population is given by $(3,958/3,998)^N$, and the probability that no contaminated event belongs to a single sample with 5% moderate or severe contamination in the population is given by $(3,958/4,158)^N$ in Table 5.50. For 1% moderate or severe contamination, the probability of selecting no contaminated events from the population is greater than 0.50 for samples of size $N \leq 65$. For 5% moderate or severe contamination, the probability of selecting no contaminated events from the population never exceeds 0.50. Given the well-known sensitivity of OLS regression to extreme events, it is not surprising that OLS regression yields optimistic levels of expected skill for larger samples, which are more likely to contain one or more moderate or severely contaminated events. It should be noted in Tables 5.44 and 5.49

TABLE 5.50. Probability of no contaminated values in each sample of size N.

Size	Contamination	
(N)	1%	5%
15	0.8600	0.4774
25	0.7777	0.2916
40	0.6688	0.1392
65	0.5202	0.0406
100	0.3658	0.0072
160	0.2001	0.0004
250	0.0810	4.4×10^{-6}
500	0.0066	2.0×10^{-11}

that neither OLS nor LAD regression is able to accommodate 5% severe contamination.

The single-sample estimate of shrinkage, C4, is higher for $m = 6$ predictors than for $m = 10$ predictors in Table 5.40 with LAD regression and $N \leq 160$ and with OLS regression and $N \leq 250$. This is also true for Table 5.41 with LAD regression and $N \leq 250$, and with OLS regression and $N \leq 40$. Further, the same relationship holds for both LAD and OLS regression in Table 5.42 with $N \leq 40$ and in Tables 5.43 and 5.44 with $N \leq 25$. These results illustrate the reduced influence of noninformative predictors for small N (a consequence of the smaller probabilities of selecting contaminated values). Clearly, regression models containing noninformative predictors should be avoided (Browne and Cudeck, 1992).

The standard deviations of the 10,000 $\hat{\Re}$ values comprising C2, denoted by SD($\hat{\Re}|$C2), and the standard deviations of the 10,000 drop-one values comprising C4, denoted by SD($\hat{\Re}|$C4), are given for each sample size ($N = 15, ..., 500$), Case (10 and 6 predictors), and regression model (LAD and OLS) combination in Tables 5.51 through 5.55. These standard deviations correspond to the five contamination levels of Tables 5.40 through 5.44, respectively.

In particular,

$$\mathrm{SD}(\hat{\Re}) = \left[\frac{1}{M-1} \sum_{i=1}^{M} \left(\hat{\Re}_i - \bar{\Re} \right)^2 \right]^{1/2},$$

where

$$\bar{\Re} = \frac{1}{M} \sum_{i=1}^{M} \hat{\Re}_i,$$

$M = 10,000$ in this study, and $\bar{\Re}$ applies to either C2 or C4. The standard deviations are confined to SD($\hat{\Re}|$C2) and SD($\hat{\Re}|$C4) since the associated

TABLE 5.51. Population 1: initial population of 3,958 noncontaminated events. Columns are [SD($\hat{\Re}$|C2)] standard deviations of 10,000 $\hat{\Re}$ values based on sample regression coefficients and [SD($\hat{\Re}$|C4)] standard deviations of 10,000 $\hat{\Re}$ values based on the average of $n \times 10,000$ single-sample drop-one $\hat{\Re}$ values.

N	Case	Model	SD($\hat{\Re}$|C2)	SD($\hat{\Re}$|C4)
15	10	LAD	0.07205	0.21811
		OLS	0.10145	0.20870
	6	LAD	0.10536	0.23722
		OLS	0.12495	0.21354
25	10	LAD	0.07976	0.19051
		OLS	0.09381	0.15925
	6	LAD	0.09650	0.18076
		OLS	0.10405	0.15057
40	10	LAD	0.07542	0.14298
		OLS	0.08140	0.11277
	6	LAD	0.08507	0.13386
		OLS	0.08608	0.10771
65	10	LAD	0.06600	0.10259
		OLS	0.06736	0.08098
	6	LAD	0.07015	0.09610
		OLS	0.06946	0.07882
100	10	LAD	0.05482	0.07727
		OLS	0.05479	0.06276
	6	LAD	0.05717	0.07272
		OLS	0.05582	0.06118
160	10	LAD	0.04579	0.05734
		OLS	0.04508	0.04804
	6	LAD	0.04702	0.05450
		OLS	0.04545	0.04737
250	10	LAD	0.03696	0.04148
		OLS	0.03620	0.03692
	6	LAD	0.03762	0.04071
		OLS	0.03636	0.03651
500	10	LAD	0.02695	0.02921
		OLS	0.02622	0.02684
	6	LAD	0.02717	0.02884
		OLS	0.02615	0.02679

TABLE 5.52. Population 2: contaminated population of 3,998 events consisting of the initial population of 3,958 events and 40 moderately extreme events. Columns are $[\mathrm{SD}(\hat{\Re}|\mathrm{C2})]$ standard deviations of 10,000 $\hat{\Re}$ values based on sample regression coefficients and $[\mathrm{SD}(\hat{\Re}|\mathrm{C4})]$ standard deviations of 10,000 $\hat{\Re}$ values based on the average of $n \times 10{,}000$ single-sample drop-one $\hat{\Re}$ values.

N	Case	Model	$\mathrm{SD}(\hat{\Re}|\mathrm{C2})$	$\mathrm{SD}(\hat{\Re}|\mathrm{C4})$
15	10	LAD	0.07354	0.21597
		OLS	0.10359	0.20627
	6	LAD	0.10890	0.23385
		OLS	0.12936	0.21345
25	10	LAD	0.08266	0.18894
		OLS	0.09707	0.15777
	6	LAD	0.10427	0.18602
		OLS	0.11167	0.15612
40	10	LAD	0.07913	0.14657
		OLS	0.08435	0.11843
	6	LAD	0.09503	0.14472
		OLS	0.09713	0.12155
65	10	LAD	0.07164	0.11311
		OLS	0.07299	0.09119
	6	LAD	0.08132	0.11164
		OLS	0.08418	0.09778
100	10	LAD	0.06286	0.08795
		OLS	0.06408	0.07473
	6	LAD	0.06886	0.08581
		OLS	0.07336	0.08112
160	10	LAD	0.05246	0.06648
		OLS	0.05481	0.06168
	6	LAD	0.05509	0.06478
		OLS	0.06151	0.06593
250	10	LAD	0.04379	0.05167
		OLS	0.04796	0.05224
	6	LAD	0.04497	0.04962
		OLS	0.05194	0.05471
500	10	LAD	0.03150	0.03451
		OLS	0.03697	0.03729
	6	LAD	0.03189	0.03289
		OLS	0.03864	0.03872

TABLE 5.53. Population 3: contaminated population of 3,998 events consisting of the initial population of 3,958 events and 40 very extreme events. Columns are [SD($\hat{\Re}$|C2)] standard deviations of 10,000 $\hat{\Re}$ values based on sample regression coefficients and [SD($\hat{\Re}$|C4)] standard deviations of 10,000 $\hat{\Re}$ values based on the average of $n \times 10,000$ single-sample drop-one $\hat{\Re}$ values.

N	Case	Model	SD($\hat{\Re}$|C2)	SD($\hat{\Re}$|C4)
15	10	LAD	0.07312	0.21340
		OLS	0.10296	0.20394
	6	LAD	0.10986	0.23235
		OLS	0.13057	0.21374
25	10	LAD	0.08271	0.18859
		OLS	0.09680	0.16023
	6	LAD	0.10943	0.19101
		OLS	0.11702	0.16443
40	10	LAD	0.07881	0.15062
		OLS	0.08353	0.12591
	6	LAD	0.10850	0.16098
		OLS	0.10854	0.14063
65	10	LAD	0.07311	0.12111
		OLS	0.07326	0.10234
	6	LAD	0.10760	0.14048
		OLS	0.10912	0.13000
100	10	LAD	0.07011	0.10276
		OLS	0.06856	0.09096
	6	LAD	0.09916	0.12123
		OLS	0.10987	0.12467
160	10	LAD	0.06532	0.09020
		OLS	0.06718	0.08629
	6	LAD	0.08366	0.09932
		OLS	0.10760	0.11722
250	10	LAD	0.06024	0.07645
		OLS	0.07112	0.08589
	6	LAD	0.07153	0.08012
		OLS	0.10170	0.10799
500	10	LAD	0.04760	0.05133
		OLS	0.07220	0.07339
	6	LAD	0.05308	0.05542
		OLS	0.08288	0.08283

TABLE 5.54. Population 4: contaminated population of 4,158 events consisting of the initial population of 3,958 events and 200 moderately extreme events. Columns are [SD($\hat{\Re}$|C2)] standard deviations of 10,000 $\hat{\Re}$ values based on sample regression coefficients and [SD($\hat{\Re}$|C4)] standard deviations of 10,000 $\hat{\Re}$ values based on the average of $n \times 10,000$ single-sample drop-one $\hat{\Re}$ values.

N	Case	Model	SD($\hat{\Re}$|C2)	SD($\hat{\Re}$|C4)
15	10	LAD	0.07562	0.20328
		OLS	0.10652	0.19460
	6	LAD	0.12349	0.23447
		OLS	0.14319	0.21392
25	10	LAD	0.09434	0.18918
		OLS	0.10862	0.16428
	6	LAD	0.13018	0.19988
		OLS	0.13574	0.17395
40	10	LAD	0.09796	0.16053
		OLS	0.10279	0.13597
	6	LAD	0.12286	0.16902
		OLS	0.12368	0.14667
65	10	LAD	0.09569	0.13179
		OLS	0.09648	0.11449
	6	LAD	0.11052	0.13891
		OLS	0.10641	0.11780
100	10	LAD	0.08759	0.10968
		OLS	0.08668	0.09591
	6	LAD	0.09751	0.11473
		OLS	0.09047	0.09552
160	10	LAD	0.07687	0.08986
		OLS	0.07262	0.07640
	6	LAD	0.08342	0.09390
		OLS	0.07305	0.07508
250	10	LAD	0.06777	0.07482
		OLS	0.05996	0.06017
	6	LAD	0.07159	0.07611
		OLS	0.05947	0.05962
500	10	LAD	0.05184	0.05465
		OLS	0.04164	0.04147
	6	LAD	0.05314	0.05635
		OLS	0.04148	0.04148

TABLE 5.55. Population 5: contaminated population of 4,158 events consisting of the initial population of 3,958 events and 200 very extreme events. Columns are [SD($\hat{\Re}$|C2)] standard deviations of 10,000 $\hat{\Re}$ values based on sample regression coefficients and [SD($\hat{\Re}$|C4)] standard deviations of 10,000 $\hat{\Re}$ values based on the average of $n \times 10,000$ single-sample drop-one $\hat{\Re}$ values.

N	Case	Model	SD($\hat{\Re}$|C2)	SD($\hat{\Re}$|C4)
15	10	LAD	0.07494	0.19074
		OLS	0.10476	0.18378
	6	LAD	0.12873	0.22530
		OLS	0.14899	0.20967
25	10	LAD	0.09339	0.17836
		OLS	0.10667	0.16084
	6	LAD	0.14751	0.20186
		OLS	0.15292	0.15169
40	10	LAD	0.10061	0.15998
		OLS	0.10400	0.14360
	6	LAD	0.15666	0.18604
		OLS	0.15555	0.17129
65	10	LAD	0.11479	0.14447
		OLS	0.11073	0.13048
	6	LAD	0.15084	0.15964
		OLS	0.14880	0.14895
100	10	LAD	0.11799	0.12954
		OLS	0.11559	0.12049
	6	LAD	0.13551	0.13828
		OLS	0.12614	0.12206
160	10	LAD	0.10895	0.11034
		OLS	0.10701	0.10334
	6	LAD	0.11705	0.11682
		OLS	0.09116	0.08748
250	10	LAD	0.09543	0.09467
		OLS	0.08361	0.07840
	6	LAD	0.10046	0.09831
		OLS	0.06166	0.05949
500	10	LAD	0.07177	0.06644
		OLS	0.04617	0.04218
	6	LAD	0.07518	0.07223
		OLS	0.03362	0.03134

estimable single sample values exist only for C2 and C4. For all five tables (Tables 5.51 through 5.55), SD($\hat{\Re}$|C2) is smaller than SD($\hat{\Re}$|C4) for small sample sizes. However, SD($\hat{\Re}$|C2) and SD($\hat{\Re}$|C4) become more similar to one another with increasing sample sizes. Also, for all five tables, the SD($\hat{\Re}$|C2) values are fairly similar for Cases with 10 and 6 predictors; this also holds for the SD($\hat{\Re}$|C4) values. The differences between the LAD and OLS regressions for both SD($\hat{\Re}$|C2) and SD($\hat{\Re}$|C4) are more complex. Whereas SD($\hat{\Re}$|C2) is smaller for LAD regression than for OLS regression with small sample sizes (15, 25, and 40), the SD($\hat{\Re}$|C2) and SD($\hat{\Re}$|C4) values are larger (perhaps slightly) for LAD regression than for OLS regression in Table 5.51. In Tables 5.52 and 5.53, SD($\hat{\Re}$|C2) is smaller for LAD regression than for OLS regression, whereas this observation holds for SD($\hat{\Re}$|C4) only with large sample sizes (250 and 500). In Tables 5.54 and 5.55, both SD($\hat{\Re}$|C2) and SD($\hat{\Re}$|C4) are larger for LAD regression than for OLS regression, except for SD($\hat{\Re}$|C2) with small sample sizes (15, 25, and 40).

5.6.2   Application to the Prediction of African Rainfall

An application of the LAD regression model to forecasting African rainfall is used to illustrate the analysis of temporally ordered response variables. The analysis includes the observed measure of agreement, the measure of agreement corrected for shrinkage based on drop-one cross-validation, P-values of the LAD regression model fit to the predictors, and P-values of the first-order autoregressive patterns for both the response and residual values.

Seasonal rainfall forecasting for the agriculturally dependent Sahel area within North Africa is very important. Of particular interest is an area of the western Sahel defined by Lamb (1978). Five predictors involving the stratospheric quasibiennial oscillation and previous West African precipitation data are utilized to provide the forecasts. Hindcast testing of the predictors in a cross-validation mode using LAD regression yields approximately 54 percent agreement between the predicted and observed rainfall values. The Sahel, lying between approximately 11° and 20° N latitude in Africa, is the region that separates the arid Sahara desert to the north and the rainforest along the Gulf of Guinea and Congo River basin to the south. The Sahel receives substantial precipitation during only three to five months in the summer and early fall. The Lamb (1978) index of precipitation is based on the rainfall in the area bounded by Dakar, Sénégal, on the western tip of Cape Verde at 17.27° W longitude, extending eastward to 10° E longitude and lying between 11° and 18° N latitude.

Table 5.56 lists the data for the dependent variable and five predictors by years, from 1950 to 1991. The first column in Table 5.56 lists the years, and the second column of 1 values provides for the intercept. Columns 3 through 7 contain the values for the five predictors. The first three predictors (U_{50}, U_{30}, and $|U_{50} - U_{30}|$) are based on the quasibiennial oscillation (QBO), which is the stratospheric (16 to 35 km in altitude) oscillation of equatorial east–west winds. These winds vary with a period of about 26 to 30 months, or roughly two years, typically blowing for 12 to 16 months from the east, then reversing and blowing 12 to 16 months from the west, then blowing easterly again. Predictor U_{50} is a 10-month extrapolation (November to September) of the QBO measured by zonal winds in meters per second near 10° to 15° N latitude at 50 millibars (at approximately 20 km in altitude). Predictor U_{30} is a 10-month extrapolation (November to September) of the QBO, measured in meters per second, near 10° to 15° N latitude at 30 millibars (at approximately 23 km in altitude). As a basis for comparison, the top of Mount Everest is approximately 8.85 km (a pressure of about 300 millibars); thus, 30 millibars occurs at 2.6 times the altitude of Mount Everest. Predictor $|U_{50} - U_{30}|$ is the absolute vertical shear between the two QBO measurements U_{50} and U_{30}. Predictor R_s is the August and September rainfall in the western Sahel obtained from 38 measuring stations. The values for R_s in Table 5.56 are the standard deviations from the mean for the western Sahel region between 1950 and 1991. Predictor R_g is the August to November rainfall along the Gulf of Guinea obtained from 24 measuring stations. The values for R_g in Table 5.56 are the standard deviations from the mean for the Gulf of Guinea region between 1950 and 1991. The dependent variable in the rightmost column of Table 5.56 is the April to October rainfall in the Lamb region based on recordings from 20 stations in the region for the years 1950 to 1988, 18 stations in 1989, 16 stations in 1990, and 17 stations in 1991. The values for the dependent variable in Table 5.56 are the standard deviations from the mean for the Lamb region from 1950 to 1991.

The LAD regression model predicting the 1992 Lamb seasonal rainfall is given by

$$\tilde{y} = 0.1997 + 0.01944\, U_{50} - 0.006534\, U_{30} - 0.01205\, |U_{50} - U_{30}|$$

$$+ 0.5803\, R_s + 0.4623\, R_g,$$

where U_{50}, U_{30}, R_s, and R_g denote the 1992 prediction values. Note that $\tilde{y}_I$ for $I = 1, ..., 42$ are the values obtained by substituting the predictor values (U_{50}, U_{30}, R_s, R_g) corresponding to 1950 to 1991, respectively. The MRBP analysis of the model yields $\delta_o = 0.3378$, $\mu = 0.7297$, $\sigma^2 = 0.4158 \times 10^{-2}$, and $\gamma = -0.8693 \times 10^{-1}$, where δ_o denotes the observed value of δ. The estimated measure of agreement is $\hat{\Re} = 0.5371$, and the estimated $\Re$ adjusted for shrinkage based on drop-one cross-validation is $\hat{\Re} = 0.3658$. The resampling ($L = 1,000,000$) and Pearson type III approximate P-values of the LAD regression model fit are 0.0000 and 0.9174×10^{-8}, respectively.

The first-order autoregressive resampling ($L = 1,000,000$) and Pearson type III approximate P-values (see Section 3.1) for the temporally ordered

TABLE 5.56. Lamb region rainfall precipitation by years with predictors U_{50}, U_{30}, $|U_{50} - U_{30}|$, R_s, and R_g .

| Year | Intercept | Predictor | | | | | Rainfall |
		U_{50}	U_{30}	$|U_{50} - U_{30}|$	R_s	R_g	
1950	1	−3	−3	0	−0.14	1.07	1.05
1951	1	−4	−13	9	1.68	−0.66	0.74
1952	1	−23	−26	3	0.49	0.65	1.45
1953	1	0	−18	18	0.93	0.41	0.99
1954	1	−23	−32	9	0.20	−0.16	1.12
1955	1	0	−4	4	0.60	0.64	1.07
1956	1	−19	−33	14	1.00	0.41	0.36
1957	1	−2	−3	1	0.47	−0.36	0.87
1958	1	−12	−28	16	0.58	1.03	0.86
1959	1	−9	−5	4	1.45	−0.74	0.30
1960	1	−6	−21	15	0.25	0.12	0.24
1961	1	−3	−3	0	0.23	1.05	0.20
1962	1	−12	−32	20	0.48	−0.74	0.41
1963	1	−17	−3	14	0.28	0.73	0.22
1964	1	−4	−18	14	−0.12	1.18	0.76
1965	1	−23	−32	9	0.59	−0.68	0.48
1966	1	−9	−2	7	0.75	−0.17	0.31
1967	1	−8	−25	17	0.34	−0.14	0.45
1968	1	−23	−14	9	0.72	−0.51	−0.34
1969	1	0	−9	9	−0.82	1.28	0.48
1970	1	−12	−30	18	0.38	−0.31	−0.35
1971	1	−3	−2	1	−0.45	−0.23	−0.50
1972	1	−8	−31	23	−0.19	−0.40	−0.88
1973	1	−5	−5	0	−1.10	−0.88	−0.91
1974	1	−14	−32	18	−0.72	−0.43	−0.31
1975	1	−5	−2	3	−0.04	−0.08	0.22
1976	1	−6	−21	15	0.06	−0.55	−0.18
1977	1	−21	−24	3	−0.50	−0.59	−0.96
1978	1	−2	−9	7	−0.75	−0.50	−0.05
1979	1	−19	−31	12	−0.36	−0.73	−0.41
1980	1	−5	−1	4	−0.92	0.55	−0.36
1981	1	−8	−30	22	−0.34	0.36	−0.53
1982	1	−21	−5	16	−0.44	−0.93	−0.84
1983	1	−2	−13	11	−0.90	−0.61	−1.28
1984	1	−23	−14	9	−1.24	−1.32	−1.23
1985	1	−2	−9	7	−1.23	0.04	−0.56
1986	1	−12	−32	20	−0.51	0.13	−0.71

(Table 5.56 continued on next page.)

TABLE 5.56. (continued from previous page).

Year	Intercept	Predictor					
		U_{50}	U_{30}	$|U_{50} - U_{30}|$	R_s	R_g	Rainfall
1987	1	-21	-9	12	-0.01	-0.48	-0.95
1988	1	-3	-13	10	-0.63	1.37	0.10
1989	1	-23	-32	9	0.29	0.35	-0.18
1990	1	-1	-2	1	0.10	0.19	-0.76
1991	1	-12	-30	18	-0.79	-0.57	-0.40

response variables $(y_1, ..., y_{42})$ and residuals $(\tilde{e}_1, ..., \tilde{e}_{42})$ are $(0.0000$ and $0.3837 \times 10^{-7})$ and $(0.6922$ and $0.6945)$, respectively, where $\tilde{e}_I = y_I - \tilde{y}_I$ for $I = 1, ..., 42$ denote the 42 residuals of the LAD regression model. Thus, the LAD regression model compensates for the strong first-order autoregressive pattern of the temporally ordered sequence of response variables.

5.6.3   Linear and Nonlinear Multivariate Regression Models

Consider r response (i.e., dependent) and m predictor (i.e., independent) regression model variables for each of N observable cases. Thus, $r + m$ values are associated with each of N cases. While rm parameters are associated with a linear regression model, assume that t parameters are associated with a nonlinear regression model. The linear and nonlinear regression models are given by

$$\mathbf{Y} = \mathbf{XB} + \mathbf{E}$$

and .

$$\mathbf{Y} = \mathbf{H}(\boldsymbol{\gamma}, \mathbf{X}) + \mathbf{E},$$

respectively, where $\mathbf{Y} = \{y_{Ik}\}$ is an $N \times r$ response matrix, $\mathbf{B} = \{\beta_{jk}\}$ is an $m \times r$ parameter matrix, $\mathbf{X} = \{x_{Ij}\}$ is an $N \times m$ predictor matrix, $\mathbf{H} = \{h_{Ik}\}$ is an $N \times r$ nonlinear matrix of parametric functions, $\boldsymbol{\gamma} = (\gamma_1, ..., \gamma_t)$ is a set of t parameters, and $\mathbf{E} = \{e_{Ik}\}$ is an $N \times r$ error matrix (Mielke and Berry, 1997b, 2003).

Let L_p^v denote the regression model that includes values of $\mathbf{B}$ and γ that minimize

$$\left[\sum_{I=1}^{N} \left(\sum_{k=1}^{r} |e_{Ik}|^p \right)^{v/p} \right]^{1/v},$$

where $p \geq 1$ and $v \geq 1$. In this context, the LAD (LSED) and OLS regression models are associated with L_2^1 and L_2^2, respectively. Since (1) regressions are invariant under rotation only when $p = 2$ and (2) regressions possess metric-based interpretations only when $v = 1$, graphically interpretable results in an r-dimensional Euclidean space occur only when

$p = 2$ and $v = 1$ (Mielke, 1987; Mielke and Berry, 2003). The algorithm by Kaufman et al. (2002) yields the L_2^1 linear regression prediction model.

If $\mathbf{Y}$ and $\tilde{\mathbf{Y}} = \{\tilde{y}_{Ik}\}$ denote the observed and predicted r-dimensional response values for N cases, respectively, then the average Euclidean distance between $\mathbf{Y}$ and $\tilde{\mathbf{Y}}$ is given by

$$\delta = \frac{1}{N} \sum_{I=1}^{N} \left[\sum_{k=1}^{r} (y_{Ik} - \tilde{y}_{Ik})^2 \right]^{1/2}.$$

The chance-corrected measure of agreement between $\mathbf{Y}$ and $\tilde{\mathbf{Y}}$ is given by

$$\Re = 1 - \frac{\delta}{\mu},$$

where μ is the expected value of δ under H_0 that all of the $N!$ sequences occur with equal probability. This is obtained by comparing the observed sequence of r-dimensional row vectors $\mathbf{y}_1, ..., \mathbf{y}_N$ with the $N!$ permutations of the predicted sequence of r-dimensional row vectors $\tilde{\mathbf{y}}_1, ..., \tilde{\mathbf{y}}_N$. Thus, μ is given by

$$\mu = \frac{1}{N!} \sum_{i=1}^{N!} \delta_i,$$

where δ_i denotes the ith among $N!$ values of δ. Note that $\Re = 1$ implies perfect agreement between the observed and model-predicted response vectors and the expected value of $\Re$ is 0 under H_0, i.e., chance corrected. Since the present permutation structure is a special case of MRBP where $b = 2$ and $g = N$, an efficient algorithm for computing μ is given in Section 4.1. In addition, the P-value associated with the observed values of $\Re$ and δ ($\Re_o$ and δ_o) is given by

$$P\left(\Re \geq \Re_o \mid H_0\right) = P\left(\delta \leq \delta_o \mid H_0\right),$$

and either a resampling or a Pearson type III P-value approximation is given in Section 4.1.

The exact P value regarding how extreme δ_o is relative to the $N!$ equally likely δ values under H_0 is given by

$$P\text{-value} = \frac{\text{number of } \delta \text{ values} \leq \delta_o}{N!}.$$

Since $N!$ is usually very large, approximate P-values may be based on either (1) a resampling approximation involving L random samples of the $N!$ equally likely pairings of the observed and model-predicted vectors under H_0, or (2) a moment approximation based on the Pearson type III distribution that is characterized by the exact mean, denoted by μ, variance, and skewness of δ under H_0.

TABLE 5.57. Example data set for multivariate multiple prediction with response variables SAT–V (y_{I1}) and SAT–M (y_{I2}) and predictor variables intercept (x_{I1}), urban high school (x_{I2}), suburban high school (x_{I3}), and GPA (x_{I4}).

| | Variables | | | | | |
| | Response | | Predictor | | | |
Student	y_{I1}	y_{I2}	x_{I1}	x_{I2}	x_{I3}	x_{I4}
1	400	450	1	1	0	2.35
2	620	460	1	1	0	3.16
3	410	420	1	1	0	2.11
4	450	440	1	1	0	2.57
5	480	580	1	1	0	2.50
6	490	410	1	1	0	3.13
7	510	460	1	1	0	3.15
8	540	600	1	1	0	3.76
9	490	580	1	0	1	2.62
10	520	680	1	0	1	2.40
11	530	660	1	0	1	3.61
12	680	700	1	0	1	3.74
13	700	640	1	0	1	3.72
14	720	740	1	0	1	3.93
15	520	600	1	0	1	2.86
16	440	510	1	0	0	2.36
17	520	650	1	0	0	2.84
18	500	500	1	0	0	3.12
19	530	480	1	0	0	3.20
20	600	480	1	0	0	3.01

TABLE 5.58. Unstandardized regression coefficients for two response variables and four predictor variables.

j	$\tilde{\beta}_{j1}$	$\tilde{\beta}_{j2}$
1	166.1	421.9
2	−16.7	−61.4
3	63.3	142.2
4	116.5	31.9

TABLE 5.59. Observed (y_{Ik}) and model-predicted $(\hat{y}_{Ik})$ response variables based on four predictors $(x_{I1}, ..., x_{I4})$ and the estimated unstandardized regression coefficients $(\hat{\beta}_{jk})$ in Table 5.58.

| | Response Variable | | | |
| | SAT–V | | SAT–M | |
Student	y_{I1}	$\hat{y}_{I1}$	y_{I2}	$\hat{y}_{I2}$
1	400	423.0	450	435.5
2	620	517.4	460	461.3
3	410	395.1	420	427.8
4	450	448.7	440	442.5
5	480	440.5	580	440.3
6	490	513.9	410	460.4
7	510	516.2	460	461.0
8	540	587.3	600	480.5
9	490	534.5	580	647.7
10	520	508.9	680	640.7
11	530	649.9	660	679.3
12	680	665.0	700	683.5
13	700	662.7	640	682.8
14	720	687.1	740	689.5
15	520	562.5	600	655.4
16	440	440.9	510	497.2
17	520	496.8	650	512.5
18	500	529.4	500	521.4
19	530	538.8	480	524.0
20	600	516.6	480	517.9

Example

To illustrate a prediction utilizing multivariate multiple regression, consider a simple example to predict verbal and mathematics SAT scores (SAT–V, SAT–M) for 20 high school seniors based on location of high school (Urban, Suburban, Rural) and high school grade point average (GPA). In this instance, $N = 20$, $r = 2$, $m = 4$, y_{I1} and y_{I2} are the SAT–V and SAT–M scores, respectively, $x_{I1} = 1$ for the intercept, $x_{I2} = 1$ if the Ith student attends an urban high school and 0 otherwise, $x_{I3} = 1$ if the Ith student attends a suburban high school and 0 otherwise, and x_{I4} is the high school GPA for $I = 1, ..., 20$. Table 5.57 lists the $r = 2$ response and $m = 4$ predictor variables for the 20 selected high school seniors. The $\hat{\beta}_{jk}$ estimated unstandardized regression coefficients for the model-predicted values of y_{Ik} are given in Table 5.58 for $j = 1, 2, 3, 4$, $k = 1, 2$, and $I = 1, ..., 20$. Table 5.59 lists the model-predicted values $\hat{y}_{I1}$ and $\hat{y}_{I2}$ based on the estimated unstandardized regression coefficients for $I = 1, ..., 20$. The analysis of the data in Table 5.57 yields $\delta_o = 63.15$, $\mu = 158.11$, $\Re_o = 0.60$, and a P-value of $.2083 \times 10^{-5}$, using the Pearson type III approximation, where δ_o and $\Re_o$ are the observed values of δ and $\Re$, respectively. Due to the small P-value, a resampling approximation would require a very large number of random samples to obtain even a few significant digits.

The chance-corrected measure of agreement ($\Re$) and MRBP provide a basis for improving the fit of exceedingly complicated nonlinear multivariate regression model predictions with observed data. In the field of atmospheric science, examples include mesoscale, satellite imagery, land ecosystem–atmosphere feedback, geopotential height, and precipitation model predictions (Cotton et al., 1994; Kelly et al., 1989; Lee et al., 1996; Tucker et al., 1989).

6
Goodness-of-Fit Tests

Goodness-of-fit techniques are essential for determining whether or not hypothetical models fit observed data. When at all reasonable, exact goodness-of-fit tests are preferred to either nonasymptotic or, especially, asymptotic tests. In addition, the structures of these goodness-of-fit tests yield entirely different detection capabilities for varying alternatives. A selection of techniques is considered for both discrete and continuous data, along with examples and simulations intended to emphasize the differences in detection capabilities. The discrete data tests are further partitioned into exact tests (including Fisher's exact test) and approximate tests, including those based on the Pearson (1900) χ^2 and Zelterman (1987) statistics. Specific concerns regarding these discrete data tests are described. Continuous data tests due to Greenwood–Moran (Greenwood, 1946; Moran, 1947), Kendall–Sherman (Kendall, 1946; Sherman, 1950), Kolmogorov (1933), Smirnov (1939a), and Fisher (1929) are included. Simulated comparisons of the Kendall–Sherman and Kolmogorov tests are given.

6.1 Discrete Data Goodness-of-Fit Tests

Consider the random assignment of n objects to k cells where the probability that any of the n objects occurs in the ith cell is $p_i > 0$ $(i = 1, ..., k)$. Then the probability that o_i objects occur in the ith cell for $i = 1, ..., k$ is the multinomial probability given by

$$P\left(o_i \mid n, \, p_i\right) = P\left(o_1, ..., o_k \mid n, \, p_1, ..., p_k\right) = \left(n! \bigg/ \prod_{i=1}^{k} o_i!\right) \prod_{i=1}^{k} p_i^{o_i},$$

where

$$\sum_{i=1}^{k} p_i = 1$$

and

$$\sum_{i=1}^{k} o_i = n.$$

The discrete goodness-of-fit tests presented here are applicable even when the values of $p_1, ..., p_k$ are estimated by fitting population model parameters from the sample data.

6.1.1   Fisher's Exact Tests

The P-value associated with Fisher's exact test is the sum of all distinct $P(o_i \mid n, \, p_i)$ values that are as small or smaller than the value of $P(o_i \mid n, \, p_i)$ associated with a set of observed cell frequencies. The null hypothesis (H_0) states that $p_1, ..., p_k$ are known positive values. Under H_0, $P(o_i \mid n, \, p_i)$ is a statistic. If a P-value is sufficiently small (e.g., less than 0.01), then it may be reasonable to reject H_0. Efficient programs exist for finding P-values when $k \leq 6$ (Mielke and Berry, 1993).[1] The efficiency of these programs involves (1) a recursive procedure over the

$$M = \binom{n + k - 1}{k - 1}$$

distinct configurations for $P(o_i \mid n, \, p_i)$, (2) initialization of the recursive procedure at an arbitrary starting value such as 10^{-200}, and (3) the require-ment that the recursive procedure depends only on elementary addition, subtraction, multiplication, and division operations. The only reason for not obtaining P-values in this manner for all discrete data goodness-of-fit tests is the amount of computational time when M becomes excessively large. In addition to Fisher's exact test, other exact tests may be obtained by summing all values of $P(o_i \mid n, \, p_i)$ associated with a selected statistic (e.g., the Pearson χ^2, Zelterman, and likelihood-ratio statistics) that are as extreme or more extreme than the observed value of the selected statistic.

---

[1] Adapted and reprinted with permission of Sage Publications, Inc. from P.W. Mielke, Jr. and K.J. Berry. Exact goodness-of-fit probability tests for analyzing categorical data. *Educational and Psychological Measurement*, 1993, 53, 707–710. Copyright © 1993 by Sage Publications, Inc.

However, the choice of $P(o_i \,|\, n,\, p_i)$ as the selected statistic seems far more intuitive for the present purpose than any other statistic.

The multinomial algorithm description is illustrated with $k = 4$. Let $o_1 = x$, $o_2 = y$, $o_3 = z$, and $o_4 = n - x - y - z$. Since n and $k = 4$ are fixed, the cell frequencies are totally described by x, y, and z. If the order specification of x, y, and z implies that z depends on x and y, and y depends on x, then the following bounds hold for x, y, and z:

$$0 \leq x \leq n,$$

$$0 \leq y \leq n - x,$$

and

$$0 \leq z \leq n - x - y.$$

In accordance with the defined order specification of x, y, and z, the conditional recursively-defined probability adjustments from (x_1, y_1, z_1) in step 1 of the recursion to (x_2, y_2, z_2) in step 2 of the recursion are given by

$$\frac{P\left(x_2,\, y_2,\, z_2 \,|\, n,\, p_1,\, p_2,\, p_3\right)}{P\left(x_1,\, y_1,\, z_1 \,|\, n,\, p_1,\, p_2,\, p_3\right)},$$

where

$$P\left(x,\, y,\, z \,|\, n,\, p_1,\, p_2,\, p_3\right) = \frac{n!\, p_1^x\, p_2^y\, p_3^z\, \left(1 - p_1 - p_2 - p_3\right)^{n-x-y-z}}{x!\, y!\, z!\, (n - x - y - z)!}.$$

Starting with an arbitrarily-defined machine-dependent initial value (e.g., 10^{-200}), the algorithm consists of two distinct steps. The first step involves $n - o_k$ recursions to obtain the value associated with the observed frequency configuration, and the second step involves M recursions to obtain the exact P-value. For $k = 4$, the first step obtains the value

$$H\left(x_o,\, y_o,\, z_o\right) = D \times P\left(x_o,\, y_o,\, z_o \,|\, n,\, p_1,\, p_2,\, p_3\right),$$

where D is the initial value, and x_o, y_o, and z_o are the observed values of x, y, and z, respectively. The second step determines (1) the conditional sum, S, of the recursively defined values of

$$H\left(x,\, y,\, z\right) = D \times P\left(x,\, y,\, z \,|\, n,\, p_1,\, p_2,\, p_3\right)$$

satisfying $H(x,\, y,\, z) \leq H(x_o,\, y_o,\, z_o)$, and (2) the unconditional sum, T, of all M values of $H(x,\, y,\, z)$. The exact P-value associated with the observed frequencies x_o, y_o, and z_o is given by S/T.

Example

To illustrate the multinomial algorithm, consider an example where $n = 10$ learning-disabled elementary school children are classified into $k = 4$ categories of learning disability with $o_1 = 4$, $o_2 = 3$, $o_3 = 2$, and $o_4 = 1$. Previous research indicates the expected proportions to be $p_1 = 0.18$, $p_2 = 0.12$, $p_3 = 0.40$, and $p_4 = 0.30$. Under the null hypothesis of no difference between the observed and expected frequencies, the exact P-value is 0.3613×10^{-1}.

Category

	1	2	3	4
o_i	4	3	2	1
p_i	0.18	0.12	0.40	0.30

6.1.2   Exact Test When $p_i = 1/k$ for $i = 1, ..., k$

If $p_i = 1/k$ for $i = 1, ..., k$, then the computation for exact tests can be made much more efficient (Berry et al., 2004).[2] This improved efficiency is based on a 1748 result by Euler that provides a generating function for the number of decompositions of n into integer summands without regard to order using the recurrence relation

$$\psi(n) = \sum_{j=1}(-1)^{j-1}\psi\left[n - \left(3j^2 \pm j\right)/2\right],$$

where $\psi(0) = 1$ and j is a positive integer satisfying $2 \leq 3j^2 \pm j \leq 2n$ (Euler, 1748/1988, pp. 256–282). Note that if $n = 1$, then $j = 1$ with only the − sign allowed; if $2 \leq n \leq 4$, then $j = 1$ with both the + and − signs allowed; if $5 \leq n \leq 6$, then $j = 1$ with both the + and − signs allowed; and $j = 2$ with only the − sign allowed; and so forth. As defined, $\psi(n)$ denotes the number of partitions of n into distinct parts. Incidentally, Hardy and Ramanujan (1918) obtained the asymptotic approximation for $\psi(n)$ and Rademacher (1937) obtained an exact infinite sum for $\psi(n)$.

---

[2]Adapted and reprinted with permission of Perceptual and Motor Skills from K.J. Berry, J.E. Johnston, and P.W. Mielke, Jr. Exact goodness-of-fit tests for unordered equiprobable categories. *Perceptual and Motor Skills*, 2004, 98, 909–919. Copyright © 2004 by Perceptual and Motor Skills.

Given the observed categorical frequencies $o_1, ..., o_k$, the multinomial weight W associated with each of the $\psi(n)$ partitions is given by

$$W = \frac{k!}{\prod\limits_{i=1}^{m} f_i!},$$

where f_i is the frequency for the ith of m distinct numbers comprising a partition. For example, if the observed partition is $\{3\ 2\ 2\ 1\ 0\ 0\}$ where $n = 8$, $k = 6$, and $m = 4$, then $f_1 = 1$, $f_2 = 2$, $f_3 = 1$, $f_4 = 2$, and $W = 180$. If $k \geq n$, then the number of distinct partitions is $\psi(n)$. If $k < n$, then the number of distinct partitions is less than $\psi(n)$ since those partitions where the number of positive values exceeds k are eliminated. For example, if $k = 3$ and $n = 5$, then the two partitions $\{2\ 1\ 1\ 1\}$ and $\{1\ 1\ 1\ 1\ 1\}$ cannot be considered since they contain four and five positive partition values that exceed $k = 3$, respectively. The sum of the values of W for the included distinct partitions is equal to M.

Three Examples

In the first example, suppose that $n = k = 8$. If the eight observed categorical frequencies are $o_1 = o_2 = 3$, $o_3 = 2$, and $o_4 = o_5 = o_6 = o_7 = o_8 = 0$, then the number of distinct ordered configurations is $M = 6{,}435$. Here, H_0 specifies that $p_i = 1/8$ for $i = 1, ..., 8$. Table 6.1 lists the $\psi(8) = 22$ distinct unordered partitions of the $n = 8$ events and $k = 8$ categories, the partition probabilities, the multinomial weight for each partition, and the weighted partition probabilities.

For the second example, let $n = 45$ and $k = 20$. If the 20 observed categorical frequencies are $o_1 = o_2 = o_3 = 6$, $o_4 = 5$, $o_5 = 4$, $o_6 = 3$, $o_7 = 2$, and $o_8 = \cdots = o_{20} = 1$, then the number of distinct ordered configurations is $M \doteq 0.8720 \times 10^{16}$. Now H_0 implies that $p_i = 1/20$ for $i = 1, ..., 20$, and $\psi(45) = 89{,}134$ exceeds the number of included distinct unordered partitions given by 81,801 since $k < n$.

The third example considers $n = 10$ and $k = 50$. If the $k = 50$ observed categorical frequencies are $o_1 = 4$, $o_2 = 3$, $o_3 = 2$, $o_4 = 1$, and $o_5 = \cdots = o_{50} = 0$, then the number of distinct ordered configurations is $M \doteq 0.6283 \times 10^{11}$. In this example, H_0 states that $p_i = 1/50$ for $i = 1, ..., 50$ and the number of distinct unordered partitions is $\psi(10) = 42$ since $k > n$.

6.1.3 Nonasymptotic Tests

Approximate tests in the present nonasymptotic context include the resampling and Pearson type III P-value approximations (see Section 2.3). While the resampling P-value approximation based on L random replications is reasonable when a P-value is not too small (say, at least 0.001),

TABLE 6.1. Partitions, exact partition probabilities, multinomial weights, and exact weighted probabilities for $n = 8$ and $k = 8$.

Number	Partition	Partition Probability	Multinomial Weight	Weighted Probability
1	1 1 1 1 1 1 1 1	$.2403 \times 10^{-2}$	1	$.2403 \times 10^{-2}$
2	2 1 1 1 1 1 1 0	$.1202 \times 10^{-2}$	56	$.6729 \times 10^{-1}$
3	2 2 1 1 1 1 0 0	$.6008 \times 10^{-3}$	420	$.2523$
4	2 2 2 1 1 0 0 0	$.3004 \times 10^{-3}$	560	$.1682$
5	2 2 2 2 0 0 0 0	$.1502 \times 10^{-3}$	70	$.1051 \times 10^{-1}$
6	3 1 1 1 1 1 0 0	$.4005 \times 10^{-3}$	168	$.6729 \times 10^{-1}$
7	3 2 1 1 1 0 0 0	$.2003 \times 10^{-3}$	1120	$.2243$
8	3 2 2 1 0 0 0 0	$.1001 \times 10^{-3}$	840	$.8411 \times 10^{-1}$
9	3 3 1 1 0 0 0 0	$.6676 \times 10^{-4}$	420	$.2804 \times 10^{-1}$
*10	3 3 2 0 0 0 0 0	$.3338 \times 10^{-4}$	168	$.5608 \times 10^{-2}$
11	4 1 1 1 1 0 0 0	$.1001 \times 10^{-3}$	280	$.2804 \times 10^{-1}$
12	4 2 1 1 0 0 0 0	$.5007 \times 10^{-4}$	840	$.4206 \times 10^{-1}$
13	4 2 2 0 0 0 0 0	$.2503 \times 10^{-4}$	168	$.4206 \times 10^{-2}$
14	4 3 1 0 0 0 0 0	$.1669 \times 10^{-4}$	336	$.5608 \times 10^{-2}$
15	4 4 0 0 0 0 0 0	$.4172 \times 10^{-5}$	28	$.1168 \times 10^{-3}$
16	5 1 1 1 0 0 0 0	$.2003 \times 10^{-4}$	280	$.5608 \times 10^{-2}$
17	5 2 1 0 0 0 0 0	$.1001 \times 10^{-4}$	336	$.3365 \times 10^{-2}$
18	5 3 0 0 0 0 0 0	$.3338 \times 10^{-5}$	56	$.1869 \times 10^{-3}$
19	6 1 1 0 0 0 0 0	$.3338 \times 10^{-5}$	168	$.5608 \times 10^{-3}$
20	6 2 0 0 0 0 0 0	$.1669 \times 10^{-5}$	56	$.9346 \times 10^{-4}$
21	7 1 0 0 0 0 0 0	$.4768 \times 10^{-6}$	56	$.2670 \times 10^{-4}$
22	8 0 0 0 0 0 0 0	$.5960 \times 10^{-7}$	8	$.4768 \times 10^{-6}$

*Observed categorical frequencies for Example 1 are identified with an asterisk.

the Pearson type III approximation requires the possibility of obtaining the exact mean, variance, and skewness of a selected statistic under H_0. For example, consider the broad class of statistics indexed by λ (Cressie and Read, 1984) given by

$$2I^{\lambda} = \frac{2}{\lambda(\lambda + 1)} \sum_{i=1}^{k} o_i \left[\left(\frac{o_i}{e_i} \right)^{\lambda} - 1 \right],$$

where $e_i = np_i$ is the expected value of o_i under H_0 and λ is a real number. Approximate P-value estimates may be obtained with a resampling algorithm for any discrete goodness-of-fit test. Whereas the limit of $2I^{\lambda}$ is the log-likelihood-ratio test for the case when $\lambda \to 0$, and many other well-known tests are included for special cases of λ, only $\lambda = 1$ (where $2I^{\lambda}$ is the Pearson χ^2 statistic) yields a case where the exact mean, variance, and skewness of $2I^{\lambda}$ have been obtained under H_0. The exact mean, variance, and skewness under H_0 of a statistic outside the previous class (Zelterman,

1987) have also been obtained. Convenient representations of the Pearson χ^2 and Zelterman statistics (Mielke and Berry, 1988) are given by

$$T = \sum_{i=1}^{k} \frac{o_i^2}{e_i}$$

and

$$S = \sum_{i=1}^{k} \frac{o_i (o_i - 1)}{e_i},$$

respectively. Under H_0, the asymptotic distribution of both $\chi^2 = T - n$ and $\zeta = S + k - n$ is chi-squared with $k - 1$ degrees-of-freedom. The exact mean, variance, and skewness of T under H_0 are given by

$$\mu_T = k + n - 1,$$

$$\sigma_T^2 = 2(k - 1) + \left[3 - (k + 1)^2 + \sum_{i=1}^{k} p_i^{-1} \right] \Big/ n,$$

and

$$\gamma_T = \frac{A}{\sigma_T^3},$$

respectively, where

$$A = 8(k - 1) - \left[2n(3k - 2)(3k + 8) - 2(k + 3)(k^2 + 6k - 4) \right.$$

$$\left. - (22n - 3k - 22) \sum_{i=1}^{k} p_i^{-1} - \sum_{i=1}^{k} p_i^{-2} \right] \Big/ n^2.$$

The exact mean, variance, and skewness of S under H_0 are given by

$$\mu_S = n - 1,$$

$$\sigma_S^2 = \frac{2(n - 1)(k - 1)}{n},$$

and

$$\gamma_S = \frac{B}{\sigma_S^3},$$

respectively, where

$$B = 4(n - 1) \left[2n(k - 1) - 7k + 6 + \sum_{i=1}^{k} p_i^{-1} \right] \Big/ n^2.$$

If T_o and S_o denote observed values of T and S, then the approximate P-values given by

$$P\left(T \geq T_o \mid H_0\right)$$

and

$$P\left(S \geq S_o \mid H_0\right),$$

respectively, utilize the Pearson type III distribution for evaluation (Berry and Mielke, 1994). A choice between T and S is suggested by calculating the mean of each statistic under an alternative hypothesis (H_1). Suppose the probability under H_1 that any of the n objects occurs in cell i is $r_i \geq 0$ $(i = 1, ..., k)$, where

$$\sum_{i=1}^{k} r_i = 1.$$

Then, the mean of T under H_1 is

$$E\left[T \mid H_1\right] = n + k - 1 + \sum_{i=1}^{k} (r_i - p_i)\left[1 + (n-1)(r_i - p_i)\right] p_i^{-1},$$

and the mean of S under H_1 is

$$E\left[S \mid H_1\right] = n - 1 + (n-1)\sum_{i=1}^{k} (r_i - p_i)^2 p_i^{-1}.$$

If H_0 and H_1 are specifically defined by $p_i = \epsilon/(k-1)$, $r_i = 0$ for $i = 1, ..., k-1$, $p_k = 1 - \epsilon$, and $r_k = 1$, where $0 < \epsilon < 1$, then $E[T \mid H_1] = \epsilon n/(1-\epsilon) < n + k - 1$ when $0 < \epsilon < (k-1)/(n+k-1)$ and $E[S \mid H_1] = (n-1)/(1-\epsilon) > n - 1$ for all ϵ. Although $E[S \mid H_1] > \mu_S$ is always true, the fact that $E[T \mid H_1] < \mu_T$ can occur provides a reason to choose S over T.

The exact, nonasymptotic, and asymptotic discrete goodness-of-fit tests considered here are inappropriate for continuous data because (1) the selection of k is subjective, and (2) the placement of $k - 1$ partition values is subjective after k is selected. Thus, objectively defined goodness-of-fit tests are essential for cases involving continuous data.

The classical asymptotic Pearson χ^2 goodness-of-fit test is known to perform poorly for cases with small expected category frequencies. A nonasymptotic algorithm for statistics T and S can be constructed to test for goodness-of-fit between the observed category frequencies and the corresponding a priori category probabilities (Berry and Mielke, 1994). The algorithm begins by first calculating the observed values of T and S, designated T_o and S_o, and then calculating the exact mean (μ_T, μ_S), variance (σ_T^2, σ_S^2), and skewness term (γ_T, γ_S) of T and S under H_0, respectively. Finally, the algorithm computes the P-values associated with T and S under H_0 given by

$$P_{T_o} = P\left(T \geq T_o \mid H_0\right)$$

and

$$P_{S_o} = P\left(S \geq S_o \mid H_0\right),$$

respectively, based on the Pearson type III distribution.

The adjustments for the nonasymptotic goodness-of-fit tests based on the statistics T and S involving the three exact cumulants under H_0 obviate the usual concerns regarding small expected category frequencies when using the commonly employed asymptotic version of T (i.e., the Pearson χ^2 distributions and their degrees-of-freedom conditions), even when parameters are fit from the observed frequency data. Furthermore, the use of Fisher's exact goodness-of-fit test also eliminates these concerns.

Despite the fact that T and S appear quite similar, they behave very differently when small sample sizes are encountered. Whenever

$$\binom{n+k-1}{k-1}$$

is not too large, Fisher's exact goodness-of-fit test (Mielke and Berry, 1993) should be used. However, when

$$\binom{n+k-1}{k-1}$$

is large, the test based on statistic S rather than statistic T may be preferred for the reason noted earlier regarding the expected value of T under H_1. A subsequent example in this section illustrates a concern pertaining to tests based on statistic S. The exact and nonasymptotic tests analogous to T and S (Berry and Mielke, 1989; Mielke and Berry, 1988, 1993) for analyzing independence in r-way contingency tables also eliminate the degrees-of-freedom problem inherent in the classical asymptotic Pearson χ^2 goodness-of-fit test.

To illustrate the use of statistics T and S, consider an example where $n = 208$ northern European adults are classified into $k = 7$ categorical blood groupings on the Rh system (Berry and Mielke, 1994). Table 6.2 lists seven Rh blood groupings using the Fisher–Race notation, along with the category probabilities (Race and Sanger, 1975, p. 184). Because the Rh haplotype CdE has such a low expected value among northern Europeans, it has been dropped from the list of eight possible Fisher–Race categories for this example. Let T_o and S_o denote the observed values of T and S, respectively. Under the null hypothesis of no difference between the observed and expected frequencies, $T_o = 221.1010$, $\mu_T = 214.0000$, $\sigma_T^2 = 14.8495$, $\gamma_T = 2.0217$, and $P_{T_o} = 0.5829 \times 10^{-1}$, while $S_o = 212.7500$, $\mu_S = 207.0000$, $\sigma_S^2 = 11.9423$, $\gamma_S = 1.4407$, and $P_{S_o} = 0.6898 \times 10^{-1}$. The corresponding approximate resampling P-values associated with T_o and S_o are 0.5275×10^{-1} and 0.6101×10^{-1}, respectively, based on $L = 1{,}000{,}000$.

TABLE 6.2. Observed frequencies and expected probabilities for seven blood groupings on the Rh System for 208 northern European adults using the Fisher–Race notation.

Haplotype	Observed frequency	Expected probability
CDe	98	0.4205
cDE	24	0.1411
cDe	12	0.0257
CDE	1	0.0024
Cde	1	0.0098
cdE	2	0.0119
cde	70	0.3886

6.1.4 Informative Examples

For the case in which $k = 3$, $N = 26$, $p_1 = 0.9$, $p_2 = 0.099$, and $p_3 = 0.001$, Table 6.3 shows that the four different exact goodness-of-fit tests treat the same frequency array in disparate ways. For example, the P-values vary from 0.01890 for the exact χ^2 test to 1.00000 for the exact Zelterman test in frequency array $(22, 3, 1)$. In addition, the P-values associated with the Fisher exact, exact likelihood-ratio, and exact χ^2 tests vary drastically, with minor changes in the frequency arrays. Examination of the frequency arrays of Table 6.3 shows, first, that the Zelterman tests are questionable due to their inability to distinguish between frequency values of 0 and 1 and, second, that the asymptotic χ^2 P-values may be off by large orders of magnitude from the corresponding exact χ^2 P-values. Besides the fact that the nonasymptotic χ^2 test may be much better than the asymptotic χ^2 test, the nonasymptotic χ^2 P-value may also differ from the exact χ^2 P-value when extreme frequency and probability configurations are encountered. The results of Table 6.3 show that, whenever possible, exact tests should be used when discrepant frequency arrays and/or probabilities are involved. In contrast, Table 6.4 with $k = 3$, $p_1 = 0.5$, $p_2 = 0.3$, and $p_3 = 0.2$ indicates that all the exact and nonasymptotic P-values converge quite rapidly to the asymptotic χ^2 P-value with larger frequency values and when discrepant conditions are not encountered.

6.2 Continuous Data Goodness-of-Fit Tests

Three types of objectively-defined goodness-of-fit tests are described for the analysis of continuous data. The null hypothesis (H_0) for each test specifies that $F(x)$ is a known cumulative distribution function for the continuous data in question. The first type is a matching test due to Smirnov (1939a), the second type is a test based on the empirical cumulative distribution

TABLE 6.3. P-value comparisons among Fisher's exact (FE), exact likelihood-ratio (ELR), exact χ^2 (Eχ^2), exact Zelterman (EZ), nonasymptotic χ^2 (Nχ^2), nonasymptotic Zelterman (NZ), and asymptotic χ^2 (Aχ^2) for three data sets specified by (o_1, o_2, o_3) when $k = 3$, $p_1 = 0.9$, $p_2 = 0.099$, and $p_3 = 0.001$.

Test	$(24, 2, 0)$	$(23, 3, 0)$	$(22, 3, 1)$
FE	1.00000	0.74592	0.02165
ELR	0.77641	1.00000	0.02993
Eχ^2	0.77641	1.00000	0.01890
EZ	0.75373	0.97892	1.00000
Nχ^2	1.00000	1.00000	0.00785
NZ	1.00000	1.00000	1.00000
Aχ^2	0.91879	0.94964	0.11×10^{-7}

TABLE 6.4. P-value comparisons among Fisher's exact (FE), exact likelihood-ratio (ELR), exact χ^2 (Eχ^2), exact Zelterman (EZ), nonasymptotic χ^2 (Nχ^2), nonasymptotic Zelterman (NZ), and asymptotic χ^2 (Aχ^2) for three data sets specified by (o_1, o_2, o_3) when $k = 3$, $p_1 = 0.5$, $p_2 = 0.3$, and $p_3 = 0.2$.

Test	$(10, 10, 10)$	$(20, 20, 20)$	$(30, 30, 30)$
FE	0.09762	0.01282	0.00150
ELR	0.14446	0.01663	0.00193
Eχ^2	0.11851	0.01155	0.00134
EZ	0.14522	0.01453	0.00160
Nχ^2	0.10666	0.01158	0.00126
NZ	0.13381	0.01414	0.00152
Aχ^2	0.10837	0.01174	0.00127

function due to Kolmogorov (1933), and the third type involves a class of coverage tests (Greenwood, 1946) that includes both the Kendall–Sherman and Greenwood–Moran tests along with a maximum coverage test due to Fisher (1929).

6.2.1 Smirnov Matching Test

The Smirnov (1939a) matching test is based on the order statistics $(x_{1,n} < \cdots < x_{n,n})$ associated with a random sample of size n from continuous data that obeys $F(x)$ under H_0. Let $(w_{i-1}, w_i]$ be a collection $(i = 1, ..., n)$ of n disjoint intervals such that $F(w_j) = j/n$ for $j = 0, ..., n$. A match occurs when $x_{i,n}$ is contained in $(w_{i-1}, w_i]$ and the matching statistic (T) is the total number of matches given by

$$T = \sum_{i=1}^{n} \Phi_i,$$

where

$$\Phi_i = \begin{cases} 1 & \text{if } x_{i,n} \in (w_{i-1}, w_i], \\ 0 & \text{otherwise.} \end{cases}$$

Since $1 \le T \le n$ and H_0 is rejected for small values of T, the exact P-value is given by

$$P(T \le T_o \mid H_0) = 1 - \prod_{j=1}^{T_o} \left(1 - \frac{j}{n}\right),$$

where $1 \le T_o \le n$ and T_o is the observed value of T (Siddiqui, 1982). A shortcoming of the Smirnov matching test is the fact that its exact P-value is never less than $1/n$. This deficiency is due to the loss of available information caused by collapsing continuous data into n ordered intervals. The subsequent tests overcome this defect and are recommended over this matching test for most applications.

6.2.2 Kolmogorov Goodness-of-Fit Test

The Kolmogorov (1933) goodness-of-fit test is based on the empirical cumulative distribution function defined by

$$F_n(x) = \frac{\text{number of } y_i \text{ values} \le x}{n},$$

where $(y_i, ..., y_n)$ is a random sample of size n from continuous data that obeys $F(x)$ under H_0. The associated test statistic is given by

$$D_n = \sup_x \left| F_n(x) - F(x) \right|,$$

and H_0 is rejected for large values of D_n. If $Z = \sqrt{n}\, D_n$ and z is an observed value of Z, then the asymptotic P-value based on random variable Z (Kolmogorov, 1933), as $n \to \infty$ is given by

$$P(Z \ge z \mid H_0) = 2 \sum_{j=1}^{\infty} (-1)^{j-1} e^{-2j^2 z^2}.$$

When n is at least 20, an approximate P-value based on random variable Z (Conover, 1999, see p. 547) occurs when z is replaced with z^*, where

$$z^* = z \left[1 + (10n)^{-1/2}\right]^{1/2}.$$

If n is small, a bootstrap P-value based on L independent simulated values of D_n under H_0 is given by

$$P(D_n \ge D_o \mid H_0) = \frac{\text{number of } D_n \text{ values} \ge D_o}{L},$$

where D_o is the observed value of D_n.

6.2.3   Goodness-of-Fit Tests Based on Coverages

Assuming a random sample of size n is obtained from continuous data that obey $F(x)$ under H_0, a class of goodness-of-fit tests based on coverages (also termed spacings) is described. Let $n+1$ coverages associated with the n order statistics $x_{1,n} < \cdots < x_{n,n}$ be defined for $i = 1, ..., n+1$ by

$$C_i = F(x_{i,n}) - F(x_{i-1,n}),$$

where $F(x_{0,n}) = 0$, $F(x_{n+1,n}) = 1$, and $E[C_i \mid H_0] = (n+1)^{-1}$. Consider the class of goodness-of-fit tests based on the test statistic given by

$$T = \sum_{i=1}^{n+1} \left| C_i - \frac{1}{n+1} \right|^v,$$

where $v > 0$. A bootstrap P-value based on L independent simulated values of T under H_0 is given by

$$P(T \geq T_o \mid H_0) = \frac{\text{number of } T \text{ values} \geq T_o}{L},$$

where T_o is the observed value of T.

Kendall–Sherman and Greenwood–Moran Tests

Specifically, T is the Kendall–Sherman test statistic when $v = 1$, and T is the Greenwood–Moran test statistic when $v = 2$ (Greenwood, 1946). M.G. Kendall (1946) suggests the Kendall–Sherman test in his discussion of this paper on pp. 103–105. In contrast to the Kolmogorov test, the Pearson type III distribution yields approximate P-values by evaluating $P(T \geq T_o \mid H_0)$, where T_o is the observed value of T and the exact mean, variance, and skewness of T are known under H_0. Sherman (1950) obtained the exact mean, variance, and skewness of the Kendall–Sherman test statistic under H_0 given by

$$\mu_T = 2 \left(\frac{n}{n+1} \right)^{n+1},$$

$$\sigma_T^2 = \frac{4}{n+2} \left[2 \left(\frac{n}{n+1} \right)^{n+2} + n \left(\frac{n-1}{n+1} \right)^{n+2} \right] - \mu_T^2,$$

and

$$\gamma_T = \frac{E}{\sigma_T^3},$$

where

$$E = \frac{8}{(n+2)(n+3)} \left\{ 6 \left[\left(\frac{n}{n+1} \right)^{n+3} + n \left(\frac{n-1}{n+1} \right)^{n+3} \right] \right.$$

$$\left. + n(n-1) \left(\frac{n-2}{n+1} \right)^{n+3} \right\} - 3\sigma_T^2 \mu_T - \mu_T^3.$$

However, Sherman (1950) obtained the exact P-value for an observed Kendall–Sherman statistic given by

$$\sum_{i=0}^{n-r-1} \sum_{j=0}^{i} (-1)^{i-j} \binom{n}{j} \binom{n+1}{i+1} \binom{n+i-j}{n} \left(\frac{n-i}{n+1} \right)^j \left(\frac{n-i}{n+1} - x \right)^{n-j},$$

where $x = T_o/2$ and $r = [x(n+1)]$ is the largest integer $\leq x(n+1)$. Moran (1947) obtained the exact mean, variance, and skewness of the Greenwood–Moran test statistic under H_0 given by

$$\mu_T = \frac{n}{(n+1)(n+2)},$$

$$\sigma_T^2 = \frac{4n}{(n+2)^2(n+3)(n+4)},$$

and

$$\gamma_T = \frac{F}{\sigma_T^3},$$

where

$$F = \frac{16n(5n-2)}{(n+2)^3(n+3)(n+4)(n+5)(n+6)}.$$

Gato and Jammalamadaka (1999) obtained saddlepoint P-value approximations for various one-sample spacing tests that include the Greenwood–Moran test. The saddlepoint P-value approximation is better than the simple Pearson type III P-value approximation. Incidentally, a test closely related to the Kendall–Sherman test for investigating H_0 that points are uniformly spaced about a circle is given by Rao (1976). Also, tables of exact critical values for the Kendall–Sherman and Greenwood–Moran statistics have been obtained by Russell and Levington (1997) and Burrows (1979), respectively.

Fisher's Maximum Coverage Test

Let $U_1 \leq \cdots \leq U_{n+1}$ denote the order statistics of the coverages denoted by $C_1, ..., C_{n+1}$. Fisher's maximum coverage test (Fisher, 1929) evaluates whether U_j is too large relative to $U_1, ..., U_{j-1}$ for $j = 2, ..., n + 1$. Under H_0, the distribution of U_j $(j = 2, ..., n + 1)$ is given by

$$
P\left(U_j \le y \mid H_0\right) = \begin{cases} 0 & \text{if } y < j^{-1}, \\[2ex] \displaystyle\sum_{i=0}^{[y^{-1}]} \binom{j}{i} (-1)^i (1 - iy)^{j-1} & \text{if } j^{-1} \le y \le 1, \\[2ex] 1 & \text{if } 1 \le y, \end{cases}
$$

where y is the observed value of $U_j / \sum_{i=1}^{j} U_j$ and $[y^{-1}]$ is the largest integer less than or equal to y^{-1}. Thus, the P-value of Fisher's maximum coverage test associated with U_j $(j = 2, ..., n + 1)$ is given by

$$
\sum_{i=1}^{[y^{-1}]} \binom{j}{i} (-1)^{i-1} (1 - iy)^{j-1}
$$

for $j^{-1} \le y \le 1$. As an example, suppose $n = 16$ (i.e., the unit interval is partitioned into 17 parts), $U_{17} = 0.52$, $U_{16} = 0.21$, and $U_{15} = 0.06$. The P-value for U_{17} is 0.1350×10^{-3}, the P-value for $U_{16}/(1 - U_{17})$ is 0.2857×10^{-2}, and the P-value for $U_{15}/(1 - U_{16} - U_{17})$ is 0.4168. The sequential procedure is terminated with U_{15} since the conditional P-value given U_{16} and U_{17} is large. An application of this procedure involving wintertime orographic cloud seeding experiments is given in Mielke et al. (1972).

6.2.4 Power Comparisons of the Kolmogorov and Kendall–Sherman Tests

In order to compare the Kolmogorov test with a test based on coverages, power comparisons of the Kolmogorov and Kendall–Sherman tests are made to provide a cursory investigation of performance differences between the Kolmogorov test and a test based on coverages. It is presently believed that (1) the Greenwood–Moran coverage test is better than the Kendall–Sherman coverage test for most cases and (2) the Kolmogorov empirical distribution function test is usually superior to both of these coverage tests. The purpose of the following simulation study is intended to indicate types of alternatives where the Kendall–Sherman (and likely the Greenwood–Moran) coverage test performs better than the Kolmogorov empirical distribution function test. The Kolmogorov and Kendall–Sherman statistics are denoted by D_n and T_n, respectively, in this section.

Using the 0.05 and 0.01 level $N(0, 1)$ distribution critical values 1.6449 and 2.3263 and using the standardized Kendall–Sherman statistic given by

$$
Z_n = \frac{T_n - \mu_{T_n}}{\sigma_{T_n}},
$$

10,000,000 simulations under H_0 yield the corresponding simulated significance values 0.05510 and 0.01313 (0.05378 and 0.01229) for $n = 10$ ($n = 20$), respectively, using the Pearson type III distribution. The matched 0.05510 and 0.01315 (0.05378 and 0.01229) level critical values of the Kolmogorov statistic D_n, also based on 10,000,000 simulations under H_0, are 0.4039 and 0.4764 (0.2911 and 0.3455) for $n = 10$ ($n = 20$), respectively. If X is a random variable having the cumulative distribution function $F(x)$, then random variable $Y = F^{-1}(X)$ is a uniform random variable on $(0, 1)$ with density function given by

$$f_Y(y) = \begin{cases} 1 & \text{if } 0 < y < 1, \\ 0 & \text{otherwise,} \end{cases}$$

under H_0. Each alternative hypothesis (H_1) considered here is based on a transformed random variable W of random variable Y denoted by $W = h(Y)$. The form of each transformed random variable, $W = h(Y)$, and the associated density function, $f_W(w)$, are given by the following.

A1(c): Asymmetric Distribution 1 $(c > -1)$

$$W = Y^{\frac{1}{c+1}},$$

$$f_W(w) = (c+1)w^c,$$

where $0 \le w \le 1$.

A2(c): Asymmetric Distribution 2 $(c > -1)$

$$W = 1 - (1 - Y)^{\frac{1}{c+1}},$$

$$f_W(w) = (c+1)(1-w)^c,$$

where $0 \le w \le 1$. Note that A1(c) and A2(c) are reflective about $w = 0.5$.

SUS(c): Symmetric U-Shaped Distribution $(c > -1)$

$$W = \begin{cases} 0.5 - 0.5|2Y - 1|^{\frac{1}{c+1}} & \text{if } 0 \le Y \le 0.5, \\ 0.5 + 0.5|2Y - 1|^{\frac{1}{c+1}} & \text{if } 0.5 \le Y \le 1, \end{cases}$$

$$f_W(w) = (c+1)|2w - 1|^c,$$

where $0 \le w \le 1$.

SMS(c): Symmetric Mound-Shaped Distribution $(c > -1)$

$$W = \begin{cases} 0.5(2Y)^{\frac{1}{c+1}} & \text{if } 0 \le Y \le 0.5, \\ 1 - 0.5[2(1 - Y)]^{\frac{1}{c+1}} & \text{if } 0.5 \le Y \le 1, \end{cases}$$

$$f_W(w) = \begin{cases} (c+1)(2w)^c & \text{if } 0 \le w \le 0.5, \\ (c+1)[2(1-w)]^c & \text{if } 0.5 \le w \le 1. \end{cases}$$

STS(k): Symmetric k-Teeth Distribution $(k = 1, 2, 3, \dots)$

$$W = \begin{cases} \dfrac{k}{2k-1}Y & \text{if } 0 \le Y \le \dfrac{1}{k}, \\[2ex] \dfrac{2}{2k-1} + \dfrac{k}{2k-1}\left(Y - \dfrac{1}{k}\right) & \text{if } \dfrac{1}{k} < Y \le \dfrac{2}{k}, \\[1ex] \vdots & \vdots \\[1ex] \dfrac{2k-2}{2k-1} + \dfrac{k}{2k-1}\left(Y - \dfrac{k-1}{k}\right) & \text{if } \dfrac{k-1}{k} < Y \le 1, \end{cases}$$

$$f_W(w) = \begin{cases} \dfrac{2k-1}{k} & \text{if } 0 \le w \le \dfrac{1}{2k-1}, \\[2ex] \dfrac{2k-1}{k} & \text{if } \dfrac{2}{2k-1} \le w \le \dfrac{3}{2k-1}, \\[1ex] \vdots & \vdots \\[1ex] \dfrac{2k-1}{k} & \text{if } \dfrac{2k-2}{2k-1} \le w \le 1, \\[2ex] 0 & \text{otherwise.} \end{cases}$$

Each of the simulated power comparisons between the Kolmogorov and Kendall–Sherman tests in Tables 6.5, 6.6, 6.7, and 6.8 are based on $L = 1{,}000{,}000$ simulations. The specific variations of H_1 included in each table are A1(c), A2(c), SUS(c), and SMS(c) for $c = -0.5$, 1, and 2 along with STS(2) and STS(3). Note that A1(0), A2(0), SUS(0), SMS(0), and STS(1) represent H_0. Tables 6.5 and 6.6 (6.7 and 6.8) are based on $\alpha = 0.01315$ and 0.05510 ($\alpha = 0.01229$ and 0.05378) when $n = 10$ ($n = 20$), respectively.

Power comparisons of the Kolmogorov and Kendall–Sherman tests yield very similar results. Three distinct features of the results in Tables 6.5, 6.6, 6.7, and 6.8 are described. First, the Kolmogorov test is more powerful than the Kendall–Sherman test for the asymmetric alternatives. Second, the Kendall–Sherman test is more powerful than the Kolmogorov test for all the symmetric alternatives; the STS(3) result in Table 6.8 indicates the existence of major advantages for the Kendall–Sherman test over the Kolmogorov test. Third, a comparison of the A1(c) and A2(c) results in Tables 6.5, 6.6, 6.7, and 6.8 indicates that the power of neither the Kolmogorov test nor the Kendall–Sherman test exhibits any directional dependence.

TABLE 6.5. Simulated power comparisons between the Kolmogorov and the Kendall–Sherman tests for 14 alternatives based on 1,000,000 simulations with $\alpha = 0.01315$ and $n = 10$.

Alternative	Simulated power	
	Kolmogorov	Kendall–Sherman
A1(−0.5)	0.22527	0.15278
A1(1)	0.18633	0.05973
A1(2)	0.57556	0.24413
A2(−0.5)	0.22516	0.15228
A2(1)	0.18607	0.05946
A2(2)	0.57651	0.24383
SUS(−0.5)	0.01434	0.07142
SUS(1)	0.08138	0.13303
SUS(2)	0.18054	0.42062
SMS(−0.5)	0.07174	0.21198
SMS(1)	0.00569	0.01926
SMS(2)	0.00711	0.09900
STS(2)	0.10847	0.14195
STS(3)	0.04770	0.19300

TABLE 6.6. Simulated power comparisons between the Kolmogorov and the Kendall–Sherman tests for 14 alternatives based on 1,000,000 simulations with $\alpha = 0.05510$ and $n = 10$.

Alternative	Simulated power	
	Kolmogorov	Kendall–Sherman
A1(−0.5)	0.41768	0.31447
A1(1)	0.40264	0.16947
A1(2)	0.81912	0.46887
A2(−0.5)	0.41679	0.31395
A2(1)	0.40362	0.16957
A2(2)	0.82025	0.47001
SUS(−0.5)	0.07981	0.18330
SUS(1)	0.21127	0.30241
SUS(2)	0.39165	0.66321
SMS(−0.5)	0.19346	0.39455
SMS(1)	0.05188	0.07548
SMS(2)	0.10150	0.25667
STS(2)	0.23942	0.37111
STS(3)	0.17124	0.44808

TABLE 6.7. Simulated power comparisons between the Kolmogorov and the Kendall–Sherman tests for 14 alternatives based on 1,000,000 simulations with $\alpha = 0.01229$ and $n = 20$.

| Alternative | Simulated power | |
	Kolmogorov	Kendall–Sherman
A1(−0.5)	0.45679	0.23831
A1(1)	0.44796	0.11360
A1(2)	0.93772	0.50941
A2(−0.5)	0.45499	0.23773
A2(1)	0.44952	0.11381
A2(2)	0.93801	0.51173
SUS(−0.5)	0.05534	0.16190
SUS(1)	0.13529	0.19197
SUS(2)	0.36004	0.65619
SMS(−0.5)	0.11569	0.29849
SMS(1)	0.02178	0.05977
SMS(2)	0.09273	0.35112
STS(2)	0.18639	0.34749
STS(3)	0.09175	0.52921

TABLE 6.8. Simulated power comparisons between the Kolmogorov and the Kendall–Sherman tests for 14 alternatives based on 1,000,000 simulations with $\alpha = 0.05378$ and $n = 20$.

| Alternative | Simulated power | |
	Kolmogorov	Kendall–Sherman
A1(−0.5)	0.67727	0.43597
A1(1)	0.70786	0.27561
A1(2)	0.98945	0.74271
A2(−0.5)	0.67517	0.43443
A2(1)	0.70977	0.27658
A2(2)	0.98936	0.74458
SUS(−0.5)	0.22402	0.33229
SUS(1)	0.32819	0.39785
SUS(2)	0.67107	0.84917
SMS(−0.5)	0.29617	0.50740
SMS(1)	0.13697	0.17419
SMS(2)	0.43682	0.59930
STS(2)	0.41630	0.66315
STS(3)	0.24196	0.82598

Now mentioned are some large sample efficiency properties. The Kolmogorov test is known to be better than either the Kendall–Sherman or Greenwood–Moran tests in most cases. However, Jammalamadaka and Zhou (1989) show that the Kendall–Sherman test has the best Bahadur efficiency for certain alternatives. Also, Sethuraman and Rao (1970) show that the Greenwood–Moran tests has the best Pitman efficiency for specific alternatives.

7
Contingency Tables

Analysis of contingency tables are discussed in this chapter. Various topics are addressed after obtaining the exact hypergeometric distribution of r-way contingency tables conditioned on fixed marginal frequency totals. These topics include Fisher's exact test for a few small contingency tables; approximate nonasymptotic tests for general r-way contingency tables; comparisons among exact, nonasymptotic, and asymptotic tests under the null hypothesis (H_0) of r independent categories; consideration of asymptotic log-linear analyses of contingency tables when sparse data are encountered; exact tests for interactions of 2^r contingency tables; and the relationship between the Pearson (1900) χ^2 symmetric statistic and the Goodman and Kruskal (1954) t_a and t_b asymmetric statistics.

7.1 Hypergeometric Distribution for r-Way Contingency Tables

Exact and nonasymptotic analyses of contingency tables are investigated in this section. For large sparse r-way contingency tables, nonasymptotic procedures are shown to yield very close approximations to the exact P-values for selected tests when the number of reference tables is large. The hypergeometric distribution conditioned on fixed marginal frequency totals is the basis for r-way contingency table analyses.

Consider an r-way contingency table consisting of $n_1 \times n_2 \times \cdots \times n_r$ cells where the observed frequency of the $(j_1, ..., j_r)$th cell is denoted by $o_{j_1,...,j_r}$, the marginal frequency total associated with subscript j_i of category i is denoted by

$$\langle i \rangle_{j_i} = \sum_{* \mid j_i} o_{j_1,\ldots,j_r}$$

for $j_i = 1, \ldots, n_i$, $i = 1, \ldots, r$, and $\sum_{* \mid j_i}$ is the partial sum over all cells with subscript j_i fixed. Then, the frequency total of the entire r-way contingency table is

$$N = \sum_{j_i=1}^{n_i} \langle i \rangle_{j_i}$$

for $i = 1, \ldots, r$. If $p_{j_1,\ldots,j_r} \geq 0$ is the probability that any of the N total events occurs in the $(j_i, \ldots, j_r)$th cell, then the multinomial probability is given by

$$P\left(o_{j_1,\ldots,j_r}\right) = \left(N! \bigg/ \prod_{i=1}^{r} \prod_{j_i=1}^{n_i} o_{j_1,\ldots,j_r}! \right) \left(\prod_{i=1}^{r} \prod_{j_i=1}^{n_i} p_{j_1,\ldots,j_r}^{o_{j_1,\ldots,j_r}} \right),$$

where $0^0 = 1$. The assumed positive marginal probability associated with subscript j_i is given by

$$[i]_{j_i} = \sum_{* \mid j_i} p_{j_1,\ldots,j_r}$$

for $j_i = 1, \ldots, n_i$, $i = 1, \ldots, r$, and

$$\sum_{j_i=1}^{n_i} [i]_{j_i} = 1$$

for $i = 1, \ldots, r$. Then, the marginal multinomial probability associated with category i is given by

$$P\left(\langle i \rangle_{j_i}\right) = \left(N! \bigg/ \prod_{j_i=1}^{n_i} \langle i \rangle_{j_i}! \right) \left(\prod_{j_i=1}^{n_i} [i]_{j_i}^{\langle i \rangle_{j_i}} \right)$$

for $i = 1, \ldots, r$. The H_0 that the r categories are independent specifies that

$$p_{j_1,\ldots,j_r} = \prod_{i=1}^{r} [i]_{j_i} > 0$$

and the conditional distribution function of the r-way contingency table under H_0 is given by

$$P\left(o_{j_1,\ldots,j_r} \mid \langle 1 \rangle_{j_1}, \ldots, \langle r \rangle_{j_r}, H_0\right) = \frac{P\left(o_{j_1,\ldots,j_r} \mid H_0\right)}{\displaystyle\prod_{i=1}^{r} P\left(\langle i \rangle_{j_i}\right)}.$$

Algebraic manipulation then yields the hypergeometric distribution function given by

$$P\left(o_{j_1,\ldots,j_r} \mid \langle 1 \rangle_{j_1}, \ldots, \langle r \rangle_{j_r}, H_0\right) = \frac{\displaystyle\prod_{i=1}^{r}\prod_{j_i=1}^{n_i} \langle i \rangle_{j_i}!}{\left(N!\right)^{r-1}\displaystyle\prod_{i=1}^{r}\prod_{j_i=1}^{n_i} o_{j_1,\ldots,j_r}!},$$

which is independent of any unknown probabilities under H_0 (Mielke, 1997; Mielke and Berry, 1988). Thus, the marginal frequency totals, $\langle i \rangle_{j_i}$, are sufficient statistics for the marginal multinomial probabilities, $[\,i\,]_{j_i}$, under H_0. This hypergeometric distribution function provides the basis for testing the independence of categories for any r-way contingency table.

7.2   Exact Tests

As indicated in Section 6.1, the use of the previously-derived conditional distribution function in Section 7.1 for an r-way contingency table as the primary statistic is more intuitive than alternative statistics, e.g., the Pearson χ^2 test statistic discussed in Section 7.3. The Fisher exact test P-value is the probability of having a conditional distribution function equal to or smaller than the observed conditional distribution function under H_0 (Fisher, 1934). Since the number of conditional loops associated with the computational algorithm for an r-way contingency table is the number of degrees-of-freedom given by

$$\prod_{i=1}^{r} n_i + r - 1 - \sum_{i=1}^{r} n_i,$$

efficient computational algorithms have been obtained for 2×2, 3×2, 4×2, 5×2, 6×2, 3×3, and $2 \times 2 \times 2$ contingency tables, which are the only r-way contingency tables with five or fewer conditional loops (Mielke and Berry, 1992; Mielke et al., 1994; Zelterman et al., 1995). The degrees-of-freedom for an r-way contingency table is the direct extension of the $(n_1 - 1)(n_2 - 1)$ degrees-of-freedom due to Fisher (1922) for a two-way contingency table. The efficiency of these programs depends on recursive procedures over all distinct table configurations that utilize an arbitrary starting value and elementary arithmetic operations as described in Section 6.1 for goodness-of-fit tests.

Efficient exhaustive enumeration algorithms are based on a technique developed by Quetelet (1849, pp. 254–269) to calculate binomial probability values. Beginning with an arbitrary initial value, a recursion procedure generates relative frequency values for all possible contingency tables, given the observed marginal frequency totals. The required probability value is obtained by summing the relative frequency values equal to or less than the observed relative frequency value and dividing by the unrestricted relative frequency total. Because no computed initial values are required and because simple recursion functions are utilized to obtain the required probability values, these algorithms are faster than other algorithms based on exhaustive enumeration. In addition, no factorials, logarithms, or log-factorial values are used, and the accuracy of these algorithms is limited only by the intrinsic precision of the computer employed.

If only two-way contingency tables are considered, Mehta and Patel (1983, 1986a, 1986b) have developed an exceedingly efficient network algorithm that circumvents the problem of exhaustively enumerating the entire reference set of contingency tables. Consequently, Mehta and Patel (1983, 1986a, 1986b) have extended exact analyses of two-way contingency tables far beyond the previously mentioned restriction of no more than five conditional loops. This highly efficient approach does not address r-way contingency tables when $r \geq 3$. Most r-way contingency tables encountered in practice are inherently sparse since the number of r-dimensional cells is large relative to N. Although an algorithm to closely approximate Fisher's exact test for large sparse r-way contingency tables does not yet exist when $r \geq 3$, an algorithm is subsequently described that closely approximates the exact χ^2 and Zelterman tests for large sparse r-way contingency tables (Mielke and Berry, 1988). As mentioned by Mehta and Patel (1983), all of the exact tests in question here converge to the asymptotic χ^2 test as the cell expectations become large. Booth and Butler (1999) and Caffo and Booth (2001) provide iterative algorithms that converge to the exact P-values of tests based on sufficient statistics for general hypotheses including the independence of r-way contingency tables, i.e., the Pearson χ^2, Zelterman, and likelihood-ratio tests.

Early work by Barnard (1945, 1947a, 1947b) and Pearson (1947) placed contingency tables into one of three cases (I, II, or III) depending on whether none, one, or both of the row and column marginal frequency totals, respectively, were fixed. It was widely held for many years that Fisher's exact probability test was limited to Case III contingency tables, where both marginal frequency totals were fixed (Fisher, 1934). Later research by Yates (1984) has shown this belief to be fallacious. To the contrary, Yates (1984) convincingly argued that Fisher's exact probability test is the preferred test for all three cases. Yates (1984) is supported in his arguments by Barnard, Bartlett, Cox, Mantel, and others (see the discussion section of Yates, 1984) and by Greenland (1991). Consequently, Fisher's exact probability test enjoys tremendous potential in contemporary research. For critics of tests conditioned on the marginal frequency totals, see Berkson (1978), D'Agostino et al. (1988), Grizzle (1967), Haviland (1990), and Upton (1982).

Examples of such applications include, first, Case I (the correlational model with neither marginal fixed), where, for example, students in a sample survey may be classified as to academic class (undergraduate or graduate) and premarital sexual experience (yes or no). A second application may be illustrated by Case II (the experimental model with one marginal fixed), where, for example, rats may be classified as to sex (female or male) and then tested for speed through a maze, measured as above or below the median elapsed time. A third potential application is illustrated by Case III (the randomization model with both marginals fixed), where, for example, a class of 50 students (20 male and 30 female) will be assigned grades at the end of the semester (10 each of As, Bs, Cs, Ds, and Fs). Efficient exhaustive enumeration algorithms for Fisher's exact test are illustrated with analyses of 2×2, 3×2, 3×3, and $2 \times 2 \times 2$ tables.

7.2.1   Analysis of a 2×2 Table

Consider a 2×2 contingency table of n cases, where x_0 denotes the observed frequency of any cell and r and c represent the row and column marginal frequencies, respectively, corresponding to x_0. If $H(x \mid N, r, c)$ is a recursively-defined positive function in which

$$H(x \mid N, r, c) = D \times \frac{\binom{r}{x}\binom{N-r}{c-x}}{\binom{N}{c}}$$

$$= \frac{D\, r!\, c!\, (N-r)!\, (N-c)!}{N!\, x!\, (r-x)!\, (c-x)!\, (N-r-c+x)!},$$

where $D > 0$ is an unknown constant, then solving the recursive relation

$$H(x+1 \mid N, r, c) = H(x \mid N, r, c) \cdot g(x)$$

yields

$$g(x) = \frac{(r-x)(c-x)}{(x+1)(N-r-c+x+1)}.$$

This algorithm may then be employed to enumerate all values of

$$H(x \mid N, r, c),$$

where $a \leq x \leq b$, $a = \max(0, r+c-N)$, $b = \min(r, c)$, and $H(a \mid N, r, c)$ is initially set to some small value, e.g., 10^{-200} (see Berry and Mielke, 1985b). The total (T) over the entire distribution may be found by

$$T = \sum_{k=a}^{b} H(k \mid N, r, c).$$

To calculate the P-value x_o, given the marginal frequency totals, the point probability of the observed table must be determined. This value, designated by $U_2 = H(x \mid N, r, c)$, is found recursively. Next, the tail associated with U_2 must be identified. Let

$$U_1 = \begin{cases} H(x_o - 1 \mid N, r, c) & \text{if } x_o > a, \\ 0 & \text{if } x_o = a, \end{cases}$$

and

$$U_3 = \begin{cases} H(x_o + 1 \mid N, r, c) & \text{if } x_o < b, \\ 0 & \text{if } x_o = b. \end{cases}$$

If $U_1 > U_3$, U_2 is in the right tail of the distribution; otherwise, U_2 is defined to be in the left tail of the distribution, and the one-tailed (S_1) and two-tailed (S_2) subtotals may be found by

$$S_1(x_o \mid N, r, c) = \sum_{k=a}^{b} K_k H(k \mid N, r, c)$$

and

$$S_2(x_o \mid N, r, c) = \sum_{k=a}^{b} L_k H(k \mid N, r, c),$$

respectively, where

$$K_k = \begin{cases} 1 & \text{if } U_1 \leq U_3 \text{ and } k \leq x_o \text{ or } U_1 > U_2 \text{ and } k \geq x_o, \\ 0 & \text{otherwise}, \end{cases}$$

and

$$L_k = \begin{cases} 1 & \text{if } H(k \mid N, r, c) \leq U_2, \\ 0 & \text{otherwise}, \end{cases}$$

for $k = a, ..., b$. The one-tailed (P_1) and two-tailed (P_2) probability values are then given by $P_1 = S_1/T$ and $P_2 = S_2/T$, respectively.

A 2×2 Example

Consider a 2×2 table

6	3	9
2	9	11
8	12	20

TABLE 7.1. Example of recursion with an arbitrary origin.

x	Probability	$H(x \mid N, r, c)$	$H(x \mid N, r, c)/T$
0	0.001310	1	0.001310
1	0.023577	18	0.023577
2	0.132032	100.8	0.132032
3	0.308073	235.2	0.308073
4	0.330079	252	0.330079
5	0.165039	126	0.165039
6	0.036675	28	0.036675
7	0.003144	2.4	0.003144
8	0.000071	0.054545	0.000071
Total	1.000000	763.454545	1.000000

where $x_o = 6$, $r = 9$, $c = 8$, $N = 20$,

$$a = \max(0, r + c - N) = \max(0, 9 + 8 - 20) = \max(0, -3) = 0,$$

$$b = \min(r, c) = \min(9, 8) = 8,$$

and $b - a + 1 = 8 - 0 + 1 = 9$ possible table configurations, given the fixed marginal frequency totals.

Table 7.1 contains the nine possible values of x, given the contingency table s. The second column of Table 7.1 lists the exact point probability values for $x = 0, ..., 8$ calculated from the preceding factorial expression. The third column of Table 7.1 contains the recursion where, for $x = 0$, the initial value is arbitrarily set to 1 for this example analysis. Then,

$$1 \left[\frac{(9)(8)}{(1)(4)} \right] = 18,$$

$$18 \left[\frac{(8)(7)}{(2)(5)} \right] = 100.8,$$

$$\vdots$$

$$2.4 \left[\frac{(2)(1)}{(8)(11)} \right] = 0.054545.$$

The total (T) of $H(x \mid N, r, c)$ for $x = 0, ..., 8$ is 763.454545. The fourth column of Table 7.1 corrects the entries of the third column by dividing each entry by T. For these data,

$$U_2 = H(x_o \mid N, r, c) = H(6 \mid 20, 9, 8) = 28,$$

$$U_1 = H(x_o - 1 \mid N, r, c) = H(5 \mid 20, 9, 8) = 126$$

because $x_o > a$ (i.e., $6 > 1$), and

$$U_3 = H(x_o + 1 \mid N, r, c) = H(7 \mid 20, 9, 8) = 2.4$$

because $x_o < b$, i.e., $6 < 8$. Thus, $U_2 = 28$ is located in the right tail since $U_1 > U_3$, i.e., $126 > 2.4$. Then,

$$S_1 = 28 + 2.4 + 0.054545 = 30.454545,$$

$$S_2 = 1 + 18 + 28 + 2.4 + 0.054545 = 49.454545,$$

$$P_1 = \frac{S_1}{T} = \frac{30.454545}{763.454545} = 0.3989 \times 10^{-1},$$

and

$$P_2 = \frac{S_2}{T} = \frac{49.454545}{763.454545} = 0.6478 \times 10^{-1}.$$

7.2.2 Analysis of a 3×2 Table

Consider a 3×2 contingency table of N cases, where x_o denotes the observed frequency of the cell in the first row and first column, y_o denotes the observed frequency of the cell in the second row and first column, and r_1, r_2, and c_1 are the observed frequency totals in the first row, second row, and first column, respectively. If $H(x, y)$, given N, r_1, r_2, and c_1, is a recursively-defined positive function, then solving the recursive relation

$$H(x, y + 1) = H(x, y) \cdot g_1(x, y)$$

yields

$$g_1(x, y) = \frac{(c_1 - x - y)(r_2 - y)}{(1 + y)(N - r_1 - r_2 - c_1 + 1 + x + y)}.$$

If $y = \min(r_2, c_1 - x)$, then $H(x + 1, y) = H(x, y) \cdot g_2(x, y)$, where

$$g_2(x, y) = \frac{(c_1 - x - y)(r_1 - x)}{(1 + x)(N - r_1 - r_2 - c_1 + 1 + x + y)},$$

given that $\max(0, r_1 + r_2 + c_1 - N - x) = 0$. However, if $y = \min(r_2, c_1 - x)$ and $\max(0, r_1 + r_2 + c_1 - N - x) > 0$, then $H(x+1, y-1) = H(x, y) \cdot g_3(x, y)$, where

$$g_3(x, y) = \frac{y(r_1 - x)}{(1 + x)(r_2 + 1 - y)}.$$

These three recursive formulae may be employed to enumerate completely the distribution of $H(x, y)$, where $a \le x \le b$, $a = \max(0, r_1 + c_1 - N)$, $b = \min(r_1, c_1)$, $c(x) \le y \le d(x)$, $c(x) = \max(0, r_1 + r_2 + c_1 - N - x)$, $d(x) = \min(r_2, c_1 - x)$, and $H[a, c(x)]$ is set initially to some small value, e.g., 10^{-200} (see Berry and Mielke, 1987).[1] The total (T) over the completely enumerated distribution may be found by

$$T = \sum_{x=a}^{b} \sum_{y=c(x)}^{d(x)} H(x,y).$$

To calculate the P-value of (x_o, y_o), given the marginal frequency totals, the point probability of the observed contingency table must be calculated; this value is found recursively. Next, the probability of a result this extreme or more extreme must be found. The subtotal (S) is given by

$$S = \sum_{x=a}^{b} \sum_{y=c(x)}^{d(x)} J_{x,y} H_{x,y},$$

where

$$J_{x,y} = \begin{cases} 1 & \text{if } H(x, y) \leq H(x_o, y_o), \\ 0 & \text{otherwise}, \end{cases}$$

for $x = a, ..., b$ and $y = c(x), ..., d(x)$. The exact P-value for independence associated with the observed frequencies x_o and y_o is given by S/T.

A 3×2 Example

Consider a 3×2 contingency table

5	8	13
3	4	7
2	7	9
10	19	29

where $x_o = 5$, $y_o = 3$, $r_1 = 13$, $r_2 = 7$, $c_1 = 10$, and $N = 29$. For these data, the exact P-value for independence is 0.6873. There are 59 tables consistent with the observed marginal frequency totals. Exactly 56 of these tables have probabilities equal to or less than the point probability of the observed table (0.8096×10^{-1}).

---

[1] Adapted and reprinted with permission of Sage Publications, Inc. from K.J. Berry and P.W. Mielke, Jr. Exact chi-square and Fisher's exact probability test for 3 by 2 cross-classification tables. *Educational and Psychological Measurement*, 1987, 47, 631–636. Copyright © 1987 by Sage Publications, Inc.

7.2.3 Analysis of a 3 × 3 Table

Consider a 3 × 3 contingency table of N cases, where w_o, x_o, y_o, and z_o denote the observed frequencies in the first row–first column, first row–second column, second row–first column, and second row–second column positions of the 3×3 table, respectively. Also, let r_1, r_2, c_1, c_2, and N denote the first row, second row, first column, second column, and overall marginal frequency totals of the 3 × 3 table, respectively. If the order specification of w, x, y, and z implies that z depends on w, x, and y, y depends on w and x, and x depends on w, then the following conditional bounds hold for w, x, y, and z:

$$\max\left(0,\, K - r_2 - c_2\right) \leq w \leq \min\left(r_1, c_1\right),$$

$$\max\left(0,\, K - r_2 - w\right) \leq x \leq \min\left(r_1 - w, c_2\right),$$

$$\max\left(0,\, K - c_2 - w\right) \leq y \leq \min\left(r_2, c_1 - w\right),$$

and

$$\max\left(0,\, K - w - x - y\right) \leq z \leq \min\left(r_2 - y, c_2 - x\right),$$

where $K = r_1 + r_2 + c_1 + c_2 - N$ (Mielke and Berry, 1992).[2] In accordance with the defined order specification of w, x, y, and z, the conditional recursively-defined probability adjustments from (w_1, x_1, y_1, z_1) on Step 1 of the recursion to (w_2, x_2, y_2, z_2) on Step 2 of the recursion are given by

$$\frac{P(w_2, x_2, y_2, z_2 \mid r_1, r_2, c_1, c_2, N)}{P(w_1, x_1, y_1, z_1 \mid r_1, r_2, c_1, c_2, N)},$$

where

$$P(w, x, y, z \mid r_1, r_2, c_1, c_2, N) =$$

$$\left[r_1!\, r_2!\, (N - r_1 - r_2)!\, c_1!\, c_2!\, (N - c_1 - c_2)! \,/\, N!\right] \Big/$$

$$\left[w!\, x!\, y!\, z!\, (r_1 - w - x)!\, (r_2 - y - z)!\, (c_1 - w - y)!\right.$$

$$\left. (c_2 - x - z)!\, (w + x + y + z - K)!\right].$$

Starting with an arbitrarily-defined initial value (e.g., 10^{-200}), the procedure depends on two sets of recursively-defined loops. The first set of

---

[2]Adapted and reprinted with permission of Sage Publications, Inc. from P.W. Mielke, Jr. and K.J. Berry. Fisher's exact probability test for cross-classification tables. *Educational and Psychological Measurement*, 1992, 52, 97–101. Copyright © 1992 by Sage Publications, Inc.

loops is a conditional set that obtains the value of

$$H(w_o, x_o, y_o, z_o) = D \times P(w_o, x_o, y_o, z_o \mid r_1, r_2, c_1, c_2, N),$$

where D is a constant that depends on the initial value. The second set of loops is an unconditional set that determines (1) the conditional sum, S, of the recursively-defined values of

$$H(w, x, y, z) = D \times P(w, x, y, z \mid r_1, r_2, c_1, c_2, N)$$

satisfying

$$H(w, x, y, z) \leq H(w_o, x_o, y_o, z_o),$$

and (2) the unconditional sum, T, of all the values of $H(w, x, y, z)$. Then, the exact P-value for independence associated with the observed frequencies w_o, x_o, y_o, and z_o is given by S/T. Although this approach can conceptually be extended to any r-way contingency table, the execution time may be substantial for contingency tables with six or more degrees-of-freedom, even when moderately-sized marginal frequency totals are involved.

A 3×3 Example

Consider a 3×3 contingency table

3	5	2	10
2	9	3	14
8	2	6	16
13	16	11	40

where $w_o = 3$, $x_o = 5$, $y_o = 2$, $z_o = 9$, $r_1 = 10$, $r_2 = 14$, $c_1 = 13$, $c_2 = 16$, and $N = 40$. For these data, the exact P-value for independence is 0.4753×10^{-1}. There are 4,818 tables consistent with the observed marginal frequency totals. Exactly 3,935 of these tables have probabilities equal to or less than the point probability of the observed table (0.1159×10^{-3}).

7.2.4 Analysis of a $2 \times 2 \times 2$ Table

Consider a $2 \times 2 \times 2$ contingency table where o_{ijk} denotes the cell frequency of the ith row, jth column, and kth slice ($i = 1, 2$; $j = 1, 2$; $k = 1, 2$). Let $A = o_{1..}$, $B = o_{.1.}$, $C = o_{..1}$, and $N = o_{...}$ denote the observed frequency totals of the first row, first column, first slice, and entire table, respectively, such that $1 \leq A \leq B \leq C \leq N/2$. Also, let $w = o_{111}$, $x = o_{112}$, $y = o_{121}$, and $z = o_{211}$ denote the cell frequencies of the contingency table. Then, the probability for any w, x, y, and z is given by

$$P(w, x, y, z \,|\, A, B, C, N) =$$

$$A!\,(N-A)!\,B!\,(N-B)!\,C!\,(N-C)!\,/$$

$$[(N!)^2\,w!\,x!\,y!\,z!\,(A-w-x-y)!\,(B-w-x-z)!$$

$$(C-w-y-z)!\,(N-A-B-C+2w+x+y+z)!]$$

(Mielke et al., 1994).[3] The nested looping structure involves two distinct passes. The first pass yields the exact probability, U, of the observed table and is terminated when U is obtained. The second pass yields the exact P-value of all tables with probabilities equal to or less than the point probability of the observed table. The four nested loops within each pass are over the cell frequency indexes w, x, y, and z, respectively. The bounds for w, x, y, and z in each pass are

$$0 \leq w \leq M_w,$$

$$0 \leq x \leq M_x,$$

$$0 \leq y \leq M_y,$$

and

$$L_z \leq z \leq M_z,$$

respectively, where $M_w = A$, $M_x = A - w$, $M_y = A - w - x$, $M_z = \min(B-w-x, C-w-y)$, and $L_z = \max(0, A+B+C-N-2w-x-y)$.

The recursion method is illustrated with the fourth (inner) loop over z given w, x, y, A, B, C, and N because this inner loop yields both U on the first pass and the P-value on the second pass. Let $H(w, x, y, z)$ be a recursively-defined positive function given A, B, C, and N, satisfying

$$H(w, x, y, z+1) = H(w, x, y, z)\,g(w, x, y, z),$$

where

$$g(w, x, y, z) = \frac{(B-w-x-z)\,(C-w-z)}{(z+1)\,(N-A-B-C+2w+x+y+z+1)}.$$

---

[3]Adapted and reprinted with permission of Sage Publications, Inc. from P.W. Mielke, Jr., K.J. Berry, and D. Zelterman. Fisher's exact test of mutual independence for $2 \times 2 \times 2$ cross-classification tables. *Educational and Psychological Measurement*, 1994, 54, 110–114. Copyright © 1994 by Sage Publications, Inc.

TABLE 7.2. Cross-classification of responses, categorized by year and region.

	Region			
	North		South	
Year	No	Yes	No	Yes
1963	410	56	126	31
1946	439	374	64	163

The remaining three loops of each pass initialize $H(w, x, y, z)$ for continued enumerations. Let $I_z = \max(0, A + B + C - N)$ and set the initial value of $H(0, 0, 0, I_z)$ to an arbitrary small constant, such as 10^{-200}. Then, the total, T, over the completely enumerated distribution is found by

$$T = \sum_{w=0}^{M_w} \sum_{x=0}^{M_x} \sum_{y=0}^{M_y} \sum_{z=L_z}^{M_z} H(w, x, y, z).$$

If w_o, x_o, y_o, and z_o are the values of w, x, y, and z in the observed contingency table, then U and the exact P-value are given by

$$U = H(w_o, x_o, y_o, z_o)/T$$

and

$$P\text{-value} = \sum_{w=0}^{M_w} \sum_{x=0}^{M_x} \sum_{y=0}^{M_y} \sum_{z=L_z}^{M_z} H(w, x, y, z)\psi(w, x, y, z)/T,$$

respectively, where

$$\psi(w, x, y, z) = \begin{cases} 1 & \text{if } H(w, x, y, z) \leq H(w_o, x_o, y_o, z_o), \\ 0 & \text{otherwise.} \end{cases}$$

A $2 \times 2 \times 2$ Example

The data in Table 7.2 are cited in Pomar (1984), where 1,663 respondents were asked if they agreed with the statement that minorities should have equal job opportunity (No, Yes). The respondents were then classified by region of the country (North, South) and by year of the survey (1946, 1963). There are 3,683,159,504 tables consistent with the observed marginal frequency totals, and exactly 2,761,590,498 of these tables have probabilities equal to or less than the point probability of the observed table (0.1860×10^{-72}). Thus, the exact P-value associated with Table 7.2 is 0.1684×10^{-65}.

7.3   Approximate Nonasymptotic Tests

Nonasymptotic resampling and Pearson type III P-value algorithms for r-way contingency tables are considered. For the Fisher exact, Pearson χ^2, Zelterman, and likelihood-ratio tests, resampling algorithms involve a comparison of L random tables with an observed table. Since the marginal probabilities depend on the marginal totals, the construction of each random table is based on adjusting the marginal probabilities of the reduced tables after each of the N contingency table events is sequentially selected (see Section A.6). For r-way contingency table analyses, the resampling with $L = 1,000,000$ and Pearson type III P-value approximations are usually very similar for the Pearson (1900) χ^2 and Zelterman (1987) tests. The only r-way contingency table Pearson type III P-value algorithms presented here are for the Pearson χ^2 and Zelterman tests. As noted in Section 6.1, a test statistic's exact mean, variance, and skewness under H_0 needed to implement the Pearson type III procedure for obtaining P-values are not available for many tests, including the Fisher exact test, log-likelihood-ratio test, and most of the Cressie and Read (1984) class of tests. The present representations of the Pearson χ^2 and Zelterman test statistics (Mielke and Berry, 1988) are given by

$$T = \sum_{j_1=1}^{n_1} \cdots \sum_{j_r=1}^{n_r} \left(o^2_{j_1,\ldots,j_r} \Big/ \prod_{i=1}^{r} \langle i \rangle_{j_i} \right)$$

and

$$S = \sum_{j_1=1}^{n_1} \cdots \sum_{j_r=1}^{n_r} \left(o^{(2)}_{j_1,\ldots,j_r} \Big/ \prod_{i=1}^{r} \langle i \rangle_{j_i} \right),$$

respectively, where

$$c^{(m)} = \prod_{i=1}^{m} (c + 1 - i).$$

Here, S is the obvious extension of a statistic due to Zelterman (1987) for a two-way contingency table. If $U = n_1 \times \cdots \times n_r$ and $V = n_1 + \cdots + n_r$, then the asymptotic distribution under H_0 of both $\chi^2 = TN^{r-1} - N$ and $\zeta = SN^{r-1} + U - N$ is chi-squared with $U - V + r - 1$ degrees-of-freedom. Incidentally, under H_0 the likelihood-ratio test statistic, termed G^2 in Section 7.5.2, is asymptotically distributed as chi-squared with $U - V + r - 1$ degrees-of-freedom. The exact mean, variance, and skewness of T under H_0 (μ_T, σ_T^2, and γ_T) are defined by

$$\mu_T = E[T],$$

$$\sigma_T^2 = E[T^2] - \mu_T^2,$$

and

$$\gamma_T = \frac{E[T^3] - 3\sigma_T^2 \mu_T - \mu_T^3}{\sigma_T^3},$$

respectively, and are obtained from the first three moments about the origin under H_0 ($E[T]$, $E[T^2]$, and $E[T^3]$), given by

$$E[T] = \left[\prod_{i=1}^{r} (N - n_i) + (N-1)^{r-1} \prod_{i=1}^{r} n_i \right] \Big/ \left(N^{(2)} \right)^{r-1},$$

$$
\begin{aligned}
E\left[T^2\right] = & \left\{ \prod_{i=1}^{r} \left(\langle i \rangle_{4,1} + \langle i \rangle_{4,2} \right) + 2N_{1,1}^{r-1} \left[2 \prod_{i=1}^{r} \langle i \rangle_{3,1} \right. \right. \\
& \left. + \prod_{i=1}^{r} \left(\langle i \rangle_{3,1} + \langle i \rangle_{3,2} \right) \right] \\
& + N_{2,1}^{r-1} \left[6 \prod_{i=1}^{r} \langle i \rangle_{2,1} + \prod_{i=1}^{r} \left(\langle i \rangle_{2,1} + \langle i \rangle_{2,2} \right) \right] \\
& + N_{3,1}^{r-1} \prod_{i=1}^{r} \langle i \rangle_{1,1} \Bigg\} \Big/ N_{4,1}^{r-1},
\end{aligned}
$$

and

$$
\begin{aligned}
E\left[T^3\right] = & \left\{ \prod_{i=1}^{r} \left(\langle i \rangle_{6,3} + 3\langle i \rangle_{6,4} + \langle i \rangle_{6,6} \right) \right. \\
& + 3N_{1,2}^{r-1} \left[4 \prod_{i=1}^{r} \left(\langle i \rangle_{5,3} + \langle i \rangle_{5,4} \right) \right. \\
& \left. + \prod_{i=1}^{r} \left(\langle i \rangle_{5,3} + 2\langle i \rangle_{5,4} + \langle i \rangle_{5,5} + \langle i \rangle_{5,6} \right) \right] \\
& + N_{2,2}^{r-1} \left[32 \prod_{i=1}^{r} \langle i \rangle_{4,3} + 18 \prod_{i=1}^{r} \left(\langle i \rangle_{4,3} + \langle i \rangle_{4,4} \right) \right. \\
& + 12 \prod_{i=1}^{r} \left(\langle i \rangle_{4,3} + \langle i \rangle_{4,5} \right) \\
& \left. + 3 \prod_{i=1}^{r} \left(\langle i \rangle_{4,3} + \langle i \rangle_{4,4} + 2\langle i \rangle_{4,5} + \langle i \rangle_{4,6} \right) \right]
\end{aligned}
$$

$$+ N_{3,2}^{r-1} \left[68 \prod_{i=1}^{r} \langle i \rangle_{3,3} + 3 \prod_{i=1}^{r} \left(\langle i \rangle_{3,3} + \langle i \rangle_{3,4} \right) \right.$$

$$\left. + 18 \prod_{i=1}^{r} \left(\langle i \rangle_{3,3} + \langle i \rangle_{3,5} \right) + \prod_{i=1}^{r} \left(\langle i \rangle_{3,3} + 3 \langle i \rangle_{3,5} + \langle i \rangle_{3,6} \right) \right]$$

$$+ N_{4,2}^{r-1} \left[28 \prod_{i=1}^{r} \langle i \rangle_{2,3} + 3 \prod_{i=1}^{r} \left(\langle i \rangle_{2,3} + \langle i \rangle_{2,5} \right) \right]$$

$$\left. + N_{5,2}^{r-1} \prod_{i=1}^{r} \langle i \rangle_{1,3} \right\} \Big/ N_{6,2}^{r-1},$$

where, for $m = 1, \ldots, 4$,

$$N_{m,1} = \prod_{j=1}^{m} (N + j - 4);$$

for $m = 1, \ldots, 6$,

$$N_{m,2} = \prod_{j=1}^{m} (N + j - 6);$$

and, using $i = 1, \ldots, r$ in the remaining expressions, for $m = 1, \ldots, 4$,

$$\langle i \rangle_{m,1} = \sum_{j=1}^{n_i} \langle i \rangle_j^{(m)} \Big/ \langle i \rangle_j^2;$$

$$\langle i \rangle_{2,2} = n_i^{(2)};$$

$$\langle i \rangle_{3,2} = (n_i - 1)(N - n_i);$$

$$\langle i \rangle_{4,2} = \sum_{j=1}^{n_i} \left(\langle i \rangle_j - 1 \right) \left(N - \langle i \rangle_j - n_i + 1 \right);$$

for $m = 1, \ldots, 6$,

$$\langle i \rangle_{m,3} = \sum_{j=1}^{n_i} \langle i \rangle_j^{(m)} \Big/ \langle i \rangle_j^3;$$

for $m = 3, ..., 6,$

$$\langle i \rangle_{m,4} = \sum_{j=1}^{n_i} \langle i \rangle_j^{(m-2)} \left(N - \langle i \rangle_j - n_i + 1 \right) / \langle i \rangle_j^2;$$

for $m = 2, ..., 5,$

$$\langle i \rangle_{m,5} = (n_i - 1) \sum_{j=1}^{n_i} \langle i \rangle_j^{(m-1)} / \langle i \rangle_j^2;$$

$$\langle i \rangle_{3,6} = n_i^{(3)};$$

$$\langle i \rangle_{4,6} = (n_i - 1)(n_i - 2)(N - n_i);$$

$$\langle i \rangle_{5,6} = (n_i - 2) \sum_{j=1}^{n_i} \left(\langle i \rangle_j - 1 \right) \left(N - \langle i \rangle_j - n_i + 1 \right);$$

and

$$\langle i \rangle_{6,6} = \sum_{j=1}^{n_i} \left(\langle i \rangle_j - 1 \right) \left(N - \langle i \rangle_j - n_i + 1 \right) \left(N - 2\langle i \rangle_j - n_i + 2 \right).$$

In the same manner that μ_T, σ_T^2, and γ_T are obtained, the corresponding values for μ_S, σ_S^2, and γ_S are obtained from $E[S]$, $E[S^2]$, and $E[S^3]$ given by

$$E[S] = \prod_{i=1}^{r} (N - n_i) \bigg/ \left(N^{(2)} \right)^{r-1},$$

$$E\left[S^2\right] = \left[\prod_{i=1}^{r} \left(\langle i \rangle_{4,1} + \langle i \rangle_{4,2} \right) + 4 N_{1,1}^{r-1} \prod_{i=1}^{r} \langle i \rangle_{3,1} \right.$$

$$\left. + 2 N_{2,1}^{r-1} \prod_{i=1}^{r} \langle i \rangle_{2,1} \right] \bigg/ N_{4,1}^{r-1},$$

and

$$E\left[S^3\right] = \left\{ \prod_{i=1}^{r} \left(\langle i \rangle_{6,3} + 3\langle i \rangle_{6,4} + \langle i \rangle_{6,6}\right) + 12 N_{1,2}^{r-1} \prod_{i=1}^{r} \left(\langle i \rangle_{5,3} + \langle i \rangle_{5,4}\right) \right.$$

$$+ N_{2,2}^{r-1} \left[6 \prod_{i=1}^{r} \left(\langle i \rangle_{4,3} + \langle i \rangle_{4,4}\right) + 32 \prod_{i=1}^{r} \langle i \rangle_{4,3} \right]$$

$$\left. + 32 N_{3,2}^{r-1} \prod_{i=1}^{r} \langle i \rangle_{3,3} + 4 N_{4,2}^{r-1} \prod_{i=1}^{r} \langle i \rangle_{2,3} \right\} \bigg/ N_{6,2}^{r-1}.$$

If T_o and S_o denote the observed values of T and S, respectively, then the P-values of T and S are given by

$$P\left(T \geq T_o \,|\, H_0\right)$$

and

$$P\left(S \geq S_o \,|\, H_0\right),$$

which utilize the Pearson type III procedure for evaluation purposes. A computer program based on these results (Berry and Mielke, 1989) yields P-values for both the Pearson χ^2 and Zelterman test statistics, T and S, respectively. The arguments for a choice between T and S in Section 6.1 remain valid. As subsequently indicated for large sparse contingency tables, the Pearson type III P-values associated with T and S are very close to the corresponding exact P-values. It is important to note that Bartlett (1937), Haldane (1940), and Lewis et al. (1984) obtained μ_T, σ_T^2, and γ_T, respectively, for two-way contingency tables under the conditional permutation distribution.

An example involving a $3 \times 4 \times 5$ contingency table is used to compare P-values obtained with the nonasymptotic resampling ($L = 1{,}000{,}000$) and Pearson type III methods and the asymptotic method for the Fisher's exact, likelihood-ratio, Pearson χ^2, and Zelterman tests, when applicable. The raw frequency data are presented in Table 7.3 and the P-values are given in Table 7.4.

7.4   Exact, Nonasymptotic, and Asymptotic Comparisons of the P-Values

It is often necessary to test null hypotheses of independence or homogeneity for two categorical variables, given a sample of N observations arranged in a sparse two-way contingency table. It is well known that when expected cell frequencies are small, probability values based on the asymptotic χ^2

TABLE 7.3. Data for $3 \times 4 \times 5$ contingency table example.

	A_1				A_2				A_3			
	B_1	B_2	B_3	B_4	B_1	B_2	B_3	B_4	B_1	B_2	B_3	B_4
C_1	0	3	1	3	4	0	0	0	2	1	4	1
C_2	0	0	0	2	1	4	1	0	3	1	3	4
C_3	4	1	0	3	1	3	4	0	0	0	2	1
C_4	3	4	0	0	0	2	1	4	1	0	3	1
C_5	2	1	4	1	0	3	1	3	4	0	0	0

TABLE 7.4. Nonasymptotic resampling P-values for Fisher's exact, likelihood-ratio, Pearson χ^2, and Zelterman tests; Pearson type III P-values for Pearson χ^2 and Zelterman tests; and asymptotic P-values for likelihood-ratio, Pearson χ^2, and Zelterman tests.

Test	Nonasymptotic		Asymptotic
	Resampling	Pearson type III	
Fisher's exact	0.000180	———	———
Likelihood-ratio	0.000010	———	0.000014
Pearson χ^2	0.001425	0.001321	0.001563
Zelterman	0.001423	0.001319	0.001561

probability distributions may be erroneous (Delucchi, 1983). The problem arises because asymptotic χ^2 probability distributions provide only approximate estimates of the underlying exact multinomial probabilities, and the quality of these approximations depends on (1) the sample size, (2) the marginal probabilities in the population, (3) the number of cells in the two-way contingency table, and (4) the significance level (Bradley et al., 1979). Although there is no universal agreement as to what constitutes a small expected cell frequency, most contemporary textbooks recommend a minimum expected cell frequency of five for two-way contingency tables with degrees-of-freedom greater than one. Monte Carlo studies have provided minimum expected cell frequencies for such tables ranging from less than one (Slakter, 1966) to 10 (Roscoe and Byars, 1971), depending on the underlying structure. Tate and Hyer (1973) suggested that minimum expected cell frequencies of 20 are necessary to ensure accurate approximations under all conditions. Although several researchers have concluded that the asymptotic χ^2 test of independence is sufficiently robust so that these limitations on minimum expected cell frequencies may be relaxed (Bradley et al., 1979; Bradley and Cutcomb, 1977; Camilli and Hopkins, 1978, 1979), many researchers continue to encounter situations in which even these very lax constraints cannot be met (Agresti and Wackerly, 1977). The constraints described for two-way contingency tables are magnified for r-way contingency tables, since large r-way contingency tables are almost always sparse. For example, a $4 \times 7 \times 3 \times 2$ contingency table contains 168 cells and, therefore, N must be very large for the four-way contingency table to possess sufficiently large expected cell frequencies for each of the 168 cells. Additional simulated comparisons among commonly-used nonasymptotic and asymptotic analyses for two-way contingency tables are given by Berry and Mielke (1988c).

In Table 7.6, P-value comparisons are made among (1) the exact χ^2 test, (2) the nonasymptotic χ^2 test of Mielke and Berry (1985) with a Pearson type III distribution, (3) the asymptotic χ^2 test with a χ^2 sampling distribution, and (4) Fisher's exact test for 16 sparse two-way contingency tables. The P-value comparisons among the exact χ^2, nonasymptotic χ^2, asymptotic χ^2, and Fisher's exact tests are based on the 16 sparse two-way contingency tables listed in Table 7.5. Six of these contingency tables (Cases 7, 11, 13, 14, 15, and 16) are taken directly from Mehta and Patel (1983, 1986a). The four P-values corresponding to each of the 16 contingency tables in Table 7.5 are given in Table 7.6. The last column in Table 7.6 is the exact number of reference tables specified by the fixed marginal frequency totals for each case. For any contingency table with $r \leq 3$ and specified fixed marginal frequency totals, an approximation for the number of reference tables is given by Gail and Mantel (1977). The major features of Table 7.6 are (1) the asymptotic χ^2 test P-value is always larger, much larger in Cases 1, 2, 3, 5, 6, 8, 9, and 10, than the exact and nonasymptotic χ^2 test P-values; (2) the exact χ^2 and Fisher's exact test P-values differ considerably for all contingency tables except Cases 1 and 2; and (3) the exact and nonasymptotic χ^2 test P-values are essentially the same when the number of distinct reference tables for fixed marginal frequency totals is large, e.g., at least 1,000,000. With the exception of 2^3 and 2^4 contingency tables (Mielke et al., 1994; Zelterman et al., 1995), few algorithms have been developed for obtaining exact test P-values for r-way contingency tables when $r \geq 3$. Since the number of cells associated with most r-way contingency tables is very large when $r \geq 3$, the expected values of cell frequencies are usually quite small; consequently, such contingency tables are often very sparse. However, the number of reference tables associated with r-way contingency tables is usually very large when $r \geq 3$ and, as with large sparse two-way contingency tables, the exact and nonasymptotic χ^2 test P-values will probably be very similar (analogous similarities hold for the exact and nonasymptotic Zelterman test P-values). Therefore, the nonasymptotic χ^2 and the nonasymptotic Zelterman test P-values provide excellent simply-obtained P-value approximations to the exact χ^2 and exact Zelterman tests, respectively, for large sparse contingency tables.

To demonstrate variations in the exact P-values among different techniques, consider the 5×5 contingency table (Case 12) in Table 7.5. The exact P-values for Fisher's exact, Pearson χ^2, Zelterman, and likelihood-ratio tests are 0.02855, 0.04446, 0.05358, and 0.05579, respectively.

TABLE 7.5. Sixteen sparse two-way contingency tables.

Case	Table	Case	Table
1	0 0 6 0 2 0	10	7 7 2 0 0
	5 2 0 1 0 4		2 2 1 3 3
2	0 0 0 0 2 0		7 7 2 0 0
	0 2 0 1 0 0	11	2 0 1 2 6
	0 0 1 1 0 0		1 3 1 1 1
	1 0 0 0 0 2		1 0 3 1 0
3	2 3 6 1 4 0		1 2 1 2 0
	5 1 1 4 0 3	12	2 2 1 1 0
4	12 9 3		0 0 2 3 0
	5 8 2		1 1 1 2 7
	4 1 10		1 2 0 0 0
5	2 0 0 1 0		1 1 1 1 0
	0 1 1 0 0	13	2 0 1 2 6 5
	0 0 2 0 1		1 3 1 1 1 2
	0 0 0 2 0		1 0 3 1 0 0
	0 0 0 0 3		1 2 1 2 0 0
6	0 7 0 0 0 0 0 1 1	14	1 1 1 0 0 0 1 2 4
	1 1 1 1 1 1 1 0 0		4 4 4 5 5 5 6 5 0
	0 8 0 0 0 0 0 1 1		1 1 1 0 0 0 1 2 4
7	1 1 1 0 0 0 1 3 3	15	1 2 2 1 1 0
	4 4 4 4 4 4 4 1 1		2 0 0 2 3 0
8	4 0 2 0 0 1 0 3 0 1 0 2		0 1 1 1 2 7
	1 1 0 2 2 2 1 0 3 0 2 1		1 1 2 0 0 0
9	1 0 0 2 0 0		0 1 1 1 1 0
	0 3 0 0 1 0	16	1 2 2 1 1 0 1
	0 0 2 0 0 3		2 0 0 2 3 0 0
	1 0 1 1 1 0		0 1 1 1 2 7 3
			1 1 2 0 0 0 1
			0 1 1 1 1 0 0

To compare the exact χ^2 and Fisher's exact test P-values given in Table 7.6 with P-values obtained from resampling, a resampling algorithm for generating random two-way contingency tables with fixed row and column totals is utilized (Patefield, 1981). Table 7.7 contains exact and resampling P-value comparisons for all 16 cases in Table 7.5. The resampling P-values

TABLE 7.6. P-values for (1) the exact χ^2 test, (2) the nonasymptotic χ^2 test, (3) the asymptotic χ^2 test, (4) Fisher's exact test, and (5) the number of reference tables for the 16 contingency tables listed in Table 7.5.

Case	(1)	(2)	(3)	(4)	(5)
1	0.00004	0.00004	0.00125	0.00004	379
2	0.02476	0.01186	0.03981	0.02476	3,076
3	0.00542	0.00638	0.01227	0.00908	3,345
4	0.00095	0.00101	0.00130	0.00210	13,576
5	0.00360	0.00292	0.01324	0.00584	20,959
6	0.04112	0.04297	0.16895	0.01480	26,108
7	0.05358	0.04740	0.06046	0.06796	35,353
8	0.01445	0.01321	0.05391	0.01919	110,688
9	0.00932	0.00909	0.01970	0.00594	123,170
10	0.00453	0.00458	0.00888	0.02432	184,100
11	0.08652	0.08782	0.09320	0.09112	3,187,528
12	0.04446	0.04492	0.05552	0.02855	29,760,752
13	0.05726	0.05820	0.06659	0.04537	97,080,796
14	0.08336	0.08473	0.09353	0.03535	1,326,849,651
15	0.06625	0.06729	0.07710	0.02584	2,159,651,513
16	0.11103	0.11269	0.12130	0.03929	108,712,356,901

based on $L = 1,000,000$ given in Table 7.7 closely approximate the exact P-values for all 16 cases.

7.5   Log-Linear Analyses of Sparse Contingency Tables

Asymptotic P-values resulting from log-linear analyses of sparse contingency tables are often much too large. Asymptotic P-values for chi-squared and likelihood-ratio statistics are compared to nonasymptotic and exact P-values for selected log-linear models (Mielke et al., 2004a).[4] The asymptotic P-values are all too often substantially larger than the exact P-values for the analysis of sparse contingency tables. An exact nondirectional permutation method is used to analyze combined independent multinomial distributions. Exact nondirectional permutation methods to analyze hypergeometric distributions associated with r-way contingency tables are confined to $r = 2$.

[4]Adapted and reprinted with permission of Psychological Reports from P.W. Mielke, Jr., K.J. Berry, and J.E. Johnston. Asymptotic log-linear analysis: Some cautions concerning sparse frequency tables. *Psychological Reports*, 2004, 94, 19–32. Copyright © 2004 by Psychological Reports.

TABLE 7.7. Exact and resampling P-values with $L = 1,000,000$ for the exact χ^2 test and Fisher's exact test for the 16 contingency tables listed in Table 7.5.

	χ^2 P-values		Fisher P-values	
Case	Exact	Resampling	Exact	Resampling
1	0.00004	0.00005	0.00004	0.00005
2	0.02476	0.02483	0.02476	0.02483
3	0.00542	0.00547	0.00908	0.00915
4	0.00095	0.00094	0.00210	0.00212
5	0.00360	0.00363	0.00584	0.00586
6	0.04112	0.04095	0.01480	0.01468
7	0.05358	0.05382	0.06796	0.06821
8	0.01445	0.01443	0.01919	0.01931
9	0.00932	0.00935	0.00594	0.00595
10	0.00453	0.00456	0.02432	0.02418
11	0.08652	0.08621	0.09112	0.09097
12	0.04446	0.04425	0.02855	0.02842
13	0.05726	0.05732	0.04537	0.04557
14	0.08336	0.08335	0.03535	0.03507
15	0.06625	0.06627	0.02584	0.02572
16	0.11103	0.11119	0.03929	0.03905

Log-linear models are appropriate for contingency tables, often termed cross-classification or frequency tables, composed of two or more categorical variables (Agresti, 1990; Agresti and Finlay, 1997; Bishop et al., 1975; Goodman, 1970; Haberman, 1978, 1979; Howell, 1997). Each log-linear model for a contingency table contains a set of expected frequencies that perfectly satisfy the model (Agresti and Finlay, 1997, p. 594). The goodness-of-fit of a specified model is typically tested with one of two chi-squared statistics: the Pearson (1900) chi-squared statistic (χ^2) or the Wilks (1935, 1938) likelihood-ratio statistic (G^2). Whenever sparse contingency tables are encountered, P-values obtained from the asymptotic chi-squared distribution may be inaccurate, either for χ^2 or G^2 (Agresti, 1990, pp. 49, 246–247; Agresti and Finlay, 1997, p. 595; Berry and Mielke, 1988c). An asymptotic test necessarily depends on expected frequencies that are not small. The small expected frequencies associated with sparse contingency tables result in test statistics that are not distributed as chi-squared and, thus, the obtained P-values can be either liberal or conservative (Agresti, 1990, pp. 246–247). In this section, exact, nonasymptotic, and asymptotic approaches for log-linear analysis of sparse contingency tables are described and compared. Sparse contingency tables occur when the sample size is small, or when the sample size is large but there is a large number of cells in the contingency table. While many authors have suggested that asymptotic chi-squared analyses of contingency tables are questionable when expected cell frequencies are less than five (Gravetter and Wallnau, 2004, p. 599; Hays, 1988, p. 781; Howell, 2002, p. 159), this stated threshold is fuzzy at best. However, the concern regarding asymptotic chi-squared analyses becomes more serious for studies involving increasingly sparse contingency tables. Since analyses commonly occur for very sparse contingency tables with expected cell frequencies less than one, the concern may be monumental. There appears to be a continuum of greater concern with increasingly sparse contingency tables. As an example, suppose that $N = 400$ subjects are assigned to a 4-way contingency table where the number of partitions are 3, 4, 6, and 7. Since the total number of cells is 504, the expected cell frequency would be only 0.79 if the marginal frequency totals for each of the four variables were equal.

Two methods associated with multinomial and hypergeometric models are considered. The multinomial and hypergeometric approaches provide exact alternative permutation analyses for specific subsets of log-linear models. These two methods provide comparisons between exact and corresponding asymptotic log-linear analysis P-values.

7.5.1   Multinomial Analyses

The subset of log-linear models considered here involves partitioning of the data into k levels of specified variables. Asymptotic, nonasymptotic, and exact P-values are calculated for each of the k levels. Each of the k independent P-values is based on the g cells of a multinomial distribution, where H_0 states that each of m events occurs in a cell with equal chance, i.e., $1/g$. Then, the distribution of the m events under H_0 is multinomial with the point probability given by

$$m! \left/ \left(g^m \prod_{i=1}^{g} o_i! \right) \right.$$

where o_i is the observed frequency for the ith of g cells and

$$m = \sum_{i=1}^{g} o_i.$$

Also, the χ^2 and G^2 test statistics corresponding to each of the k frequency configurations are given by

$$\chi^2 = \sum_{i=1}^{g} \frac{(o_i - e_i)^2}{e_i}$$

and

$$G^2 = 2 \sum_{i=1}^{g} o_i \ln \left(\frac{o_i}{e_i} \right),$$

respectively, where the expected frequency of the ith cell under H_0 is

$$e_i = \frac{m}{g}$$

for $i = 1, ..., g$. Note that m may differ for each of the k frequency configurations.

The sum of independent χ^2 or G^2 values is asymptotically distributed as chi-squared with degrees-of-freedom equal to the sum of the individual degrees-of-freedom. Consequently, for both χ^2 and G^2, the degrees-of-freedom and test statistics for each of the k frequency configurations sum to the corresponding degrees-of-freedom and test statistics associated with the asymptotic log-linear model.

Fisher (1934, pp. 103–105) described a method for combining k independent probabilities $(P_1, ..., P_k)$ from continuous distributions based on the statistic

$$-2 \sum_{i=1}^{k} \ln P_i,$$

which is distributed as chi-squared with $2k$ degrees-of-freedom. The method of Fisher requires that the k probabilities be independent uniform random variables from 0 to 1 and is not appropriate for discontinuous probability distributions where only a few different events are possible (Lancaster, 1949; also see Section 9.1). As shown, the method of Fisher provides conservative results, i.e., the compound P-value will be too large (Gordon et al., 1952). The nonasymptotic P-values are based on the k combined nonasymptotic goodness-of-fit P-values for χ^2 (Mielke and Berry, 1988; also see Section 6.1.3) using the method of Fisher (1934). Nonasymptotic P-values for G^2 are undefined because logarithmic functions of frequencies preclude the computation of expected values.

Described next is a nondirectional permutation method to obtain an exact combined P-value for k discontinuous probability distributions. This method is a special case of a recently-described technique for combining P-values associated with independent discrete probability distributions (Mielke et al., 2004b; also see Section 9.1). Recall that the analogous nondirectional method described by Fisher (1934) to obtain an exact combined P-value was for k continuous probability distributions. In the present context, k multinomial distributions are considered. Because the test statistic values and the probabilities are not monotonic (Agresti and Wackerly, 1977; Berry and Mielke, 1985b; Radlow and Alf, 1975), each of the k multinomial probability distributions must be based on the ordered magnitudes of the test statistics, not the ordered probabilities. In this context, the probability distributions are ordered by either the χ^2 or G^2 values.

Let m_i be the total number of events in the ith of k levels and let o_{ij} be the number of events in the jth of g cells within the ith of k levels. Thus,

$$m_i = \sum_{j=1}^{g} o_{ij}$$

and the expected value of o_{ij} under H_0 is m_i/g for $i = 1, ..., k$. Also, let

$$L = \sum_{i=1}^{k} m_i$$

be the total number of events over the k levels. If each of the m_i events within the ith of k levels is perceived as distinguishable, then there are

$$M = g^L$$

equally-likely distinguishable configurations over the k levels under H_0. Let χ_l^2 and G_l^2 denote the respective sums of the k χ^2 and G^2 test statistic values for the lth of M configurations. In addition, let χ_o^2 and G_o^2 denote the respective sums of the k χ^2 and G^2 test statistic values for the observed configuration. If P_A and P_B denote the exact χ^2 and G^2 P-values for the k combined levels, respectively, then

$$P_A = \frac{1}{M} \sum_{l=1}^{M} A_l$$

and

$$P_B = \frac{1}{M} \sum_{l=1}^{M} B_l,$$

where

$$A_l = \begin{cases} 1 & \text{if } \chi_l^2 \geq \chi_o^2, \\ 0 & \text{otherwise,} \end{cases}$$

and

$$B_l = \begin{cases} 1 & \text{if } G_l^2 \geq G_o^2, \\ 0 & \text{otherwise,} \end{cases}$$

respectively. While M can be extremely large, an algorithm that assumes the M configurations are equally likely with a partitioning of the χ^2 and G^2 test statistic values into a reduced number of equivalence classes yields P_A and P_B in an efficient manner under H_0, respectively (Euler, 1748/1988; also see Section 6.1.2). An alternative exact permutation method for combining P-values for discontinuous probability distributions due to Wallis

(1942) is not applicable here, as the method of Wallis is based on k cumulative distribution functions, and is therefore directional. Moreover, whenever the observed P-value is tied with other nonobserved P-values, different combined P-values will result, depending on which of the tied P-values is considered as the observed P-value.

7.5.2 Hypergeometric Analyses

Following the opening notation of this chapter and Mielke and Berry (1988, 2002c), consider an r-way contingency table with $n_1 \times \cdots \times n_r$ cells where $o_{j_1,...,j_r}$ is the observed frequency of the $(j_1, ..., j_r)$th cell, $n_i \geq 2$ is the number of ith partitions for variables $i = 1, ..., r$, $\langle i \rangle_{j_i}$ is the marginal frequency total for the ith variable in the j_ith partition for $j_i = 1, ..., n_i$, and

$$N = \sum_{j_i=1}^{n_i} \langle i \rangle_{j_i}$$

is the frequency total for the r-way contingency table. This notation accommodates all r-way contingency tables, i.e., $r \geq 2$. Under the H_0 that the r variables are independent, the exact distribution conditioned on the fixed marginal frequency totals is hypergeometric with the point probability given by

$$\prod_{i=1}^{r} \prod_{j_i=1}^{n_i} \langle i \rangle_{j_i}! \left[(N!)^{r-1} \prod_{i=1}^{r} \prod_{j_i=1}^{n_i} o_{j_1,...,j_r}! \right]^{-1}.$$

The χ^2 and G^2 test statistics for independence of r variables are given by

$$\chi^2 = N^{r-1} \left[\sum_{i=1}^{r} \sum_{j_i=1}^{n_i} \left(o_{j_1,...,j_r}^2 \bigg/ \prod_{k=1}^{r} \langle k \rangle_{j_k} \right) \right] - N$$

and

$$G^2 = 2 \sum_{i=1}^{r} \sum_{j_i=1}^{n_i} o_{j_1,...,j_r} \ln \left(N^{r-1} o_{j_1,...,j_r} \bigg/ \prod_{k=1}^{r} \langle k \rangle_{j_k} \right),$$

respectively.

Under the H_0 that the r variables of an r-way contingency table are independent, three methods to obtain P-values for χ^2 and G^2 can be defined, given fixed marginal frequency totals: asymptotic, nonasymptotic, and exact. The asymptotic method is a large sample approximation that assumes that all expected cell frequencies are at least five (Agresti and Finlay, 1997, p. 595) and the asymptotic distribution of both χ^2 and G^2 is chi-squared with

$$\prod_{i=1}^{r} n_i - \sum_{i=1}^{r} (n_i - 1) - 1$$

degrees-of-freedom under H_0.

The nonasymptotic method obtains the exact mean, variance, and skewness of χ^2, based on the exact distribution under H_0 denoted by μ, σ^2, and γ, respectively. The distribution of

$$\frac{\chi^2 - \mu}{\sigma}$$

is approximated by the Pearson type III distribution characterized by the single skewness parameter γ (Mielke and Berry, 1988; also see Section 7.1). The nonasymptotic method compensates for small expected cell frequencies and is not totally dependent on degrees-of-freedom as is the asymptotic log-linear method.

The exact method calculates both the χ^2 and G^2 test statistic values for all possible cell arrangements of the r-way contingency table, given fixed marginal frequency totals. The exact P-value is the sum of the probabilities associated with test statistic values, under H_0, equal to or greater than the observed test statistic value for the r-way contingency table. Small expected cell frequencies and a complete dependence on degrees-of-freedom are not relevant to the exact method.

The P-values of the asymptotic, nonasymptotic, and exact methods are essentially equivalent when all cell frequencies are large. However, given the small expected cell frequencies that commonly occur in a sparse r-way contingency table, a P-value obtained with the asymptotic method may differ considerably from the P-values obtained with the nonasymptotic and exact methods. While G^2 is well defined for the asymptotic and exact methods, it is not possible to obtain the exact mean, variance, and skewness of G^2 for sparse contingency tables due to the logarithmic functions of the frequencies. Consequently, unlike χ^2, G^2 is undefined for the nonasymptotic method.

7.5.3 Example

Consider the $3 \times 4 \times 5$ sparse frequency data in Table 7.8. In this example, 10 of the 17 possible unsaturated models are selected for examination. The 17 models are listed in Table 7.9 and the 10 selected models are indicated with asterisks. The notation for describing the log-linear models in Table 7.9 uses letters to stand for specific variables, enclosing letters of related variables within braces. Of these 10 models, six are multinomial: $\{A\}$, $\{B\}$, $\{C\}$, $\{AB\}$, $\{AC\}$, and $\{BC\}$. Each of the six multinomial models is disjoint with a balanced number of replicates in each partition. The 60 cells are partitioned according to one or more variables and the remaining cells within each partition consist of ordered replicates of the remaining variables. The partitioned multinomial distributions are individually tested for goodness-of-fit under the stated H_0, and the P-values are combined using either the method of Fisher (1934) or the previously-described

TABLE 7.8. Sparse $3 \times 4 \times 5$ example for log-linear analysis.

	A_1				A_2				A_3			
	B_1	B_2	B_3	B_4	B_1	B_2	B_3	B_4	B_1	B_2	B_3	B_4
C_1	0	0	2	1	1	0	0	0	0	1	0	0
C_2	0	1	0	0	1	0	0	1	0	0	1	4
C_3	0	0	0	1	0	2	1	0	1	0	0	0
C_4	1	0	0	1	0	1	2	0	1	1	0	0
C_5	0	0	2	0	1	0	0	0	0	3	0	1

nondirectional permutation method. The remaining four of the 10 models are hypergeometric: $\{AB\}\{C\}$, $\{AC\}\{B\}$, $\{BC\}\{A\}$, and $\{A\}\{B\}\{C\}$. These four hypergeometric models are both exhaustive, i.e., each of the $3 \times 20 = 4 \times 15 = 5 \times 12 = 3 \times 4 \times 5 = 60$ cells is considered in each hypergeometric model analysis, and disjoint, i.e., each of the 60 cells is considered exactly once in each analysis.

In model $\{A\}$, variables B and C are examined with equal weight given to each replicate of variables B and C under H_0 for each level of variable A. In model $\{B\}$, variables A and C are examined with equal weight given to each replicate of variables A and C under H_0 for each level of variable B. In model $\{C\}$, variables A and B are examined with equal weight given to each replicate of variables A and B under H_0 for each level of variable C. In model $\{AB\}$, variable C is examined with equal weight given to each replicate of variable C under H_0 for each combined level of variables A and B. In model $\{AC\}$, variable B is examined with equal weight given to each replicate of variable B under H_0 for each combined level of variables A and C. In model $\{BC\}$, variable A is examined with equal weight given to each replicate of variable A under H_0 for each combined level of variables B and C. In model $\{AB\}\{C\}$, all combinations of variables A and B are independent of variable C under H_0. In model $\{AC\}\{B\}$, all combinations of variables A and C are independent of variable B under H_0. In model $\{BC\}\{A\}$, all combinations of variables B and C are independent of variable A under H_0. In model $\{A\}\{B\}\{C\}$, variables A, B, and C are mutually independent under H_0.

Since models $\{A\}$, $\{B\}$, $\{C\}$, $\{AB\}$, $\{AC\}$, and $\{BC\}$ are associated with balanced replicates, these six models do not involve an exhaustive partitioning of the data, i.e., more than one of the 60 cells occurs in each level of the relevant variable or variables. On the other hand, models $\{AB\}\{C\}$, $\{AC\}\{B\}$, $\{BC\}\{A\}$, and $\{A\}\{B\}\{C\}$ do involve an exhaustive partitioning of the data because there are no replicates, i.e., exactly one cell occurs in each level of the relevant variables.

TABLE 7.9. Log-linear models for the $3 \times 4 \times 5$ sparse frequency data in Table 7.8.

Model	Interpretation
{A}*	Variable A is the only variable of interest.
{B}*	Variable B is the only variable of interest.
{C}*	Variable C is the only variable of interest.
{AB}*	All combinations of variables A and B are of interest.
{AC}*	All combinations of variables A and C are of interest.
{BC}*	All combinations of variables B and C are of interest.
{A}{B}	Variable A is independent of variable B.
{A}{C}	Variable A is independent of variable C.
{B}{C}	Variable B is independent of variable C.
{AB}{C}*	{AB} is independent of variable C.
{AC}{B}*	{AC} is independent of variable B.
{BC}{A}*	{BC} is independent of variable A.
{AB}{AC}	{AB} is independent of {AC}.
{AB}{BC}	{AB} is independent of {BC}.
{AC}{BC}	{AC} is independent of {BC}.
{A}{B}{C}*	Variables A, B, and C are mutually independent.
{AB}{AC}{BC}	{AB}, {AC}, and {BC} are mutually independent.

* The models analyzed are indicated by an asterisk.

Analyses of the Six Multinomial Models

Table 7.10 contains the test statistics and associated P-values for the asymptotic χ^2, nonasymptotic χ^2, exact χ^2, asymptotic G^2, and exact G^2 for the six multinomial models. Degrees-of-freedom are not applicable to the exact and nonasymptotic analyses in Table 7.10.

For the multinomial models {A}, {B}, and {C} in Table 7.10, the nonasymptotic χ^2 values and the exact χ^2 and G^2 values are the sums of the corresponding nonasymptotic χ^2, exact χ^2, and exact G^2 values calculated for the three, four, and five levels of variables A, B, and C, respectively. For the multinomial models {AB}, {AC}, and {BC}, the nonasymptotic χ^2 values are the sums of the nonasymptotic goodness-of-fit values of χ^2 calculated for the 12 combined levels of variables A and B, the 15 combined

TABLE 7.10. Asymptotic χ^2, nonasymptotic χ^2, exact χ^2, asymptotic G^2, and exact G^2 P-values for multinomial models {A}, {B}, {C}, {AB}, {AC}, and {BC} for the sparse data in Table 7.8.

Model	Test	Statistic	df	P value
{A}	Asymptotic χ^2	72.581	57	0.07995
	Nonasymptotic χ^2	72.581	NA*	0.07341
	Exact χ^2	72.581	NA	0.07444
	Asymptotic G^2	68.209	57	0.14698
	Exact G^2	68.209	NA	0.08705
{B}	Asymptotic χ^2	72.583	56	0.06731
	Nonasymptotic χ^2	72.583	NA	0.06035
	Exact χ^2	72.583	NA	0.05995
	Asymptotic G^2	68.215	56	0.12681
	Exact G^2	68.215	NA	0.07035
{C}	Asymptotic χ^2	72.743	55	0.05481
	Nonasymptotic χ^2	72.743	NA	0.05029
	Exact χ^2	72.743	NA	0.04659
	Asymptotic G^2	67.861	55	0.11422
	Exact G^2	67.861	NA	0.06409
{AB}	Asymptotic χ^2	57.667	48	0.16005
	Nonasymptotic χ^2	57.667	NA	0.22042
	Exact χ^2	57.667	NA	0.08374
	Asymptotic G^2	59.358	48	0.12600
	Exact G^2	59.358	NA	0.05089
{AC}	Asymptotic χ^2	55.600	45	0.13370
	Nonasymptotic χ^2	55.600	NA	0.21821
	Exact χ^2	55.600	NA	0.04684
	Asymptotic G^2	59.445	45	0.07306
	Exact G^2	59.445	NA	0.02815
{BC}	Asymptotic χ^2	53.200	40	0.07901
	Nonasymptotic χ^2	53.200	NA	0.13188
	Exact χ^2	53.200	NA	0.00342
	Asymptotic G^2	59.762	40	0.02296
	Exact G^2	59.762	NA	0.00332

*Degrees-of-freedom are not applicable (NA) for nonasymptotic and exact tests.

levels of variables A and C, and the 20 combined levels of variables B and C, respectively.

The nonasymptotic P-values for multinomial models $\{A\}$, $\{B\}$, $\{C\}$ $\{AB\}$, $\{AC\}$, and $\{BC\}$ were obtained by combining the three, four, five, 12, 15, and 20 nonasymptotic goodness-of-fit P-values for χ^2, respectively, using the method of Fisher (1934). As already noted, nonasymptotic P-values for G^2 are undefined. The exact P-values for χ^2 and G^2 of models $\{A\}$, $\{B\}$, $\{C\}$, $\{AB\}$, $\{AC\}$, and $\{BC\}$ in Table 7.10 were obtained by combining the three, four, five, 12, 15, and 20 exact goodness-of-fit P-values for χ^2 and G^2, respectively, using the previously-described nondirectional permutation method. The asymptotic P-values for χ^2 and G^2 of the six multinomial models were obtained from SPSS LOGLINEAR (SPSS, Inc., 2002).

The χ^2, G^2, and associated P-values for the six multinomial models are listed in Table 7.10. For model $\{A\}$, the asymptotic and nonasymptotic P-values for χ^2 of 0.07995 and 0.07341, respectively, are good estimates of the exact P-value for χ^2 of 0.07444. However, the asymptotic P-value for G^2 of 0.14698 overestimates the exact P-value for G^2 of 0.08705.

For model $\{B\}$, the asymptotic and nonasymptotic P-values for χ^2 of 0.06731 and 0.06035, respectively, are close to the exact P-value for χ^2 of 0.05995. The asymptotic P-value for G^2 of 0.12681 again overestimates the exact P-value for G^2 of 0.07035.

For model $\{C\}$, the asymptotic and nonasymptotic P-values for χ^2 of 0.05481 and 0.05029, respectively, slightly overestimate the exact P-value for χ^2 of 0.04659. It should be noted that, in this case, the asymptotic and nonasymptotic P-values for χ^2 are slightly above the nominal value of $\alpha = 0.05$ and the exact P-value for χ^2 is slightly below $\alpha = 0.05$. The asymptotic P-value for G^2 of 0.11422 once again overestimates the exact P-value for G^2 of 0.06409 as with models $\{A\}$ and $\{B\}$.

For model $\{AB\}$, the asymptotic and nonasymptotic P-values for χ^2 of 0.16005 and 0.22042, respectively, severely overestimate the exact P-value for χ^2 of 0.08374, and the asymptotic P-value for G^2 of 0.12600 is more than twice as large as the exact P-value for G^2 of 0.05089. The poor asymptotic and nonasymptotic P-values are likely due to the sparse number of discrete arrangements to be approximated by a continuous distribution. In particular, four of the 12 combined levels of variables A and B contain only a single event, e.g., $\{0\ 1\ 0\ 0\ 0\}$.

For model $\{AC\}$, the asymptotic and nonasymptotic P-values for χ^2 of 0.13370 and 0.21821, respectively, severely overestimate the exact P-value for χ^2 of 0.04684, and the asymptotic P-value for G^2 of 0.07306 overestimates the exact P-value for G^2 of 0.02815. Here, the poor approximate P-values for χ^2 may be because four of the 15 combined levels of variables A and C contain only a single event and three of the 15 combined levels contain only two events.

TABLE 7.11. Asymptotic χ^2, nonasymptotic χ^2, exact χ^2, asymptotic G^2, and exact G^2 P-values for hypergeometric models {AB}{C}, {AC}{B}, {BC}{A}, and {A}{B}{C} for the sparse data in Table 7.8.

Model	Test	Statistic	df	P value
{AB}{C}	Asymptotic χ^2	54.232	44	0.13875
	Nonasymptotic χ^2	54.232	NA	0.09047
	Exact χ^2	54.232	NA	0.08988
	Asymptotic G^2	58.216	44	0.07398
	Exact G^2	58.216	NA	0.03406
{AC}{B}	Asymptotic χ^2	56.178	42	0.07055
	Nonasymptotic χ^2	56.178	NA	0.02021
	Exact χ^2	56.178	NA	0.02017
	Asymptotic G^2	58.657	42	0.04536
	Exact G^2	58.657	NA	0.01824
{BC}{A}	Asymptotic χ^2	53.631	38	0.04770
	Nonasymptotic χ^2	53.631	NA	0.00155
	Exact χ^2	53.631	NA	0.00131
	Asymptotic G^2	58.967	38	0.01618
	Exact G^2	58.967	NA	0.00240
{A}{B}{C}*	Asymptotic χ^2	67.406	50	0.05084
	Nonasymptotic χ^2	67.406	NA	0.04179
	Exact χ^2	———	——	———
	Asymptotic G^2	66.279	50	0.06133
	Exact G^2	———	——	———

*This table configuration does not allow for computation of exact P values.

For model {BC}, the asymptotic and nonasymptotic P-values for χ^2 of 0.07901 and 0.13188, respectively, substantially overestimate the exact P-value for χ^2 of 0.00342, and the asymptotic P-value for G^2 of 0.02296 likewise overestimates the exact P-value for G^2 of 0.00332. Since 12 of the 20 combined levels of variables B and C contain only a single event, it is not surprising that the asymptotic P-values are such poor estimates of the exact P-values.

Analyses of the Four Hypergeometric Models

Table 7.11 contains the test statistics and associated P-values for the asymptotic χ^2, nonasymptotic χ^2, exact χ^2, asymptotic G^2, and exact G^2 for the four hypergeometric models. Degrees-of-freedom are not applicable to the exact and nonasymptotic analyses in Table 7.11.

For the hypergeometric models {AB}{C}, {AC}{B}, {BC}{A}, and {A}{B}{C} in Table 7.11, the nonasymptotic χ^2 and associated P-values for models $\{AB\}\{C\}$, $\{AC\}\{B\}$, and $\{BC\}\{A\}$ were obtained using the r-way contingency table analysis of Mielke and Berry (1988, 2002c). The exact P-values for χ^2 and G^2 values were obtained using a StatXact algorithm (Cytel Software Corp., 2002). Presently, no algorithm exists to obtain the exact P-value of model $\{A\}\{B\}\{C\}$. The asymptotic P-values for χ^2 and G^2 of the four hypergeometric models were obtained using SPSS LOGLINEAR (SPSS, Inc., 2002).

The χ^2, G^2, and associated P-values for the four hypergeometric models are listed in Table 7.11. For model $\{AB\}\{C\}$, the asymptotic P-value for χ^2 of 0.13875 overestimates the exact P-value for χ^2 of 0.08988. Similarly, the asymptotic P-value for G^2 of 0.07398 overestimates the exact P-value for G^2 of 0.03406. On the other hand, the nonasymptotic P-value for χ^2 of 0.09047 is very close to the exact P-value for χ^2 of 0.08988.

For model $\{AC\}\{B\}$, the asymptotic P-value for χ^2 of 0.07055 overestimates the exact P-value for χ^2 of 0.02017. The asymptotic P-value for G^2 of 0.04536 also overestimates the exact P-value for G^2 of 0.01824. The nonasymptotic P-value for χ^2 of 0.02021 is again very close to the exact P-value for χ^2 of 0.02017.

For model $\{BC\}\{A\}$, the asymptotic P-value for χ^2 of 0.04770 severely overestimates the exact P-value for χ^2 of 0.00131. Similarly, the asymptotic P-value for G^2 of 0.01618 is almost an order of magnitude greater than the exact P-value for G^2 of 0.00240. However, the nonasymptotic P-value for χ^2 of 0.00155 is once again close to the exact P-value for χ^2 of 0.00131 as with models $\{AB\}\{C\}$ and $\{AC\}\{B\}$.

Model $\{A\}\{B\}\{C\}$ yields a $3 \times 4 \times 5$ contingency table that presently does not allow the computation of an exact P-value. Although the P-values for the asymptotic χ^2, nonasymptotic χ^2, and asymptotic G^2 for model $\{A\}\{B\}\{C\}$ do not differ greatly, it is interesting to note that the asymptotic P-values for χ^2 and G^2 of 0.05084 and 0.06133, respectively, are slightly above the nominal value of $\alpha = 0.05$ and the nonasymptotic P-value for χ^2 of 0.04179 is slightly below $\alpha = 0.05$. For hypergeometric models, the nonasymptotic P-values for χ^2 are close to the exact P-values for χ^2 for all examples that allow a comparison (Mielke and Berry, 2002c; also see Section 7.4).

7.5.4   Discussion

It is evident from Tables 7.10 and 7.11 that exceedingly inaccurate asymptotic P-values for both the χ^2 and G^2 test statistics in log-linear analyses are associated with sparse contingency tables. Although the results indicate that asymptotic chi-squared P-values for sparse contingency tables often severely overestimate the exact P-values, Agresti (1990, pp. 246–249) notes that asymptotic chi-squared P-values may either overestimate or underestimate exact P-values, leading to both conservative and liberal estimates of the true P-values. Although the exact approach is obviously preferable, it is not computationally feasible for any but the simplest log-linear analyses. While the nonasymptotic approach provides excellent approximations to exact P-values for χ^2 of hypergeometric log-linear models, the nonasymptotic approach yields poor approximations to the exact P-values of multinomial log-linear models with sparse frequency configurations. These poor approximations may result, in part, from the method to combine P-values from continuous distributions due to Fisher (1934). In addition, the functional form involving logarithms prohibits the nonasymptotic approach for G^2. Also, the exact and nonasymptotic approaches are limited to log-linear models that are both disjoint and exhaustive. In particular, exact and nonasymptotic analyses were not given for log-linear models $\{A\}\{B\}$, $\{A\}\{C\}$, and $\{B\}\{C\}$, since these models are not exhaustive. Nonasymptotic analyses were not given for models $\{AB\}\{AC\}$, $\{AB\}\{BC\}$, $\{AC\}\{BC\}$, and $\{AB\}\{AC\}\{BC\}$, since these models are not disjoint (Goodman, 1970; Williams, 1976a). Development of appropriate exact analyses for models other than the simple multinomial and hypergeometric models considered here is encouraged. While exact methods for many analyses associated with log-linear models are unknown, the concerns detailed in the tractable comparisons given in this chapter likely hold for all comparisons.

It is somewhat disquieting to consider that conventional log-linear methods may produce erroneous conclusions when contingency tables are sparse. As contingency tables become larger, e.g., with four or five dimensions, then sparseness is increasingly likely, the likelihood of zero marginal frequency totals increases, and the potential for errors is exacerbated. While the problem with the use of asymptotic P-values in log-linear analysis was confined to a 3-way contingency table, the situation only becomes worse for log-linear analyses of r-way contingency tables when $r \geq 4$ (Bishop et al., 1975; Goodman, 1970; Haberman, 1978, 1979).

The most popular log-linear method involves hierarchical analyses. In hierarchical log-linear analyses, forward or backward elimination is used to find the best fitting log-linear model. The process fits an initial model, then adds or subtracts interaction terms based on the significance of either χ^2 or G^2. The process continues in a tree-like fashion until the resulting model is the one with the least number of interaction terms necessary to fit the observed contingency table. Should the asymptotic P-values underestimate or overestimate the specified nominal level of significance, the hierarchical process may continue up the wrong branch of the decision tree, or fail to go down the correct branch, resulting in an erroneous final model for the data. Until better methods are developed for log-linear analyses of sparse contingency tables, the results of conventional log-linear analyses should be considered suspect.

7.6   Exact Tests For Interaction in 2^r Tables

If the null hypothesis of independence is rejected for an r-way contingency table (r is an integer ≥ 2), then the cause for this lack of independence is in question. In the case of 2^r contingency tables, this question is addressed by individually analyzing the $2^r - r - 1$ interactions in order to identify the cause. Although this approach extends to other r-way contingency tables, the present discussion is confined to 2^r contingency tables.

Let $p_{i_1 \cdots i_r}$ denote the probability associated with the $(i_1 \cdots i_r)$th cell of a 2^r contingency table where index $i_j = 1$ or 2 for $j = 1, \ldots, r$. For the marginal probability values, one or more indices are replaced by dot notation, i.e., the indices are summed over 1 and 2. For a 2×2 (i.e., 2^2) contingency table, the H_0 that there is no interaction of order 1 is

$$p_{11} \, p_{22} = p_{12} \, p_{21}. \tag{7.1}$$

The H_0 that there is no interaction of order 1 in a 2^2 contingency table is equivalent to the H_0 that the two classifications are independent. For a $2 \times 2 \times 2$ (i.e., 2^3) contingency table, the H_0 that there is no interaction of order 2 is

$$p_{111} \, p_{221} \, p_{122} \, p_{212} = p_{112} \, p_{222} \, p_{121} \, p_{211} \tag{7.2}$$

(Bartlett, 1935), and the three H_0s that there is no interaction of order 1 are

$$p_{11.} \, p_{22.} = p_{12.} \, p_{21.},$$

$$p_{1.1} \, p_{2.2} = p_{1.2} \, p_{2.1}, \tag{7.3}$$

and

$$p_{.11} \, p_{.22} = p_{.12} \, p_{.21}.$$

In general, the H_0 that there is no interaction of order $r - 1$ in a 2^r contingency table may be obtained recursively from the H_0 that there is no interaction of order $r - 2$ in a 2^{r-1} contingency table in the following manner. The first (second) set of terms on the left side of H_0 that there is no interaction of order $r-1$ in a 2^r contingency table are the left (right) side terms of H_0 that there is no interaction of order $r-2$ in a 2^{r-1} contingency table where a 1 (2) is appended to the right side of each term's subscript. Similarly, the first (second) set of terms on the right side of H_0 that there is no interaction of order $r-1$ in a 2^r contingency table are the left (right) side terms of H_0 that there is no interaction of order $r-2$ in a 2^{r-1} contingency table where a 2 (1) is appended to the right side of each term's subscript. As an example, compare the structure of H_0 that there is no interaction of order 2 in a 2^3 contingency table in Expression (7.2) with H_0 that there is no interaction of order 1 in a 2^2 contingency table in Expression (7.1). Thus, the H_0 that there is no interaction of order 3 in a $2 \times 2 \times 2 \times 2$ (i.e., 2^4) contingency table is obtained from the H_0 that there is no interaction of order 2 in a 2^3 contingency table in Expression (7.2) and is given by

$$p_{1111} \, p_{2211} \, p_{1221} \, p_{2121} \, p_{1122} \, p_{2222} \, p_{1212} \, p_{2112} =$$

$$p_{1112} \, p_{2212} \, p_{1222} \, p_{2122} \, p_{1121} \, p_{2221} \, p_{1211} \, p_{2111}. \tag{7.4}$$

The lower-order $\binom{r}{j+1}$ H_0s that there is no interaction of order j in a 2^r contingency table are obtained from the H_0 that there is no interaction of order j in a 2^{j+1} contingency table. This is accomplished in a manner analogous to constructing the three H_0s that there is no interaction of order 1 in a 2^3 contingency table by inserting a dot into each of the $\binom{3}{2} = 3$ distinct positions indicated in Expression (7.3). In general, $r - j - 1$ dots are inserted into the $\binom{r}{j+1}$ distinct positions associated with the 2^r contingency table $(j = 1, 2, ..., r - 2)$. As an example, consider a 2^4 contingency table. Although the H_0 that there is no interaction of order 3 is given by Expression (7.4), the $\binom{4}{2} = 6$ H_0s that there is no interaction of order 1 are

$$p_{11..} \, p_{22..} = p_{12..} \, p_{21..},$$

$$p_{1.1.} \, p_{2.2.} = p_{1.2.} \, p_{2.1.},$$

$$p_{1..1} \, p_{2..2} = p_{1..2} \, p_{2..1},$$

$$p_{.11.} \, p_{.22.} = p_{.12.} \, p_{.21.},$$

$$p_{.1.1} \, p_{.2.2} = p_{.1.2} \, p_{.2.1},$$

and

$$p_{..11} \, p_{..22} = p_{..12} \, p_{..21},$$

and the $\binom{4}{3} = 4$ H_0s that there is no interaction of order 2 are

$$p_{111.} \, p_{221.} \, p_{122.} \, p_{212.} = p_{112.} \, p_{222.} \, p_{121.} \, p_{211.},$$

$$p_{11.1} \, p_{22.1} \, p_{12.2} \, p_{21.2} = p_{11.2} \, p_{22.2} \, p_{12.1} \, p_{21.1},$$

$$p_{1.11} \, p_{2.21} \, p_{1.22} \, p_{2.12} = p_{1.12} \, p_{2.22} \, p_{1.21} \, p_{2.11},$$

and

$$p_{.111} \, p_{.221} \, p_{.122} \, p_{.212} = p_{.112} \, p_{.222} \, p_{.121} \, p_{.211}.$$

The number of distinct interactions associated with a 2^r contingency table is $2^r - r - 1$, the degrees-of-freedom for testing H_0 that the r classifications are mutually independent. The computing time needed to implement $2^r - r - 1$ single-loop exact tests for interaction is trivial relative to the computing time needed to implement the corresponding $2^r - r - 1$ loop exact test that the r classifications are mutually independent. Exact tests for the mutual independence of the r classifications in a 2^r contingency table have been constructed for $r = 3$ and $r = 4$ (Mielke et al., 1994; Zelterman et al., 1995). In addition, exact tests for the $2^r - r - 1$ interactions of a 2^r contingency table have also been constructed for $r = 3$ and $r = 4$ (Mielke and Berry, 1996b, 1998). Although extensions of exact tests for the mutual independence of r classifications appear to be computationally difficult for 2^r contingency tables with $r > 4$, extensions of exact tests concerning interactions of 2^r contingency tables beyond $r = 3$ are easily obtained and computationally feasible. The exact test for interactions is illustrated with two examples, one for a 2^3 contingency table and one for a 2^4 contingency table.

7.6.1 Analysis of a 2^3 Contingency Table

It is occasionally necessary to test the independence among three classification variables, each of which consists of two mutually exclusive classes, i.e., a 2^3 contingency table. As discussed earlier in the chapter, Mielke et al. (1994) provide an algorithm for the exact P-value for independence obtained from an examination of all possible permutations of the eight cell frequencies, conditioned on the observed marginal frequency totals, of a 2^3 contingency table. An alternative approach that may be more informative and not as computationally intensive involves the examination of the first- and second-order interactions in a 2^3 contingency table when the observed marginal frequency totals are fixed. This approach was first proposed by Bartlett (1935) and has been discussed by Darroch (1962, 1974), Haber (1983, 1984), Odoroff (1970), Plackett (1962), Pomar (1984), Simpson (1951), and Zachs and Solomon (1976). An algorithm is described here to compute the exact probabilities of the three first-order (two-variable) interactions and the one second-order (three-variable) interaction (Mielke and Berry, 1996b).[5]

The logic on which the algorithm is based is the same as for the Fisher exact contingency table tests. Beginning with a small arbitrary initial value, a simple recursion procedure generates relative frequency values for all possible 2^3 contingency tables, given the observed marginal frequency totals.

---

[5] Adapted and reprinted with permission of Sage Publications, Inc. from P.W. Mielke, Jr. and K.J. Berry. Exact probabilities for first-order and second-order interactions in $2 \times 2 \times 2$ tables. *Educational and Psychological Measurement*, 1996, 56, 843–847. Copyright © 1996 by Sage Publications, Inc.

The desired exact P-value is obtained by summing the relative frequency values equal to or less than the observed relative frequency value and dividing the resultant sum by the unrestricted relative frequency total.

Consider a sample of N independent observations arranged in a 2^3 contingency table. Let o_{ijk} denote the observed cell frequency of the ith row, jth column, and kth slice, and let p_{ijk} denote the corresponding cell probability ($i = 1, 2$; $j = 1, 2$; $k = 1, 2$). Also, let $o_{.jk}$, $o_{i.k}$, $o_{ij.}$, $o_{i..}$, $o_{.j.}$, $o_{..k}$, and $o_{...}$ indicate the observed marginal frequency totals of the 2^3 contingency table, and let the corresponding marginals over p_{ijk} be indicated by $p_{.jk}$, $p_{i.k}$, $p_{ij.}$, $p_{i..}$, $p_{.j.}$, $p_{..k}$, and $p_{...}$, respectively ($i = 1, 2$; $j = 1, 2$; $k = 1, 2$). Because the categories are mutually exclusive and exhaustive, $o_{...} = N$ and $p_{...} = 1$.

The null hypotheses for the three first-order interactions are

$$p_{.11}\, p_{.22} = p_{.12}\, p_{.21},$$

$$p_{1.1}\, p_{2.2} = p_{1.2}\, p_{2.1},$$

and

$$p_{11.}\, p_{22.} = p_{12.}\, p_{21.}.$$

(Bartlett, 1935).

The null hypothesis for the second-order interaction is

$$p_{111}\, p_{122}\, p_{212}\, p_{221} = p_{112}\, p_{121}\, p_{211}\, p_{222}$$

(Bartlett, 1935; Haber, 1984; O'Neill, 1982). For simplicity, set $w = o_{111}$, $x = o_{.11}$, $y = o_{1.1}$, $z = o_{11.}$, $A = o_{1..}$, $B = o_{.1.}$, $C = o_{..1}$, and $N = o_{...}$. The point probability of any w is then given by

$$P(w \mid x, y, z, A, B, C, N) =$$

$$A!\,(N - A)!\,B!\,(N - B)!\,C!\,(N - C)! \,/$$

$$\left[(N!)^2 w!\,(x - w)!\,(y - w)!\,(z - w)!\,(A - y - z + w)! \right.$$

$$\left. (B - x - z + w)!\,(C - x - y + w)!\,(N - A - B - C + x + y + z - w)! \right].$$

If $H(k)$, given x, y, z, A, B, C, and N, is a recursively-defined positive function, then solving the recursive relation $H(k + 1) = H(k) \cdot g(k)$ yields

$$g(k) = \frac{(x - k)(y - k)(z - k)(N - A - B - C + x + y + z - k)}{(k + 1)(A - y - z + k + 1)(B - x - z + k + 1)(C - x - y + k + 1)},$$

which is employed to enumerate the complete distribution of

$$P(k \mid x, y, z, A, B, C, N),$$

$a \leq k \leq b$, where

$$a = \max(0, \, y + z - A, \, x + z - B, \, x + y - C),$$

$$b = \min(x, \, y, \, z, \, N - A - B - C + x + y + z),$$

and where $H(v)$ is set intially to some small value, such as 10^{-200}. The total (T) over the completely enumerated distribution may be found by

$$T = \sum_{k=a}^{b} H(k).$$

The exact second-order interaction P-value is found by

$$P = \sum_{k=a}^{b} I_k H(k)/T,$$

where I_k is an indicator function given by

$$I_k = \begin{cases} 1 & \text{if } H(k) \leq H(w), \\ 0 & \text{otherwise.} \end{cases}$$

A 2^3 Contingency Table Example

Table 7.12 contains a 2^3 contingency table based on $N = 76$ responses to a question (Yes, No) classified by gender (Female, Male) in two elementary school grades (First, Fourth). The first-order interaction probabilities associated with the data in Table 7.12 are 0.8134 (Grade by Gender over Response), 0.2496 (Gender by Response over Grade), and 0.4830 (Grade by Response over Gender). The second-order interaction P-value is 0.9036×10^{-3}. The exact P-value for independence of a table this extreme or more extreme than the observed table is 0.4453×10^{-2} (Mielke et al., 1994).

7.6.2 Analysis of a 2^4 Contingency Table

Consider a test of independence among four classification variables, each of which consists of two mutually exclusive classes, i.e., a 2^4 contingency table. Zelterman et al. (1995) provide an algorithm for the exact P-value for independence obtained from an examination of all possible permutations of the 16 cell frequencies, conditioned on the observed marginal frequency

TABLE 7.12. Cross-classification of responses, categorized by gender and school grade.

	Gender			
	Females		Males	
Grade	Yes	No	Yes	No
First	10	4	2	16
Fourth	6	11	15	12

totals of a 2^4 contingency table. An alternative approach, which is not as computationally intensive, is to examine the first-, second-, and third-order interactions in a 2^4 contingency table when the observed marginal frequency totals are fixed. Here, an algorithm is described to compute the exact probabilities of the six first-order (two-variable) interactions, the four second-order (three-variable) interactions, and the one third-order (four-variable) interaction for a 2^4 contingency table (Mielke and Berry, 1998).[6]

Following Mielke (1997), let $p_{i_1 i_2 i_3 i_4}$ denote the probability of cell $i_1 i_2 i_3 i_4$ in a 2^4 contingency table, where the index $i_j = 1$ or 2 for $j = 1, ..., 4$. The six null hypotheses of no first-order interaction for a 2^4 contingency table are

$$p_{11..}\, p_{22..} = p_{12..}\, p_{21..},$$

$$p_{1.1.}\, p_{2.2.} = p_{1.2.}\, p_{2.1.},$$

$$p_{1..1}\, p_{2..2} = p_{1..2}\, p_{2..1},$$

$$p_{.11.}\, p_{.22.} = p_{.12.}\, p_{.21.},$$

$$p_{.1.1}\, p_{.2.2} = p_{.1.2}\, p_{.2.1},$$

and

$$p_{..11}\, p_{..22} = p_{..12}\, p_{..21}.$$

Thus, $p_{.1.1}$ is the sum over indices i_1 and i_3. The four null hypotheses of no second-order interaction for a 2^4 contingency table are

---

[6]Adapted and reprinted with permission of Perceptual and Motor Skills from P.W. Mielke, Jr. and K.J. Berry. Exact probabilities for first-order, second-order, and third-order interactions in $2 \times 2 \times 2 \times 2$ contingency tables. *Perceptual and Motor Skills*, 1998, 86, 760–762. Copyright © 1998 by Perceptual and Motor Skills.

TABLE 7.13. Cross-classification of responses, categorized by variables A, B, C, and D.

Variable	Value							
D	1							
C	1				2			
B	1		2		1		2	
A	1	2	1	2	1	2	1	2
	187	15	42	40	256	42	34	62
D	2							
C	1				2			
B	1		2		1		2	
A	1	2	1	2	1	2	1	2
	177	14	30	63	194	27	52	121

$$p_{111.}\, p_{221.}\, p_{122.}\, p_{212.} = p_{112.}\, p_{222.}\, p_{121.}\, p_{211.},$$

$$p_{11.1}\, p_{22.1}\, p_{12.2}\, p_{21.2} = p_{11.2}\, p_{22.2}\, p_{12.1}\, p_{21.1},$$

$$p_{1.11}\, p_{2.21}\, p_{1.22}\, p_{2.12} = p_{1.12}\, p_{2.22}\, p_{1.21}\, p_{2.11},$$

and

$$p_{.111}\, p_{.221}\, p_{.122}\, p_{.212} = p_{.112}\, p_{.222}\, p_{.121}\, p_{.211}.$$

The null hypothesis of no third-order interaction for a 2^4 contingency table is given by

$$p_{1111}\, p_{2211}\, p_{1221}\, p_{2121}\, p_{1122}\, p_{2222}\, p_{1212}\, p_{2112} =$$

$$p_{1112}\, p_{2212}\, p_{1222}\, p_{2122}\, p_{1121}\, p_{2221}\, p_{1211}\, p_{2111}.$$

A 2^4 Contingency Table Example

Table 7.13 contains a 2^4 contingency table based on $N = 1,356$ responses classified on four dichotomous variables (A, B, C, and D). The example data in Table 7.13 are adapted from Bhapkar and Koch (1968, p. 589). The first-, second-, and third-order interaction probabilities associated with the data in Table 7.13 are given in Table 7.14. In contrast with existing approximate techniques, such as log-linear analysis, the 2^4 contingency table algorithm provides exact P-values.

TABLE 7.14. Interactions and associated exact P-values.

Interaction	P-value
$A \times B$	0.3822×10^{-91}
$A \times C$	0.4891×10^{-3}
$A \times D$	0.8690×10^{-4}
$B \times C$	0.2181
$B \times D$	0.5475×10^{-5}
$C \times D$	1.0000
$A \times B \times C$	0.4491
$A \times B \times D$	0.2792×10^{-1}
$A \times C \times D$	0.7999
$B \times C \times D$	0.4021×10^{-2}
$A \times B \times C \times D$	0.6517×10^{-1}

7.7 Relationship Between Chi-Square and Goodman-Kruskal Statistics

Since the Goodman and Kruskal (1954) asymmetric statistics t_a and t_b in Section 3.2 are defined for $r = 2$, let $o_{i,j} = o_{j_1,j_2}$, $g = n_1$, $h = n_2$, $G_i = \langle 1 \rangle_i$ for $i = 1, ..., g$, and $H_j = \langle 2 \rangle_j$ for $j = 1, ..., h$. Then, the Goodman and Kruskal statistics are given by

$$t_a = \left(N \sum_{i=1}^{g} \sum_{j=1}^{h} \frac{o_{i,j}^2}{G_i} - \sum_{j=1}^{h} H_j^2 \right) \bigg/ \left(N^2 - \sum_{j=1}^{h} H_j^2 \right)$$

and

$$t_b = \left(N \sum_{i=1}^{g} \sum_{j=1}^{h} \frac{o_{i,j}^2}{H_j} - \sum_{i=1}^{g} G_i^2 \right) \bigg/ \left(N^2 - \sum_{i=1}^{g} G_i^2 \right).$$

Also, the Pearson (1900) χ^2 statistic is given by

$$\chi^2 = N \sum_{i=1}^{g} \sum_{j=1}^{h} \frac{o_{i,j}^2}{G_i H_j} - N.$$

Although t_a, t_b, and χ^2 generally differ, they are equivalent in a few cases. If $H_j = N/h$ for $j = 1, ..., h$, then $\chi^2 = N(h-1)t_a$. If $G_i = N/g$ for $i = 1, ..., g$, then $\chi^2 = N(g-1)t_b$. If $G_i = N/g$ and $H_j = N/h$ for $i = 1, ..., g$ and $j = 1, ..., h$, then $\chi^2 = N(h-1)t_a = N(g-1)t_b$. If $h = 2$, then $\chi^2 = Nt_a$. Also, if $g = 2$, then $\chi^2 = Nt_b$. Thus, if $g = h = 2$, then $\chi^2 = Nt_a = Nt_b$. Patefield (1981) provides an efficient resampling P-value algorithm for testing independence in any two-way contingency table (see Section 7.3). Resampling P-value algorithms are easily obtained for MRPP (see

Section 2.3). Since the Goodman and Kruskal (1954) asymmetric statistics are special cases of MRPP, a resampling P-value technique also exists for testing independence in two-way contingency tables when any of the above equivalences exist.

Since inferences based on t_a, t_b, and χ^2 statistics depend on distinct probability structures, the P-values associated with t_a, t_b, and χ^2 for a given two-way contingency table may be substantially different. The following example based on a test of homogeneity of proportions illustrates these differences.

The discrete data of this example consist of $N = 80$ responses arranged in a 3×5 ($g = 3$ and $h = 5$) contingency table. The exact, resampling ($L = 1,000,000$), and Pearson type III P-values associated with statistic t_a are 0.1437×10^{-2}, 0.1415×10^{-2}, and 0.1449×10^{-2}, respectively; the exact, resampling ($L = 1,000,000$), and Pearson type III P-values associated with statistic t_b are 0.5714×10^{-1}, 0.5714×10^{-1}, and 0.5829×10^{-1}, respectively; and the exact, resampling ($L = 1,000,000$), and Pearson type III P-values associated with statistic χ^2 are 0.1009×10^{-2}, 0.1055×10^{-2}, and 0.9763×10^{-3}, respectively.

4	7	2	9	0	22
1	5	2	7	6	21
4	5	10	18	0	37
9	17	14	34	6	80

7.8 Summary

Fisher's (1934) exact test is a uniformly-most-powerful unbiased test for 2^2 contingency tables (Lehmann, 1986) and is recommended for this case. Except for 2^2 contingency tables, no such optimal property exists for any other contingency table. Thus, the use of exact tests is recommended whenever possible, especially for sparse contingency tables. For large sparse r-way contingency tables where exact tests are not feasible, the nonasymptotic resampling and Pearson type III approximate tests are recommended since their corresponding P-values will be close to the P-values of the exact tests (provided the P-values are not exceedingly small, in which case the inferences will be the same). When $r \geq 2$, the Pearson type III P-value approximation pertains only to the Pearson χ^2 and Zelterman tests since their exact mean, variance, and skewness values are available. A comparison between asymptotic log-linear and exact analyses based on Pearson χ^2 and likelihood-ratio statistics for a very sparse contingency table indicates that the asymptotic log-linear P-values are much larger than the exact P-values for most cases. The implication is that asymptotic log-linear analyses should not be used to analyze sparse contingency tables. Methods to obtain all exact interaction P-values are described for 2^r tables when $r \leq 4$. Finally, the relation between Goodman-Kruskal t_a and t_b and Pearson χ^2 statistics is presented. The symmetry of the Pearson χ^2 test is shown to sometimes eliminate information associated with the asymmetrical Goodman-Kruskal t_a and t_b tests.

8

Multisample Homogeneity Tests

Homogeneity techniques are needed to identify differences between two or more data sets. As with goodness-of-fit techniques, major differences occur between discrete and continuous data. Unlike symmetric techniques such as Fisher's (1934) exact test, Pearson's (1900) χ^2 test, and Zelterman's (1987) S test, all of which are used to test homogeneity for discrete data, MRPP asymmetric techniques such as the Goodman and Kruskal (1954) t_a and t_b tests distinguish between the response categories and the possible differences among the data sets. For continuous data, the homogeneity techniques include the generalized runs test, the Kolmogorov–Smirnov test, and tests based on empirical coverages. Specific examples are given for both discrete and continuous data to show definitive differences among the operating characteristics of these techniques.

8.1   Discrete Data Tests

Consider the application of MRPP to two-way contingency tables (see Section 3.2). Let o_{ij} denote the observed frequency of the ith response ($i = 1, ..., r$) in the jth group ($j = 1, ..., g$). Then,

$$n_j = \sum_{i=1}^{r} o_{ij}$$

is the number of responses in the jth group and

$$N = \sum_{j=1}^{g} n_j,$$

i.e., $N = K$ and $n_{g+1} = 0$. Here, each response is a row vector of the form $x'_I = (x_{1I}, ..., x_{rI})$, where $x_{iI} = 1$ if the ith response occurred and the remaining $r - 1$ entries are 0 ($I = 1, ..., N$). The null hypothesis (H_0) in this case is that all of the

$$M = \frac{N!}{\displaystyle\prod_{j=1}^{g} n_j!}$$

assignments of the N discrete responses to the g groups with fixed sizes are equally likely. A natural MRPP statistic for this purpose that tests H_0 is given by

$$\delta = \sum_{j=1}^{g} C_j \xi_j,$$

where $n_j \geq 2$, $C_j = n_j/N$,

$$\xi_j = \binom{n_j}{2}^{-1} \sum_{I<J} \Delta_{I,J} \Psi_j(\omega_I) \Psi_j(\omega_J),$$

is the average distance function for all distinct pairs of objects in group S_j ($j = 1, ..., g$), $\sum_{I<J}$ is the sum over all I and J such that $1 \leq I < J \leq N$, $\Psi_j(\cdot)$ is an indicator function given by

$$\Psi_j(\omega_I) = \begin{cases} 1 \text{ if } \omega_I \in S_j, \\ 0 \text{ otherwise,} \end{cases}$$

the MRPP distance function is $\Delta_{I,J} = 1 - x'_I x_J$ (see Sections 2.1, 2.2, and 2.3), and the test statistic is given by

$$T = \frac{\delta - \mu}{\sigma}.$$

As noted in Section 3.2, this statistic is equivalent to one of the asymmetric Goodman and Kruskal (1954) statistics, t_a or t_b, when

$$C_j = \frac{n_j - 1}{N - g}.$$

Although the MRPP test is the correct choice for testing H_0, the symmetric Fisher and Pearson χ^2 statistics (see Section 7.4) have incorrectly been used for this same purpose by testing H_0 that the g group categories

TABLE 8.1. Example data set for residence type and personality type.

| Personality type | Residence type | | | Total |
	Rural	Suburban	City	
Domineering	5	7	5	17
Assertive	0	0	5	5
Passive	17	9	7	33
Submissive	4	4	1	9
Independent	9	2	2	13
Total	35	22	20	77

are independent of the r response categories in a two-way contingency table. The following example demonstrates the possibility of monumental differences among the results based on inappropriate symmetric test analyses such as the Fisher and Pearson χ^2 tests, on the one hand, and results based on appropriate asymmetric test analyses such as the Goodman and Kruskal t_a and t_b tests, on the other hand.

8.1.1 Example Using Incorrect Symmetric Tests

Consider a sample of $N = 77$ seventh-grade female students, all from complete families with three children, stratified by Residence Type (Rural, Suburban, and Inner-city). In a classroom setting, each subject is classified by a panel of trained observers into one of five Personality Types: Domineering, Assertive, Submissive, Passive, or Independent (Berry and Mielke, 2000a).[1] The data are given in Table 8.1. The null hypothesis posits that the proportions of the $r = 5$ Personality Types are the same for each of the $g = 3$ Residence Types. Thus, Residence Type is the dependent variable and Personality Type is the independent variable. Since the exact number of reference tables is 14,630,056 for the data in Table 8.1, the Fisher and Pearson χ^2 exact test P-values are 0.2083×10^{-1} and 0.4784×10^{-2}, respectively. Also the Fisher and Pearson χ^2 resampling test P-values based on $L = 1,000,000$ are 0.2097×10^{-1} and 0.4807×10^{-2}, respectively. For comparison, the nonasymptotic Pearson type III and asymptotic P-values for the Pearson χ^2 test are 0.4732×10^{-2} and 0.6297×10^{-2}, respectively (see Section 7.4). The Fisher and Pearson χ^2 tests are symmetrical tests that do not distinguish between the dependent and independent variables. Consequently, these symmetric tests are excluding important information.

---

[1] Adapted and reprinted with permission of Psychological Reports from K.J. Berry and P.W. Mielke, Jr. An asymmetric test of homogeneity of proportions. *Psychological Reports*, 2000, 87, 259–265. Copyright © 2000 by Psychological Reports.

8.1.2 Example Using Correct Asymmetric Tests

Based on the same data in Table 8.1,

$$M = \frac{77!}{35!\,22!\,20!} \doteq 0.5138 \times 10^{34}$$

and exact tests may not be feasible. However, in the context of a two-way contingency table, the number of cases reduces to only 14,630,056 probabilistically weighted reference tables. The t_b statistic designed by Goodman and Kruskal (1954) yields an asymmetric test and, under the null hypothesis $H_0 : \tau_b = 0$, $t_b(N-1)(r-1)$ is asymptotically distributed as χ^2 with $(r-1)(g-1)$ degrees-of-freedom as $N \to \infty$ (Margolin and Light, 1974). For the data in Table 8.1, $t_b = 0.0413$, the adjusted t_b value is $t_b(N-1)(r-1) = (0.0413)(77-1)(5-1) = 12.5553$ and, because $(r-1)(g-1) = (5-1)(3-1) = 8$ df, the asymptotic Margolin and Light (1974) χ^2 P-value is 0.1281. Since t_b (see Section 3.2) is just a special case of MRPP when $C_j = (n_j - 1)/(N-g)$, MRPP can be directly applied, yielding the observed value of δ given by $\delta_o = 0.7194$, the exact P-value is 0.1380, a resampling ($L = 1,000,000$) P-value is 0.1380, and, since $\mu = 0.7307$, $\sigma^2 = 0.1154 \times 10^{-3}$, $\gamma = -1.2436$, and the observed value of T is $T_o = -1.0468$, the Pearson type III P-value is 0.1402. Since the asymmetric tests interpret the Personality Type classification as a five-dimensional response and the Resident Type classification as three groups, the results are substantially different than the three symmetric tests, which do not distinguish between the response vectors and groups.

If the symmetric χ^2 test yields a low P-value, then at least one of the asymmetric t_a and t_b tests will also yield a low P-value. To demonstrate this statement, suppose Personality Type is the dependent variable and Residence Type is the independent variable. Then, for the data in Table 8.1, $t_a = 0.1339$, the adjusted t_a value is $t_a(N-1)(g-1) = (0.1339)(77-1)(3-1)$ $= 20.3555$ and, because $(r-1)(g-1) = (5-1)(3-1) = 8$ df, the asymptotic Margolin and Light (1974) χ^2 P-value is 0.9072×10^{-2}. If

$$N_i = \sum_{j=1}^{g} o_{ij}$$

for $i = 1, ..., r$, then t_a is just a special case of MRPP when

$$C_i = \frac{N_i - 1}{N - r}$$

and MRPP can be directly applied, yielding $\delta_o = 0.5968$, the exact P-value is 0.6859×10^{-2}, a resampling ($L = 1,000,000$) P-value is 0.6992×10^{-2}, and, since $\mu = 0.6528$, $\sigma^2 = 0.3027 \times 10^{-3}$, $\gamma = -0.9264$, and $T_o = -3.2195$, the Pearson type III P-value is 0.6874×10^{-2}.

Clearly, the Pearson χ^2 test of homogeneity is detecting the substantial departure from homogeneity of the row proportions. This is reflected in the

TABLE 8.2. Conditional column sample proportions for residence type and personality type.

Personality type	Residence type		
	Rural	Suburban	City
Domineering	0.1429	0.3182	0.2500
Assertive	0.0000	0.0000	0.2500
Passive	0.4857	0.4091	0.3500
Submissive	0.1143	0.1818	0.0500
Independent	0.2571	0.0909	0.1000
Total	1.0000	1.0000	1.0000

TABLE 8.3. Conditional row sample proportions for residence type and personality type.

Personality type	Residence type			Total
	Rural	Suburban	City	
Domineering	0.2941	0.4118	0.2941	1.0000
Assertive	0.0000	0.0000	1.0000	1.0000
Passive	0.5152	0.2727	0.2121	1.0000
Submissive	0.4444	0.4444	0.1111	1.0000
Independent	0.6923	0.1538	0.1538	1.0000

low P-value for t_a where the row variable (Personality Type) is considered the dependent variable. As the dependent variable of interest is the column variable (Residence Type), the Pearson χ^2 test of homogeneity yields a misleading result with an exact P-value $= 0.4784 \times 10^{-2}$ compared to the exact P-value $= 0.1380$ for t_b.

Table 8.2 displays the conditional column proportions obtained from the sample cell frequencies of Table 8.1. In Table 8.2, Personality Type is the dependent variable and the conditional column proportions are given by $p_{i|j} = n_{ij}/n_j$, e.g., $p_{1|1} = 5/35 = 0.1429$. Table 8.3 displays the conditional row proportions obtained from the sample cell frequencies of Table 8.1. In Table 8.3, Residence Type is the dependent variable and the conditional row proportions are given by $p_{j|i} = n_{ij}/N_i$, e.g., $p_{1|1} = 5/17 = 0.2941$. Even a casual visual inspection of Tables 8.2 and 8.3 shows the relative homogeneity extant among the proportions in the columns of Table 8.2, compared with the lack of homogeneity among the proportions in the rows of Table 8.3. Compare, for example, the Assertive (0.0000, 0.0000, 1.0000) and Independent (0.6923, 0.1538, 0.1538) row proportions in Table 8.3. It is this departure from homogeneity in the row proportions that produces the low P-value, i.e., 0.4784×10^{-2}, that is similar in size to the P-value of the Pearson χ^2 test.

8.2   Continuous Data Tests

Provided the samples are sufficiently large, the tests considered here can detect any nontrivial alternative to the null hypothesis (H_0) that two or more samples have been obtained from a common population of continuous data. These tests include the generalized runs test, the Kolmogorov–Smirnov test, and tests based on empirical coverages. A broader treatment of this class of tests is given by Holst and Rao (1980).

8.2.1   Generalized Runs Test

Suppose the

$$N = \sum_{i=1}^{g} n_i$$

univariate values of g samples are ordered from the smallest to the largest value. If an ordered value belongs to the ith of the g samples, the value is replaced by i ($i = 1, ..., g$). Each of the N ordered positions (i.e., nodes) of the resulting sequence is occupied by one of g distinct symbols ($1, ..., g$). Statistic R is the number of runs of distinct symbols. In terms of the generalized runs test (Section 3.5), there is only one tree ($t = 1$) where each of the two end nodes has one link and each of the remaining $N - 2$ nodes has two links. Here, the total number of links is $L = N - 1$ and the defining equation relating R and the MRPP statistic δ is given by

$$R = N - \delta \sum_{i=1}^{g} \binom{n_i}{2};$$

see Expression (3.1) in Section 3.5. Because H_0 is suspect when R is small, the exact P-value under H_0 of the MRPP test is

$$P(\delta \geq \delta_o \,|\, H_0) = \frac{\text{number of } \delta \text{ values} \geq \delta_o}{M},$$

where

$$M = \frac{N!}{\displaystyle\prod_{i=1}^{g} n_i!}$$

and δ_o is the observed value of δ.

8.2.2   Kolmogorov–Smirnov Test

If two samples of sizes n_1 and n_2 are obtained from continuous data, then the empirical cumulative distribution functions of these samples are denoted by $F_{n_1}(x)$ and $F_{n_2}(x)$, respectively (see Section 6.2). Then, the two-sample Kolmogorov–Smirnov test statistic is defined by

$$D_{n_1,n_2} = \sup_x |F_{n_1}(x) - F_{n_2}(x)|,$$

and H_0 is rejected for large values of D_{n_1,n_2} (Smirnov, 1939b). If the n of the Kolmogorov statistic D_n in Section 6.2 is equated to the largest integer less than or equal to $n_1 n_2/(n_1 + n_2)$, and D_{n_1,n_2} is treated as D_n, then either the asymptotic approach or the small-sample simulation approach described in Section 6.2 may be used to obtain P-values. These P-value approximations may be very crude when $n_1 n_2/(n_1 + n_2) < 10$. Also, the exact P-value is given by

$$\frac{2}{\displaystyle\binom{n_1 + n_2}{n_1}}$$

for the extreme case when $D_{n_1,n_2} = 1$. Exact cutoff values for $n_1 n_2 D_{n_1,n_2}$ for $1 \leq n_1 \leq n_2 \leq 25$ with $\alpha = 0.1$, 0.05, 0.025, 0.01, 0.005, and 0.001 are given in Pearson and Hartley (1972, pp. 360–363). Although asymptotic extensions of the Kolmogorov–Smirnov test exist for more than two samples (Kiefer, 1959), an analogous small-sample simulation approach is needed for application purposes.

8.2.3 Empirical Coverage Tests

A class of multisample tests that immediately extends to $g \geq 2$ samples is the collection of g-sample empirical coverage tests (Mielke and Yao, 1988, 1990). Let $x_{1,i} < \cdots < x_{n_i,i}$ be the n_i order statistics associated with the ith sample $(i = 1, ..., g)$,

$$N = \sum_{i=1}^{g} n_i,$$

$$G_N(x) = \frac{\text{number of observed } N \text{ pooled values } \leq x}{N + 1},$$

and $G_N(x) = 1$ if x is greater than or equal to the least upper bound of the domain of x. As defined, $G_N(x)$ differs slightly from the empirical distribution function of the pooled sample. The $n_i + 1$ empirical coverages associated with the n_i observed values of the ith sample $(i = 1, ..., g)$ are denoted by

$$C_{j,i} = G_N(x_{j,i}) - G_N(x_{j-1,i})$$

for $j = 1, ..., n_i + 1$, where $G_N(x_{0,i}) = 0, G_N(x_{n_i+1,i}) = 1$, and $x_{0,i}$ and $x_{n_i+1,i}$ are the greatest lower and least upper bound values of the unknown population domain of x in question under H_0, respectively. Thus,

$$\sum_{j=1}^{n_i+1} C_{j,i} = 1$$

for $i = 1, ..., g$. As an example, suppose $g = 2, n_1 = 4, n_2 = 3$, and

$$x_{1,1} < x_{2,1} < x_{3,1} < x_{1,2} < x_{4,1} < x_{2,2} < x_{3,2}$$

are the sample order statistics. The empirical coverages for this example are

$$C_{1,1} = C_{2,1} = C_{3,1} = C_{3,2} = C_{4,2} = 0.125,$$

$$C_{4,1} = C_{2,2} = 0.250,$$

$$C_{5,1} = 0.375,$$

and

$$C_{1,2} = 0.500.$$

Under H_0, the expected value of $C_{j,i}$ is $(n_i + 1)^{-1}$ for $i = 1, ..., g$. The g-sample empirical coverage test statistic is given by

$$T_v = \sum_{i=1}^{g} \sum_{j=1}^{n_i+1} \left| C_{j,i} - (n_i + 1)^{-1} \right|^v,$$

where $v > 0$. Provided the g samples are sufficiently large, this test is able to detect any nontrivial alternative to H_0. Since the total number of equally-likely events is

$$M = \frac{N!}{\prod_{i=1}^{g} n_i!},$$

the exact P-value is given by

$$P\text{-value} = \frac{\text{number of the } M \text{ events when } T_v \geq T_{vo}}{M}$$

where T_{vo} is the observed value of T_v. When M is large, approximate resampling and Pearson type III P-values are essential. The exact mean of T_v under H_0 is given by

$$\mu_v = \sum_{i=1}^{g} (n_i + 1) \sum_{j=1}^{N-n_i+1} \left| j(N+1)^{-1} - (n_i + 1)^{-1} \right|^v \binom{N-j}{n_i - 1} \Big/ \binom{N}{n_i}$$

and is easily computed. To obtain a Pearson type III P-value given by

$$P(T_v \geq T_{vo} \mid H_0),$$

the exact variance and skewness of T_v under H_0 (σ_v^2 and γ_v) are required. However, calculating σ_v^2 and γ_v is exceedingly time-consuming even for moderate sample sizes, due to the multiple looping structures involved. Consequently, a Pearson type III P-value algorithm initially obtains μ_v

and then, based on L independent simulations of T_v denoted by $T_{v1}, ..., T_{vL}$, evaluates estimators of σ_v^2 and γ_v given by

$$\tilde{\sigma}_v^2 = \frac{1}{L} \sum_{i=1}^{L} (T_{vi} - \mu_v)^2$$

and

$$\tilde{\gamma}_v = \frac{\frac{1}{L} \sum_{i=1}^{L} (T_{vi} - \mu_v)^3}{\tilde{\sigma}_v^3}.$$

Furthermore, a resampling P-value is given by

$$P\text{-value} = \frac{\text{number of the } L \text{ events when } T_{vi} \geq T_{vo}}{L}.$$

Suggested choices of v and L for routine applications of this algorithm are $v = 1$ and $L = 1,000,000$. While the resampling P-value is preferred, the Pearson type III P-value provides a crude estimate of a very small exact P-value. Incidentally, Rao and Murthy (1981) proposed the special case among this class of tests when $g = v = 2$.

8.2.4 Examples

In order to demonstrate differences among the generalized runs (GR) test, the Kolmogorov–Smirnov (KS) test, and the empirical coverage (EC) test with $v = 1$, data set 1 in Table 8.4 and data set 2 in Table 8.5 are confined to $g = 2$. In addition, data sets 1 and 2 are graphically displayed in Figures 8.1 and 8.2, respectively. To add further information for these comparisons, two versions of MRPP designated M1 and M2 (both with $\Delta_{IJ} = |x_I - x_J|$, $C_i = n_i/N$, and with respective truncation constants $B = 1.0$ and B set to ∞) are included (see Section 2.2). The P-values associated with each test and data set combination are given in Table 8.6. The number of runs associated with the GR test for data sets 1 and 2 are 7 and 16, respectively. The observed KS statistics for data sets 1 and 2 are $D_{16,15} = 0.25$ and $D_{20,17} = 0.6235$, respectively. Thus, the KS statistic P-values for data sets 1 and 2 are obtained with the Kolmogorov statistics $D_7 = 0.25$ and $D_9 = 0.6235$, respectively. The observed, expected, and standardized values of the EC statistic for data set 1 are 1.5221, 0.9677, and 3.4430, respectively. Similarly, the observed, expected, and standardized values of the EC statistic for data set 2 are 1.1621, 0.9942, and 1.1785, respectively. The standardized value and skewness value pairs of the M1 statistic for data sets 1 and 2 are $(-1.8918, -0.5485)$ and $(-0.4493, -0.4164)$, respectively. The standardized value and skewness value pairs of the M2 statistic for data sets 1 and 2 are $(0.3182, -2.3678)$ and $(-5.5488, -2.3359)$, respectively. In addition, let ECr and ECp denote the resampling approximation with

TABLE 8.4. Data set 1, consisting of two groups with sizes $n_1 = 16$ and $n_2 = 15$.

Group 1		Group 2	
42.64	60.26	45.16	59.25
43.37	60.34	45.67	59.67
44.25	60.42	47.69	59.98
48.91	60.97	48.11	61.18
49.94	67.59	48.73	61.97
50.42	68.22	54.84	62.33
50.71	68.36	55.30	67.48
51.45	69.46	58.63	

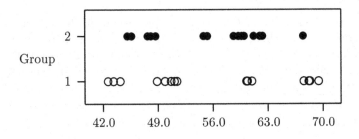

FIGURE 8.1. Plot of the data in Table 8.4.

$L = 1,000,000$ simulations and the Pearson type III approximation of the empirical coverage test, respectively. Similarly, let M1r and M2r denote the resampling approximations of MRPP with $L = 1,000,000$ simulations when $B = 1.0$ and B is ∞, respectively, and let M1p and M2p denote the Pearson type III approximations of MRPP when $B = 1.0$ and B is ∞, respectively. The results are given in Table 8.6.

In detecting the alternating pattern of response values between groups 1 and 2 comprising data set 1, the P-values of Table 8.6 indicate that the GR and EC tests are very sensitive, M1 (MRPP with $B = 1.0$) is only slightly sensitive, and the KS test and M2 (MRPP when B is ∞) are not sensitive at all to alternating patterns. For detecting the major shift in response values between groups 1 and 2 comprising data set 2, the P-values of Table 8.6 indicate that the KS test and M2 (MRPP when B is ∞) are very sensitive, the GR and EC tests are marginally sensitive, and M1 (MRPP with $B = 1.0$) is not at all sensitive to major shifts. Whereas the KS, GR, and EC tests are able to detect various group difference alternatives with increasing sample sizes, data sets 1 and 2 show that the sensitivity associated with the distinctly different structures of these tests (like any other test) varies dramatically with the alternative hypothesis in question.

TABLE 8.5. Data set 2, consisting of two groups with sizes $n_1 = 20$ and $n_2 = 17$.

Group 1		Group 2	
42.50	59.90	46.50	75.10
44.20	60.00	54.00	75.50
44.90	64.20	60.50	78.60
50.10	65.40	66.50	80.70
50.20	65.90	66.80	81.90
52.40	66.00	69.90	83.90
53.80	72.00	72.30	86.10
56.80	73.50	72.80	
57.90	75.30	74.60	
58.90	83.70	74.70	

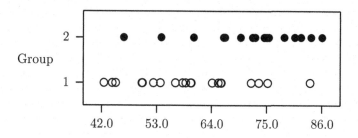

FIGURE 8.2. Plot of the data in Table 8.5.

TABLE 8.6. Comparative P-values for analyses of data sets 1 and 2 with generalized runs (GR) test, Kolmogorov–Smirnov (KS) test, empirical coverage (ECr and ECp) tests with $v = 1$, MRPP (M1r and M1p) with $B = 1.0$, and MRPP (M2r and M2p) when B is ∞.

Test	Data set 1	Data set 2
GR	0.3395×10^{-3}	0.1680
KS	0.6889	0.6970×10^{-3}
ECr	0.3360×10^{-3}	0.1171
ECp	0.2878×10^{-3}	0.1197
M1r	0.4343×10^{-1}	0.3082
M1p	0.4217×10^{-1}	0.3068
M2r	0.4980	0.2147×10^{-2}
M2p	0.4840	0.2026×10^{-2}

8.3 Summary

For discrete data, the use of symmetric techniques (e.g., Fisher's exact test, Pearson's χ^2 test, and Zelterman's test) is shown to detect group differences for small samples when appropriate asymmetric techniques (e.g., the Goodman and Kruskal τ test) for homogeneity do not detect the group differences. The continuous-data examples indicate substantially different detection capabilities for the generalized runs, Kolmogorov–Smirnov, and empirical coverage tests. Thus, the total reliance on a single test (e.g., the Kolmogorov–Smirnov test) for detecting general differences among groups of continuous data is highly suspect.

9
Selected Permutation Studies

While a multitude of permutation studies involving exact and/or random sampling with and without replacement exist, the present choice of three recent investigations is used because they yielded new and interesting results. These investigations include (1) a comparison of continuous and discrete methods for combining independent P-values, (2) the Fisher Z transformation, and (3) a method based on distance functions for comparing multivariate g-group similarity patterns between two samples. Unfortunately, many important topics such as permutation tests of ordered alternatives are omitted (Jonckheere, 1954; Mielke and Berry, 2000b; Terpstra, 1952).

9.1 A Discrete Method For Combining P-Values

An exact method to combine independent P-values that obey discrete probability distributions is introduced (Mielke et al., 2004b, 2005b).[1,2] The

---

[1] Adapted and reprinted with permission of Psychological Reports from P.W. Mielke, Jr., J.E. Johnston, and K.J. Berry. Combining probability values from independent permutation tests: A discrete analog method of Fisher's classical method. *Psychological Reports*, 2004, 95, 449–458. Copyright © 2004 by Psychological Reports.

[2] Adapted and reprinted with permission of Perceptual and Motor Skills from P.W. Mielke, Jr., K.J. Berry, and J.E. Johnston. Comparisons of continuous and discrete methods for combining probability values associated with matched-pairs t-test data. *Perceptual and Motor Skills*, 2005, 100, 799–805. Copyright © 2005 by Perceptual and Motor Skills.

exact method is the discrete analog to Fisher's classical method for combining P-values from independent continuous probability distributions. If the combination of P-values includes even one P-value that obeys a sparse discrete probability distribution, then Fisher's classical method may be grossly inadequate. Many methods for combining P-values of both independent and dependent tests are described by Pesarin (2001, see Chapters 6 and 7). Among these methods, the classical method by Fisher (1934, pp. 103–105) is known to possess excellent asymptotic properties for combining independent P-values from continuous uniform distributions (Littell and Folks, 1971, 1973). The purpose of this paper is to introduce a discrete analog of Fisher's classical method to combine independent P-values from permutation tests.

9.1.1 Fisher Continuous Method to Combine P-Values

Fisher (1934) described a method for combining k independent P-values $(P_1, ..., P_k)$ from continuous probability distributions based on the statistic

$$T = -2\ln\left(\prod_{i=1}^{k} P_i\right) = -2\sum_{i=1}^{k}\ln P_i,$$

which is distributed as chi-squared with $2k$ degrees-of-freedom under the null hypothesis (H_0) that $P_1, ..., P_k$ are independent uniform random variables between 0 and 1. If T_o is the observed value of T, then the combined P-value based on the Fisher continuous method is

$$P\left(T \geq T_o | H_0\right).$$

Consequently, while the Fisher continuous method is exact for P-values under H_0, it is not appropriate for independent P-values obeying discrete probability distributions where only a limited number of different events are possible (Lancaster, 1949; Pearson, 1950). In such cases, the Fisher continous method often yields conservative results, i.e., the combined P-value usually is too large (Edgington and Haller, 1984; Gordon et al., 1952; Kincaid, 1962; Trehub and Heilizer, 1962). Kincaid (1962, p. 11) described how even a small discontinuity in an otherwise continuous probability distribution can have a substantial effect on the combined P-value based on the Fisher continuous method.

9.1.2 A Discrete Method For Combining P-Values

A discrete analog of the Fisher (1934) continuous method for combining P-values is described for Fisher's exact, exact chi-squared, and exact log likelihood-ratio tests. Note that while the discrete method is illustrated with the exact chi-squared and exact log likelihood-ratio statistics, the choice of these statistics is arbitrary, and the discrete method is applicable to a broad spectrum of statistics. Let $p_{ij} > 0$, $\chi_{ij}^2 \geq 0$, and $G_{ij}^2 \geq 0$ denote the point probability, chi-squared statistic, and log likelihood-ratio statistic, respectively, for the ith of k specified discrete probability distributions to be combined and the jth of m_i events associated with the ith discrete probability distribution; thus, $j = 1, ..., m_i$ and $i = 1, ..., k$. Note that

$$\sum_{j=1}^{m_i} p_{ij} = 1$$

for $i = 1, ..., k$. Also, let p_{io}, χ_{io}^2, and G_{io}^2 denote the observed values of p_{ij}, χ_{ij}^2, and G_{ij}^2, respectively. The exact combined P-values corresponding to Fisher's exact, exact chi-squared, and exact log likelihood-ratio tests for the ith of k discrete probability distributions are given by

$$P_{iF} = \sum_{j=1}^{m_i} p_{ij} A_{ij},$$

$$P_{i\chi^2} = \sum_{j=1}^{m_i} p_{ij} B_{ij},$$

and

$$P_{iG^2} = \sum_{j=1}^{m_i} p_{ij} C_{ij},$$

where

$$A_{ij} = \begin{cases} 1 & \text{if } p_{ij} \leq p_{io}, \\ 0 & \text{otherwise}, \end{cases}$$

$$B_{ij} = \begin{cases} 1 & \text{if } \chi_{ij}^2 \geq \chi_{io}^2, \\ 0 & \text{otherwise}, \end{cases}$$

and

$$C_{ij} = \begin{cases} 1 & \text{if } G^2_{ij} \geq G^2_{io}, \\ 0 & \text{otherwise,} \end{cases}$$

respectively. In this context, the ith of k Fisher exact tests is uninformative when $p_{ij} = 1/m_i$ for $j = 1, ..., m_i$ since $P_{iF} = 1$. When combining P-values with either the Fisher continuous method or the discrete method, H_0 specifies that the k probability distributions are mutually independent. Again, note that

$$\sum_{j_1=1}^{m_1} \cdots \sum_{j_k=1}^{m_k} \prod_{i=1}^{k} p_{ij_i} = 1.$$

Under H_0, the exact combined P-values of the k discrete probability distributions for Fisher's exact, exact chi-squared, and exact log-likelihood-ratio tests are given by

$$P_F = \sum_{j_1=1}^{m_1} \cdots \sum_{j_k=1}^{m_k} \alpha_{j_1,...,j_k} \prod_{i=1}^{k} p_{ij_i},$$

$$P_{\chi^2} = \sum_{j_1=1}^{m_1} \cdots \sum_{j_k=1}^{m_k} \beta_{j_1,...,j_k} \prod_{i=1}^{k} p_{ij_i},$$

and

$$P_{G^2} = \sum_{j_1=1}^{m_1} \cdots \sum_{j_k=1}^{m_k} \gamma_{j_1,...,j_k} \prod_{i=1}^{k} p_{ij_i},$$

where

$$\alpha_{j_1,...,j_k} = \begin{cases} 1 & \text{if } \prod_{i=1}^{k} p_{ij_i} \leq \prod_{i=1}^{k} p_{io}, \\ 0 & \text{otherwise,} \end{cases}$$

$$\beta_{j_1,...,j_k} = \begin{cases} 1 & \text{if } \sum_{i=1}^{k} \chi^2_{ij_i} \geq \sum_{i=1}^{k} \chi^2_{io}, \\ 0 & \text{otherwise,} \end{cases}$$

and

$$
\gamma_{j_1,...,j_k} =
\begin{cases}
1 & \text{if } \sum_{i=1}^{k} G_{ij_i}^2 \geq \sum_{i=1}^{k} G_{io}^2, \\
0 & \text{otherwise,}
\end{cases}
$$

respectively. Consequently, there are

$$
M = \prod_{i=1}^{k} m_i
$$

events associated with each combined P-value of the discrete method, which converges to the Fisher continuous method for combining P-values in the following manner. Let p_i^* be the maximum value of $p_{i1}, ..., p_{im_i}$ for $i = 1, ..., k$. If the maximum value of $p_1^*, ..., p_k^*$ goes to zero as the minimum value of $m_1, ..., m_k$ goes to infinity, then the discrete method and the Fisher continuous method are equivalent. The last statement is purely hypothetical since the discrete method is computationally intractable when M is large. A modified version of the discrete method involving Euler partitions (Berry et al., 2004; also see Section 6.1.2) was used to obtain exact P-values for specific exact log-linear analyses associated with sparse contingency tables (Mielke et al., 2004a; also see Section 7.5.1).

An example follows to demonstrate the implementation of the discrete method. Consider a trinomial distribution where the cell probabilities under H_0 are 0.10, 0.35, and 0.55, along with corresponding cell frequency indices denoted by (l_1, l_2, l_3). If $l_1 + l_2 + l_3 = 2$, then the discrete density function under H_0 is

$$
\frac{2!}{l_1!\, l_2!\, l_3!}(0.10)^{l_1}(0.35)^{l_2}(0.55)^{l_3}.
$$

If the P-values for two of these trinomial distributions are combined, then $k = 2$, $m_1 = m_2 = 6$, and $M = 36$. Here $p_{1j} = p_{2j}$, $\chi_{1j}^2 = \chi_{2j}^2$, and $G_{1j}^2 = G_{2j}^2$, for $j = 1, ..., 6$. The values of p_{ij}, χ_{ij}^2, and G_{ij}^2 for the six distinct trinomial indices (l_1, l_2, l_3) are given in Table 9.1. Let $j = 5$ and 6 of Table 9.1 denote the observed values for Distributions 1 and 2, respectively. The exact P-values for Distribution 1 are $P_{1F} = P_{1\chi^2} = 0.08$ and $P_{1G^2} = 0.2025$. The exact P-values for Distribution 2 are $P_{2F} = P_{2\chi^2} = P_{2G^2} = 0.01$. Here the exact combined P-values based on the discrete method are $P_F = P_{\chi^2} = 0.00150$ and $P_{G^2} = 0.00395$. In contrast, the combined P-value estimates of P_F, P_{χ^2}, and P_{G^2} based on the Fisher continuous method are 0.00650, 0.00650, and 0.01458, respectively.

The discrete method described here is conceptually applicable to obtaining exact combined P-values for a multitude of independent permutation tests, including the Fisher–Pitman test (Berry et al., 2002; Fisher,

TABLE 9.1. Values of p_{ij}, χ_{ij}^2, and G_{ij}^2 for the six distinct trinomial indices (l_1, l_2, l_3).

j	(l_1, l_2, l_3)	p_{ij}	χ_{ij}^2	G_{ij}^2
1	(0, 0, 2)	0.3025	1.6364	2.3913
2	(0, 1, 1)	0.3850	0.3377	0.5227
3	(0, 2, 0)	0.1225	3.7143	4.1993
4	(1, 0, 1)	0.1100	3.9091	3.0283
5	(1, 1, 0)	0.0700	4.4286	3.9322
6	(2, 0, 0)	0.0100	18.0000	9.2103

1935; Pitman, 1937a, 1937b, 1938); rank tests such as the Ansari–Bradley dispersion test (Ansari and Bradley, 1960), the Brown–Mood median test (Brown and Mood, 1951), the Mood dispersion test (Mood, 1954), the Taha squared-rank test (Duran and Mielke, 1968; Grant and Mielke, 1967; Taha, 1964), and the Wilcoxon–Mann–Whitney tests (Mann and Whitney, 1947; Mielke, 1972; Wilcoxon, 1945); MRPP (see Chapters 2 and 3); MRBP (see Chapter 4); and matched-pairs tests (Berry et al., 2003), since all these tests are based on finite-discrete distributions.

9.1.3   Three Examples

The Fisher continuous method and the discrete method for combining P-values are compared for three distinct examples. The first example involves a case where the individual point probabilities are unequal, which arises when combining P-values from sparse and non-sparse contingency tables. The second example combines P-values from matched-pairs t tests where the point probabilities are equal. The third example combines P-values from two-sample t tests where, again, the point probabilities are equal.

Example 1

While sparse and non-sparse discrete distributions for various permutation tests could be used as examples to compare the discrete method and the Fisher continuous method for combining P-values, the discrete distributions of five two-way contingency tables with fixed row and column totals are employed for this purpose, under the H_0 that the rows and columns are independent (see Section 7.2). Table 9.2 contains three sparse and two non-sparse contingency tables, which are utilized to illustrate and compare the discrete method and the Fisher continuous method for combining P-values from Fisher's exact, exact chi-squared, and exact log likelihood-ratio tests. The three 3×4 tables in Table 9.2 (S1, S2, and S3) are sparse data tables and the two 2×3 tables in Table 9.2 (N1 and N2) are non-sparse data tables.

TABLE 9.2. Sparse (S) and non-sparse (N) example data tables.

Sparse Tables			Non-sparse Tables	
S1	S2	S3	N1	N2
3 0 0 2	3 0 0 2	2 0 0 2	15 9 14	15 9 14
0 2 1 1	0 3 1 1	0 2 1 1	8 16 7	8 17 7
1 0 3 0	1 0 3 0	1 0 3 0		

TABLE 9.3. Number of distinct values/maximum, observed test statistic values, and exact observed P-values for Fisher's exact probability (FEP), exact chi-squared (χ^2), and exact log likelihood-ratio (G^2) tests for data tables listed in Table 9.2.

Data table	Test statistic	Number of distinct values/maximum	Observed test statistic value	Exact observed P-value
S1	FEP	24/460	0.000533*	0.047086
	χ^2	84/460	12.837500	0.039094
	G^2	25/460	15.597147	0.047086
S2	FEP	23/706	0.000190	0.018696
	χ^2	84/706	14.816667	0.019552
	G^2	26/706	17.798045	0.018696
S3	FEP	15/360	0.001039	0.096104
	χ^2	22/360	11.500000	0.083636
	G^2	16/360	14.229844	0.096104
N1	FEP	250/416	0.002927	0.068341
	χ^2	382/416	5.773039	0.065416
	G^2	383/416	5.818275	0.068341
N2	FEP	265/429	0.002047	0.037626
	χ^2	418/429	6.458471	0.035639
	G^2	417/429	6.530206	0.037626

*The observed test statistic is the observed point probability value for the Fisher exact probability test.

Table 9.3 lists, for the five data tables in Table 9.2, the number of distinct Fisher's exact point probability, exact chi-squared statistic, and exact log likelihood-ratio statistic values among the maximum number of possible values given the fixed marginal frequencies, the observed point probability values, the observed chi-squared and log likelihood-ratio test statistics, and the exact observed P-values for Fisher's exact, exact chi-squared, and exact log likelihood-ratio tests. For example, consider the sparse data table S1. There are 24 distinct point probability values for Fisher's exact test, 84 distinct test statistic values for the exact chi-squared test, and 25 distinct test statistic values for the exact log likelihood-ratio test, each from among

TABLE 9.4. The discrete (D) and the Fisher continous (C) combined P-Values of three contingency tables for Fisher's exact, exact chi-squared, and exact log likelihood-ratio tests for data tables listed in Table 9.2.

Data	Fisher's exact		Chi-squared		Likelihood-ratio	
table	D	C	D	C	D	C
S1	0.00113	0.00545	0.00120	0.00347	0.00092	0.00545
S2	0.00008	0.00055	0.00012	0.00062	0.00008	0.00055
S3	0.00702	0.02904	0.00699	0.02116	0.00555	0.02904
N1	0.00946	0.01323	0.00801	0.01194	0.00963	0.01323
N2	0.00410	0.00316	0.00336	0.00276	0.00420	0.00316
S1 & N1	0.00622	0.00987	0.00426	0.00795	0.00448	0.00987
S1 & N2	0.00341	0.00379	0.00238	0.00298	0.00253	0.00379
S2 & N1	0.00362	0.00472	0.00204	0.00456	0.00215	0.00472
S2 & N2	0.00196	0.00178	0.00112	0.00168	0.00120	0.00178
S3 & N1	0.00913	0.01725	0.00739	0.01447	0.00755	0.01725
S3 & N2	0.00502	0.00674	0.00413	0.00552	0.00426	0.00674

the maximum of 460 values, given the fixed marginal frequency totals. In contrast, consider the non-sparse data table N1. There are 250 distinct point probability values for Fisher's exact test, 382 distinct test statistic values for the exact chi-squared test, and 383 distinct test statistic values for the exact log likelihood-ratio test, each from among the maximum of 416 values, given the fixed marginal frequency totals. The Fisher continuous method for combining P-values, assuming continuous probability distributions, is anticipated to provide better approximations for the non-sparse tables than for the sparse tables listed in Table 9.2.

Table 9.4 contains combined P-values for the discrete method and the Fisher continous method for Fisher's exact, exact chi-squared, and exact log likelihood-ratio tests. As an example, the sparse data set of data table S1 in Table 9.2, along with the corresponding results in Table 9.3, are used to compare combined P-values from the discrete method and the Fisher continous method for the three independent identical probability distributions associated with data table S1. For the discrete method, the three identical probability distributions yield the combined P-values of 0.00113, 0.00120, and 0.00092 in Table 9.4 for Fisher's exact, exact chi-squared, and exact log likelihood-ratio tests, respectively. For the Fisher continous method, the three identical observed P-values of each test in Table 9.3 yield combined P-values of 0.00545, 0.00347, and 0.00545 in Table 9.4 for Fisher's exact, exact chi-squared, and exact log likelihood-ratio tests, respectively. The discrete method and the Fisher continous method combined P-values for the three independent identical-probability distributions associated with data tables S2, S3, N1, and N2 in Table 9.2 were obtained in the same manner.

To provide results illustrating contamination of two non-sparse tables with one sparse table, combinations of three independent probability distributions based on these data tables were constructed. The combinations were based on data tables S1 and N1, S1 and N2, S2 and N1, S2 and N2, S3 and N1, and S3 and N2 in Table 9.2. In particular, consider the combined data set S1 & N1 consisting of data tables S1 and N1 in Table 9.2. For the discrete method, the two identical probability distributions of data table N1 were combined with the probability distribution of data table S1 to yield the discrete combined P-values of 0.00622, 0.00426, and 0.00448 in Table 9.4 for the Fisher's exact, exact chi-squared, and exact log likelihood-ratio tests, respectively. For the Fisher continuous method, the two identical observed P-values of data table N1 and the single observed P-value of data table S1 for each test in Table 9.3 yield the Fisher continuous method P-values of 0.00987, 0.00795, and 0.00987 in Table 9.4 for Fisher's exact, exact chi-squared, and exact log likelihood-ratio tests, respectively. The discrete method and the Fisher continuous method P-values for the three independent identical-probability distributions associated with data sets S1 & N2, S2 & N1, S2 & N2, S3 & N1, and S3 & N2 in Table 9.2 were obtained in the same manner.

The combined P-values based on the discrete method and the Fisher continuous method for Fisher's exact, exact chi-squared, and exact log likelihood-ratio tests in Table 9.4 may be compared using a standardized difference defined as the percentage change of the Fisher continuous P-value minus the corresponding discrete P-value, relative to the discrete P-value. To illustrate, for S1 and Fisher's exact test in Table 9.4, the standardized percentage difference is

$$\left(\frac{0.00545 - 0.00113}{0.00113} \right) 100 = 382.3.$$

Table 9.5 contains the standardized percentage differences for S1, S2, S3, N1, N2, S1 & N1, S1 & N2, S2 & N1, S2 & N2, S3 & N1, and S3 & N2, for Fisher's exact, exact chi-squared, and exact log likelihood-ratio tests. The standardized differences in Table 9.5 demonstrate that, for the sparse data tables S1, S2, and S3 in Table 9.2, the combined P-values of the Fisher continuous method can be very conservative. For the non-sparse data tables N1 and N2 in Table 9.2, the combined P-values of the Fisher continuous method yield improved approximations to the exact combined P-values of the discrete method. Note for data tables N1 and N2 in Table 9.2, the Fisher continuous method to combine P-values from independent continuous probability distributions exhibits both liberal and conservative results. While the Fisher continuous method to combine P-values from independent continuous probability distributions provides good results for discrete probability distributions from non-sparse data tables, when non-sparse discrete probability distributions are contaminated with a sparse

TABLE 9.5. Standardized percentage differences for Fisher's exact, exact chi-squared, and exact log likelihood-ratio tests for the paired discrete and Fisher's continuous combined P-values in Table 9.4.

Data table	Fisher's exact test	Chi-squared test	Likelihood-ratio test
S1	382.3	189.2	492.4
S2	587.5	416.7	587.5
S3	313.7	202.7	423.2
N1	39.9	49.1	37.4
N2	−22.9	−17.9	−24.8
S1 & N1	58.7	86.6	120.3
S1 & N2	11.1	25.2	49.8
S2 & N1	30.4	123.5	119.5
S2 & N2	−9.2	50.0	48.3
S3 & N1	88.9	95.8	128.5
S3 & N2	34.3	33.7	58.2

discrete probability distribution, as in S1 & N1,..., S3 & N2, the Fisher continuous method yields P-values that are usually too large.

The method introduced here to combine P-values from independent discrete probability distributions is the analog of the Fisher continuous method to combine P-values from independent continuous probability distributions. However, it is readily apparent from the standardized percentage differences in Table 9.5 that the Fisher continuous method is not appropriate for discrete probability distributions from sparse data tables such as S1, S2, and S3 in Table 9.2. Also, as is evident in the standardized percentage differences in Table 9.5 for the contaminated combinations S1 & N1,..., S3 & N2, the inclusion of even a single sparse discrete probability distribution can have a substantial effect on the Fisher continuous method to combine P-values.

If unacceptable continuous distribution assumptions such as normality are removed, then all tests are intrinsically discrete. Thus, the Fisher continuous method to combine independent P-values is at best an approximation to the discrete method when M is large.

Example 2

This example compares the Fisher continuous method and the exact discrete method for combining P-values associated with matched-pairs t test data (see Section 4.4). The exact discrete method for this example follows. Let n_i be the number of non-zero matched-pair differences for the ith of k matched-pair experiments. In the present context, $m_i = 2^{n_i}$ and $p_{ij} = 1/m_i$ for $j = 1, ..., m_i$ and $i = 1, ..., k$ designate the k discrete probability distributions in question. Therefore,

$$M = 2^N,$$

where

$$N = \sum_{i=1}^{k} n_i$$

is the pooled sample size for the k experiments. Let t_{ij} denote the matched-pairs t test statistic for the jth of the m_i outcomes associated with the ith of k combined experiments. The exact one-sided P-value for the ith of k experiments is

$$P_{it} = \sum_{j=1}^{m_i} \frac{D_{ij}}{m_i},$$

where

$$D_{ij} = \begin{cases} 1 & \text{if } t_{ij} \geq t_{io}, \\ 0 & \text{otherwise,} \end{cases}$$

and t_{io} is the observed matched-pairs t-test statistic for the ith of k experiments.

When combining P-values with the exact discrete method, H_0 specifies only that the k discrete probability distributions are independent. Under H_0, the exact combined one-sided P-value for the k discrete probability distributions is given by

$$P_t = \frac{1}{M} \sum_{j_1=1}^{m_1} \cdots \sum_{j_k=1}^{m_k} \delta_{j_1,\ldots,j_k},$$

where

$$\delta_{j_1,\ldots,j_k} = \begin{cases} 1 & \text{if } \sum_{i=1}^{k} t_{ij_i} \geq \sum_{i=1}^{k} t_{io}, \\ 0 & \text{otherwise.} \end{cases}$$

Again, in the present context,

$$\prod_{i=1}^{k} p_{ij_i} = \frac{1}{M}.$$

This comparison of the Fisher continuous method and the exact discrete method involves the combining of one-sided matched-pairs t-test P-values. The example has the property that the exact discrete method combined P-value and the exact P-value for the combined data are the same. The equality of P-values holds for the matched-pairs t test because

$$M = 2^N = \prod_{i=1}^{k} m_i = \prod_{i=1}^{k} 2^{n_i}.$$

and $1/M$ is the common probability of each event for both the combined sample P-values and the P-value of the combined sample. As demonstrated in Examples 1 and 3, this property is seldom satisfied.

The apparent difference in the size of the horizon moon when compared to a zenith moon intrigued even the earliest scientists, including Aristotle, Ptolemy, Alhazen, Roger Bacon, Leonardo da Vinci, Johann Kepler, René Descartes, and Christiaan Huyghens (Ross and Plug, 2002, pp. 4–5). Contemporary literature posits a number of hypotheses to describe why the moon appears larger at the horizon than at zenith, including atmospheric refraction and physiological or neurophysiological causes.

Holway and Boring (1940a, 1940b) introduced the "angle of regard:" the hypothesis that the moon illusion could be explained by testing whether a subject observed the moon with eyes level, i.e., the horizon moon, or with eyes raised, i.e., the zenith moon. They concluded that the size of the moon was perceived to be larger when the subject viewed the moon with eyes level and smaller with eyes raised. Further research on the moon illusion has utilized a broad range of hypotheses and experimental settings (Kaufman and Kaufman, 2000; Kaufman and Rock, 1962; Restle, 1970; Rock and Kaufman, 1962).

Consider an experiment that requires subjects to modify an adjustable "moon" projected onto an artificial horizon so that it matches the size of a standard moon at zenith. Subjects perform the task in two different positions: eyes raised and eyes level. The ratio of the diameter of the adjusted moon to the projected moon is recorded for each subject in both positions.

Data for four flights of experiments are listed in Table 9.6 where a "flight" is defined as $k = 3$ independent matched-pairs experiments with varying numbers of subjects. Flight A consists of three independent experiments with $n_1 = n_2 = n_3 = 6$ subjects. Flight B consists of three independent experiments with $n_1 = n_2 = n_3 = 7$ subjects. Flight C consists of three independent experiments with $n_1 = n_2 = n_3 = 8$ subjects. Flight D consists of three independent experiments with $n_1 = 6$, $n_2 = 7$, and $n_3 = 8$.

For each of the 12 experiments, two analyses were conducted. The first analysis was a permutation version of the matched-pairs t test (Berry et al., 2003; also see Section 4.2) that yielded an exact one-sided P-value for each of the experiments under H_0 of no difference in perception between eyes raised and eyes level. The second analysis was a conventional matched-pairs t test that yielded a classical one-sided P-value for each experiment based on the Student t distribution with $n_i - 1$ degrees-of-freedom for $i = 1, 2, 3$, which assumes normality. The exact and classical one-sided P-values for the 12 experiments are listed in Table 9.7. With two exceptions, all the P-values in Table 9.7 exceed a nominal significance level of $\alpha = 0.05$.

The exact one-sided P-values for each flight of experiments in Table 9.7 were combined using the Fisher continuous method and the exact discrete method. First, the exact one-sided P-values were combined using the exact discrete method. Second, the exact one-sided P-values were combined using

TABLE 9.6. Magnitude of the moon illusion ratio when zenith moon is viewed with eyes raised and with eyes level.

| Flight | Experiment | | | | | |
| | 1 | | 2 | | 3 | |
	Raised	Level	Raised	Level	Raised	Level
A	1.80	1.65	2.07	1.77	0.87	0.92
	1.70	1.60	1.83	1.95	1.89	1.86
	1.23	1.11	1.39	1.18	1.24	1.07
	1.05	0.87	1.08	1.24	1.55	1.68
	2.01	1.78	0.97	0.94	1.41	1.22
	0.81	1.05	1.42	1.17	1.13	0.91
B	0.99	0.97	1.97	1.65	2.08	1.88
	1.55	1.62	1.55	1.78	1.58	1.73
	1.79	1.49	0.91	0.87	1.22	1.15
	0.63	0.77	1.02	1.12	0.90	0.89
	1.13	0.99	1.35	1.17	1.19	1.11
	1.61	1.52	1.62	1.35	1.44	1.26
	1.82	1.80	1.49	1.44	1.95	1.99
C	1.94	1.70	2.10	1.99	1.69	1.70
	1.38	1.66	1.83	1.73	1.23	1.27
	1.01	0.88	1.26	1.19	2.01	1.99
	1.59	1.26	0.96	0.83	0.96	0.88
	1.88	1.84	1.44	1.23	1.25	1.08
	1.32	1.31	1.53	1.68	1.77	1.68
	1.41	1.25	1.03	1.11	1.79	1.84
	1.57	1.26	1.72	1.39	1.31	1.00
D	0.94	0.82	1.03	0.96	1.73	1.40
	1.17	1.41	1.55	1.53	1.05	1.18
	1.64	1.49	1.11	1.02	1.36	1.08
	0.91	0.81	0.88	0.90	1.60	1.36
	1.44	1.21	0.99	1.13	0.98	0.82
	1.76	1.58	1.22	0.92	1.53	1.52
			1.64	1.50	1.29	0.98
					0.97	1.01

TABLE 9.7. Exact and classical matched-pairs t-test P-values associated with experiments 1, 2, and 3 in flights A, B, C, and D.

Flight	Individual P-value	Experiment 1	2	3
A	Exact	0.1250	0.1719	0.1250
	Classical	0.1233	0.1695	0.1378
B	Exact	0.2031	0.1875	0.1563
	Classical	0.1907	0.1750	0.1613
C	Exact	0.0625	0.0742	0.0742
	Classical	0.0687	0.0686	0.0707
D	Exact	0.1250	0.1484	0.0352
	Classical	0.1233	0.1259	0.0263

TABLE 9.8. Exact discrete and the Fisher continuous combined P-values for flights A, B, C, and D.

Combining method	Individual P-value	Flight A	B	C	D
Exact discrete	———*	0.0241	0.0451	0.0040	0.0044
Fisher continuous	Exact	0.0656	0.1146	0.0140	0.0230
Fisher continuous	Classical	0.0690	0.1070	0.0137	0.0160

*The exact discrete method utilizes the $k = 3$ discrete probability distributions and individual P-values are not used.

the Fisher continuous method. Third, the classical one-sided P-values were combined using the Fisher continuous method. The combined P-values for each of the four experimental flights are listed in Table 9.8.

For Flight A in Table 9.7 with $n_1 = n_2 = n_3 = 6$, the exact discrete method yields a combined P-value that is less than $\alpha = 0.05$. In contrast, the Fisher continuous method yields results for both the exact and classical one-sided P-values that exceed $\alpha = 0.05$.

For Flight B in Table 9.7 with $n_1 = n_2 = n_3 = 7$, similar results were obtained. Note that the combined P-value for the exact discrete method is less than $\alpha = 0.05$, while the two Fisher continuous method combined P-values are both greater than $\alpha = 0.10$. For Flight C with $n_1 = n_2 = n_3 = 8$, the combined P-value for the exact discrete method is less than $\alpha = 0.01$, while the two Fisher continuous method combined P-values are greater than $\alpha = 0.01$. Similar results were obtained for Flight D with $n_1 = 6$, $n_2 = 7$, and $n_3 = 8$.

As is evident from comparing the exact combined P-values in the first row of Table 9.8 based on the exact discrete method, the combined P-values in the second and third rows based on the Fisher continuous method are

TABLE 9.9. Standardized percentage combined P-value differences from Table 9.8 for the Fisher continuous method based on exact and classical individual P-values relative to the exact discrete method.

Individual	Flight			
P-value	A	B	C	D
Exact	172.2	154.1	250.0	422.7
Classical	186.3	137.3	242.5	263.6

too large and, consequently, not appropriate for many discrete probability distributions. The differences in levels of significance between the second and third rows of Table 9.8 for the Fisher continuous method are ascribed to the second row being based on exact probabilities for each individual test and the third row being based on classical approximate P-values that assume normality. It is noted that the P-values of the second and third rows of Table 9.8 are very similar.

Standardized percentage combined P-value differences relative to the exact combined P-value between the Fisher continuous method and the exact discrete method were introduced by Mielke et al. (2004b). For the results given in Table 9.8, standardized percentage combined P-value differences relative to the exact combined P-value are given in Table 9.9. As an example, the Table 9.9 entry corresponding to Flight A and the Fisher continuous method with exact individual P-values is

$$\left(\frac{.0656 - .0241}{.0241}\right) 100 = 172.2.$$

Unfortunately, the exact discrete method is not applicable when M is very large. While the Fisher continuous method provides conservative results for each flight of discrete distributions summarized in Table 9.8, liberal results can also be obtained. A problem arises because the normality assumption intrinsic to the matched-pairs t test implies known underlying continuous distributions. Combining P-values from independent matched-pairs t tests using the Fisher continuous method compounds the problem by assuming the P-values follow independent uniform distributions on $[0, 1]$. The Fisher continuous method to combine P-values and the Fisher Z transformation (see Section 9.2) share the same problem. Neither the continuity assumption underlying the Fisher continuous method for combining P-values, i.e., the P-values are distributed as independent uniform random variables on $[0, 1]$, nor the normality assumption underlying the Fisher Z transformation is ever fulfilled in practice. Consequently, problems with the Fisher continuous method for combining P-values and the Fisher Z transformation (see Section 9.2) result from erroneous assumptions. As previously noted, neither of these statistical methods may be useful when the attendant assumptions are not satisfied. Simply stated, the assumptions of the Fisher continuous method for combining independent P-values are never satisfied in practice; either discreteness will be encountered or fabricated distributional assumptions such as normality must be invoked.

Example 3

This example compares the Fisher continuous method and the exact discrete method for combining P-values associated with two-sample t-test data (see Section 2.9). The exact discrete method for this example follows. Let n_i and o_i denote the sample sizes of Treatment 1 and Treatment 2 values for the ith of k two-sample experiments. In the present context,

$$m_i = \frac{(n_i + o_i)!}{n_i!\, o_i!}$$

and $p_{ij} = 1/m_i$ for $j = 1, ..., m_i$ and $i = 1, ..., k$ designate the k probability distributions in question. Therefore,

$$M = \prod_{i=1}^{k} m_i.$$

If

$$N = \sum_{i=1}^{k} n_i$$

and

$$O = \sum_{i=1}^{k} o_i,$$

then the exact discrete method combined P-value is not the same as the exact P-value of the combined data since

$$M \neq \frac{(N + O)!}{N!\, O!}.$$

Let t_{ij} denote the two-sample t-test statistic for the jth of the m_i outcomes associated with the ith of k combined experiments. The exact one-sided P-value for the ith of k experiments is

$$P_{it} = \sum_{j=1}^{m_i} \frac{D_{ij}}{m_i},$$

where

$$D_{ij} = \begin{cases} 1 & \text{if } t_{ij} \geq t_{io}, \\ 0 & \text{otherwise}, \end{cases}$$

and t_{io} is the observed two-sample t-test statistic for the ith of k experiments.

When combining P-values with the exact discrete method, H_0 specifies only that the k discrete probability distributions are independent. Under H_0, the exact combined one-sided P-value for the k discrete probability distributions is given by

$$P_t = \frac{1}{M} \sum_{j_1=1}^{m_1} \cdots \sum_{j_k=1}^{m_k} \delta_{j_1,\ldots,j_k},$$

where

$$\delta_{j_1,\ldots,j_k} = \begin{cases} 1 & \text{if } \sum_{i=1}^{k} t_{ij_i} \geq \sum_{i=1}^{k} t_{1o}, \\ 0 & \text{otherwise.} \end{cases}$$

Also, in the present context,

$$\prod_{i=1}^{k} p_{ij_i} = \frac{1}{M}.$$

In this example, the comparison of the Fisher continuous method and the exact discrete method involves the combining of one-sided two-sample t-test P-values.

The data for this example are given in Table 9.10 for three experiments associated with three sets of values. Here $k = 3$, $n_1 = 5$, $o_1 = 4$, $n_2 = 3$, $o_2 = 7$, and $n_3 = o_3 = 4$. For each of the three experiments, two analyses were done. The first analysis was a permutation version of the two-sample t test (see Section 2.9) that yielded an exact one-sided P-value for each experiment under H_0 of no difference between Treatment 1 and Treatment 2. The second analysis was a conventional two-sample t test that yielded the classical one-sided P-value for each experiment based on the t distribution with $n_i + o_i - 2$ degrees-of-freedom for $i = 1, 2, 3$, which assumes normality. The exact and classical one-sided P-values for the three experiments are listed in Table 9.11. All of the P-values in Table 9.11 exceed the nominal significance level of $\alpha = 0.05$. Table 9.12 contains (1) the combined exact one-sided P-values using the discrete method, (2) the combined one-sided exact P-values using the Fisher continuous method, and (3) the classical P-values using the Fisher continuous method. Although not appropriate in the present context, the exact and classical P-values for the combined data are 0.0088 and 0.0078, respectively, for the purpose of comparison. Finally, the standardized percentage combined P-value differences in Table 9.12 for the Fisher continuous method based on exact and classical P-values relative to the exact discrete method are 262.4 and 170.9, respectively (see the explanation for Table 9.9 in Example 2). In summary, the Fisher continuous method for combining P-values of independent experiments may be exceedingly conservative when small samples are encountered.

TABLE 9.10. Three data sets consisting of two treatments each.

Data set 1		Data set 2		Data set 3	
Treat. 1	Treat. 2	Treat. 1	Treat. 2	Treat. 1	Treat. 2
14	20	16	21	16	22
19	27	22	18	12	29
15	14	13	24	21	16
23	18		15	17	19
11			28		
			25		
			19		

TABLE 9.11. Exact and classical two-sample t-test P-values associated with treatments 1 and 2 for experiments 1, 2, and 3.

Individual	Experiment		
P-value	1	2	3
Exact	0.2063	0.1000	0.1143
Classical	0.1762	0.0969	0.0926

TABLE 9.12. Exact discrete and the Fisher continuous combined P-values for experiments 1, 2, and 3.

Combining method	Individual P-value	Combined P-value
Exact discrete	———*	0.0165
Fisher continuous	Exact	0.0598
Fisher continuous	Classical	0.0447

*The exact discrete method utilizes the $k = 3$ discrete probability distributions and individual P-values are not used.

9.2   Fisher Z Transformation

To attach probability statements to inferences about the Pearson product-moment correlation coefficient, it is necessary to know the sampling distribution of a statistic that relates the sample correlation coefficient r to the population parameter ρ (Berry and Mielke, 2000b).[3] Because $-1.0 \leq r \leq +1.0$, the sampling distribution of statistic r is asymmetric whenever $\rho \neq 0.0$. Given two random variables that follow the bivariate normal

[3] Adapted and reprinted with permission of Psychological Reports from K.J. Berry and P.W. Mielke, Jr. A Monte Carlo investigation of the Fisher Z transformation for normal and nonnormal distributions. *Psychological Reports*, 2000, 87, 1101–1114. Copyright © 2000 by Psychological Reports.

distribution with population parameter ρ, the sampling distribution of statistic r approaches normality as the sample size n increases; however, it converges very slowly for $|\rho| \geq 0.6$, even with samples as large as $n = 400$ (David, 1938, p. xxxiii). Fisher (1915, 1921) obtained the basic distribution of r and showed that, when bivariate normality is assumed, a logarithmic transformation of r (henceforth referred to as the Fisher Z transform) given by

$$Z = \frac{1}{2} \ln \left(\frac{1+r}{1-r} \right) = \tanh^{-1}(r)$$

becomes normally distributed with an approximate mean of

$$\frac{1}{2} \ln \left(\frac{1+\rho}{1-\rho} \right) = \tanh^{-1}(\rho)$$

and an approximate standard error of

$$\frac{1}{\sqrt{n-3}}$$

as n becomes large.

The Fisher Z transform is presented in many statistics textbooks and is available in a wide array of statistical software packages. In this section, the precision and accuracy of the Fisher Z transform are examined for a variety of bivariate distributions, sample sizes, and ρ values. If $\rho \neq 0.0$ and the distribution is not bivariate normal, then the previously stated large sample distributional properties of the Fisher Z transform fail.

There are two general applications of the Fisher Z transform. The first application comprises the computation of confidence interval limits for ρ and the second involves the testing of hypotheses about specified values of $\rho \neq 0.0$. The second application is more tractable than the first as a hypothesized value of ρ is available. The following four sections (1) describe the bivariate distributions that are examined, (2) investigate confidence intervals, (3) explore hypothesis testing, and (4) provide some general conclusions regarding research applications of the Fisher Z transform.

Seven bivariate distributions are used to study applications of the Fisher Z transform. In addition, two related techniques by Gayen (1951) and Jeyaratnam (1992) are also examined. The Gayen and Jeyaratnam techniques are characterized by simplicity, accuracy, and ease of use. For related studies, see Bond and Richardson (2004); David (1938); Hotelling (1953); Kraemer (1973); Liu et al., (1996); Mudholkar and Chaubey (1976); Pillai (1946); Ruben (1966); and Samiuddin (1970).

9.2.1 Distributions

The density function of the standardized normal, $N(0,1)$, distribution is given by

$$f(x) = (2\pi)^{-1/2} e^{-x^2/2}.$$

The density function of the generalized logistic (GL) distribution is given by

$$f(x) = \left(e^{\theta x}/\theta\right)^{1/\theta} \left(1 + e^{\theta x}/\theta\right)^{-(\theta+1)/\theta}$$

for $\theta > 0$ (Mielke, 1972; also see Section 3.6.2). The generalized logistic distribution is positively skewed for $\theta < 1$ and negatively skewed for $\theta > 1$. When $\theta = 1$, $GL(\theta)$ is the symmetric logistic distribution that closely resembles the normal distribution, with somewhat heavier tails. When $\theta = 0.1$, $GL(\theta)$ is a generalized logistic distribution with positive skewness. When $\theta = 0.01$, $GL(\theta)$ is a generalized logistic distribution with even greater positive skewness. The density function of the symmetric kappa (SK) distribution is given by

$$f(x) = 0.5\lambda^{-1/\lambda} \left(1 + |x|^{\lambda}/\lambda\right)^{-(\lambda+1)/\lambda}$$

for $\lambda > 0$ (Mielke, 1972, 1973; also see Section 3.6.2). The symmetric kappa distribution varies from an exceedingly heavy-tailed distribution as λ approaches zero to a uniform distribution as λ goes to infinity. When $\lambda = 2$, $SK(\lambda)$ is a peaked heavy-tailed distribution identical to the Student t distribution with 2 degrees-of-freedom. Thus, the variance of $SK(2)$ does not exist. When $\lambda = 3$, $SK(\lambda)$ is also a heavy-tailed distribution, but the variance exists. When $\lambda = 25$, $SK(\lambda)$ is a loaf-shaped distribution resembling a uniform distribution with the addition of very light tails. These distributions provide a variety of populations from which to sample and evaluate the Fisher Z transform and the Gayen (1951) and Jeyaratnam (1992) techniques.

The seven bivariate correlated distributions were constructed in the following manner. Let X and Y be independent identically-distributed univariate random variables from each of the seven univariate distributions, i.e., $N(0,1)$, $GL(1)$, $GL(0.1)$, $GL(0.01)$, $SK(2)$, $SK(3)$, and $SK(25)$, and define the correlated random variables U_1 and U_2 of each bivariate distribution by

$$U_1 = X\left(1 - \rho^2\right)^{1/2} + Y\rho$$

and $U_2 = Y$, where ρ is the desired Pearson product-moment correlation of random variables U_1 and U_2. Then a Monte Carlo procedure obtains random samples, corresponding to X and Y, from the normal, generalized logistic, and symmetric kappa distributions. The Monte Carlo procedure utilizes a pseudorandom number generator (Kahaner et al., 1988, pp. 410–411) to generate the simulations. Common seeds (83 for the tests of hypotheses and 91 for the confidence intervals) were used to facilitate comparisons.

9.2.2 Confidence Intervals

Monte Carlo confidence intervals are based on the seven distributions: $N(0,1)$, $GL(1)$, $GL(0.1)$, $GL(0.01)$, $SK(2)$, $SK(3)$, and $SK(25)$. Each

TABLE 9.13. Containment probability values for a bivariate $N(0,1)$ distribution with Fisher (F) and Jeyaratnam (J) $1 - \alpha$ correlation confidence intervals for $\rho = 0.0$ and $\rho = 0.4$.

$1 - \alpha$	n	$\rho = 0.0$		$\rho = 0.4$	
		F	J	F	J
0.90	10	0.9014	0.8992	0.9026	0.9004
	20	0.9012	0.9005	0.9015	0.9008
	40	0.9004	0.9001	0.9012	0.9009
	80	0.9002	0.9001	0.9000	0.9000
0.95	10	0.9491	0.9501	0.9490	0.9501
	20	0.9495	0.9502	0.9493	0.9501
	40	0.9495	0.9499	0.9497	0.9501
	80	0.9595	0.9498	0.9497	0.9499
0.99	10	0.9875	0.9900	0.9877	0.9900
	20	0.9889	0.9900	0.9888	0.9900
	40	0.9893	0.9899	0.9896	0.9901
	80	0.9896	0.9899	0.9897	0.9900

simulation is based on 1,000,000 bivariate random samples (U_1 and U_2) of size $n = 10$, 20, 40, and 80 for $\rho = 0.0$, 0.4, 0.6, and 0.8 with $1 - \alpha = 0.90$, 0.95, and 0.99. Confidence intervals obtained from two methods are considered. The first confidence interval is based on the Fisher Z transform and is defined by

$$\tanh\left[\tanh^{-1}(r) - z_{\alpha/2}/\sqrt{n-3}\right] \leq \rho \leq \tanh\left[\tanh^{-1}(r) + z_{\alpha/2}/\sqrt{n-3}\right]$$

where $z_{\alpha/2}$ is the upper 0.5α probability point of the $N(0,1)$ distribution. The second confidence interval is based on a method proposed by Jeyaratnam (1992) and is defined by

$$(r - w)/(1 - rw) \leq \rho \leq (r + w)/(1 + rw)$$

where

$$w = \frac{\left(t_{\alpha/2,\,n-2}\right)/\sqrt{n-2}}{\left[1 + \left(t_{\alpha/2,\,n-2}\right)^2/(n-2)\right]^{1/2}}$$

and $t_{\alpha/2,\,n-2}$ is the upper 0.5α probability point of the Student t distribution with $n - 2$ degrees-of-freedom.

A containment probability is the probability that a specific sample correlation value is contained in a Fisher or Jeyaratnam confidence interval of a prescribed size. The results of the Monte Carlo analyses are summarized in Tables 9.13 through 9.26, providing simulated containment probability values for the seven bivariate distributions with specified nominal value of

TABLE 9.14. Containment probability values for a bivariate $N(0,1)$ distribution with Fisher (F) and Jeyaratnam (J) $1 - \alpha$ correlation confidence intervals for $\rho = 0.6$ and $\rho = 0.8$.

		$\rho = 0.6$		$\rho = 0.8$	
$1 - \alpha$	n	F	J	F	J
0.90	10	0.9037	0.9015	0.9048	0.9025
	20	0.9009	0.9002	0.9020	0.9014
	40	0.9009	0.9006	0.9011	0.9009
	80	0.9006	0.9005	0.9008	0.9007
0.95	10	0.9497	0.9508	0.9516	0.9516
	20	0.9500	0.9507	0.9500	0.9507
	40	0.9493	0.9497	0.9502	0.9506
	80	0.9501	0.9503	0.9498	0.9500
0.99	10	0.9877	0.9901	0.9880	0.9904
	20	0.9890	0.9901	0.9891	0.9902
	40	0.9894	0.9900	0.9895	0.9901
	80	0.9897	0.9900	0.9897	0.9900

TABLE 9.15. Containment probability values for a bivariate $GL(1)$ distribution with Fisher (F) and Jeyaratnam (J) $1 - \alpha$ correlation confidence intervals for $\rho = 0.0$ and $\rho = 0.4$.

		$\rho = 0.0$		$\rho = 0.4$	
$1 - \alpha$	n	F	J	F	J
0.90	10	0.9011	0.8990	0.8930	0.8907
	20	0.9009	0.9002	0.8894	0.8886
	40	0.9007	0.9004	0.8873	0.8871
	80	0.9005	0.9004	0.8851	0.8850
0.95	10	0.9485	0.9496	0.9425	0.9437
	20	0.9491	0.9498	0.9407	0.9415
	40	0.9491	0.9496	0.9402	0.9406
	80	0.9497	0.9499	0.9394	0.9396
0.99	10	0.9873	0.9897	0.9852	0.9880
	20	0.9886	0.9897	0.9855	0.9870
	40	0.9891	0.9897	0.9861	0.9867
	80	0.9895	0.9898	0.9860	0.9864

TABLE 9.16. Containment probability values for a bivariate $GL(1)$ distribution with Fisher (F) and Jeyaratnam (J) $1 - \alpha$ correlation confidence intervals for $\rho = 0.6$ and $\rho = 0.8$.

		$\rho = 0.6$		$\rho = 0.8$	
$1 - \alpha$	n	F	J	F	J
0.90	10	0.8833	0.8809	0.8710	0.8684
	20	0.8742	0.8734	0.8565	0.8557
	40	0.8701	0.8698	0.8484	0.8481
	80	0.8677	0.8676	0.8438	0.8437
0.95	10	0.9359	0.9372	0.9273	0.9287
	20	0.9313	0.9322	0.9170	0.9181
	40	0.9274	0.9279	0.9116	0.9121
	80	0.9266	0.9269	0.9082	0.9085
0.99	10	0.9827	0.9858	0.9794	0.9832
	20	0.9821	0.9838	0.9764	0.9785
	40	0.9815	0.9823	0.9744	0.9755
	80	0.9808	0.9812	0.9729	0.9735

TABLE 9.17. Containment probability values for a bivariate $GL(0.1)$ distribution with Fisher (F) and Jeyaratnam (J) $1 - \alpha$ correlation confidence intervals for $\rho = 0.0$ and $\rho = 0.4$.

		$\rho = 0.0$		$\rho = 0.4$	
$1 - \alpha$	n	F	J	F	J
0.90	10	0.9016	0.8995	0.8878	0.8854
	20	0.9013	0.9006	0.8821	0.8813
	40	0.9010	0.9007	0.8780	0.8777
	80	0.9006	0.9004	0.8760	0.8759
0.95	10	0.9486	0.9497	0.9389	0.9401
	20	0.9495	0.9502	0.9354	0.9362
	40	0.9495	0.9499	0.9335	0.9340
	80	0.9498	0.9500	0.9320	0.9323
0.99	10	0.9871	0.9895	0.9835	0.9865
	20	0.9882	0.9895	0.9833	0.9850
	40	0.9890	0.9895	0.9833	0.9841
	80	0.9895	0.9898	0.9828	0.9832

TABLE 9.18. Containment probability values for a bivariate $GL(0.1)$ distribution with Fisher (F) and Jeyaratnam (J) $1 - \alpha$ correlation confidence intervals for $\rho = 0.6$ and $\rho = 0.8$.

		$\rho = 0.6$		$\rho = 0.8$	
$1 - \alpha$	n	F	J	F	J
0.90	10	0.8729	0.8704	0.8544	0.8516
	20	0.8593	0.8584	0.8321	0.8313
	40	0.8510	0.8507	0.8174	0.8170
	80	0.8459	0.8457	0.8081	0.8079
0.95	10	0.9281	0.9295	0.9150	0.9165
	20	0.9197	0.9206	0.8982	0.8993
	40	0.9136	0.9141	0.8871	0.8877
	80	0.9100	0.9102	0.8797	0.8800
0.99	10	0.9793	0.9830	0.9744	0.9787
	20	0.9770	0.9790	0.9674	0.9700
	40	0.9752	0.9763	0.9623	0.9637
	80	0.9737	0.9743	0.9585	0.9592

TABLE 9.19. Containment probability values for a bivariate $GL(0.01)$ distribution with Fisher (F) and Jeyaratnam (J) $1 - \alpha$ correlation confidence intervals for $\rho = 0.0$ and $\rho = 0.4$.

		$\rho = 0.0$		$\rho = 0.4$	
$1 - \alpha$	n	F	J	F	J
0.90	10	0.9019	0.8996	0.8860	0.8837
	20	0.9015	0.9008	0.8798	0.8790
	40	0.9012	0.9009	0.8754	0.8752
	80	0.9002	0.9001	0.8726	0.8724
0.95	10	0.9485	0.9496	0.9375	0.9388
	20	0.9496	0.9503	0.9337	0.9346
	40	0.9495	0.9499	0.9317	0.9321
	80	0.9500	0.9502	0.9296	0.9298
0.99	10	0.9869	0.9893	0.9829	0.9860
	20	0.9881	0.9893	0.9825	0.9842
	40	0.9889	0.9895	0.9825	0.9833
	80	0.9897	0.9897	0.9821	0.9825

TABLE 9.20. Containment probability values for a bivariate $GL(0.01)$ distribution with Fisher (F) and Jeyaratnam (J) $1 - \alpha$ correlation confidence intervals for $\rho = 0.6$ and $\rho = 0.8$.

		$\rho = 0.6$		$\rho = 0.8$	
$1 - \alpha$	n	F	J	F	J
0.90	10	0.8693	0.8667	0.8485	0.8457
	20	0.8545	0.8537	0.8243	0.8234
	40	0.8454	0.8450	0.8084	0.8080
	80	0.8394	0.8393	0.7984	0.7982
0.95	10	0.9255	0.9269	0.9106	0.9121
	20	0.9160	0.9170	0.8921	0.8932
	40	0.9092	0.9097	0.8797	0.8803
	80	0.9055	0.9057	0.8713	0.8716
0.99	10	0.9782	0.9820	0.9725	0.9771
	20	0.9752	0.9774	0.9644	0.9671
	40	0.9732	0.9743	0.9584	0.9600
	80	0.9712	0.9718	0.9540	0.9548

TABLE 9.21. Containment probability values for a bivariate $SK(2)$ distribution with Fisher (F) and Jeyaratnam (J) $1 - \alpha$ correlation confidence intervals for $\rho = 0.0$ and $\rho = 0.4$.

		$\rho = 0.0$		$\rho = 0.4$	
$1 - \alpha$	n	F	J	F	J
0.90	10	0.8961	0.8942	0.8054	0.8029
	20	0.9002	0.8996	0.7582	0.7573
	40	0.9050	0.9048	0.6968	0.6965
	80	0.9097	0.9096	0.6192	0.6191
0.95	10	0.9403	0.9413	0.8670	0.8687
	20	0.9415	0.9421	0.8257	0.8269
	40	0.9436	0.9439	0.7726	0.7732
	80	0.9461	0.9463	0.6982	0.6986
0.99	10	0.9797	0.9828	0.9357	0.9420
	20	0.9789	0.9803	0.9065	0.9102
	40	0.9788	0.9794	0.8694	0.8715
	80	0.9794	0.9797	0.8107	0.8121

TABLE 9.22. Containment probability values for a bivariate $SK(2)$ distribution with Fisher (F) and Jeyaratnam (J) $1 - \alpha$ correlation confidence intervals for $\rho = 0.6$ and $\rho = 0.8$.

$1 - \alpha$	n	$\rho = 0.6$		$\rho = 0.8$	
		F	J	F	J
0.90	10	0.7487	0.7457	0.6806	0.6774
	20	0.6650	0.6641	0.5733	0.5723
	40	0.5755	0.5752	0.4784	0.4781
	80	0.4884	0.4883	0.3942	0.3941
0.95	10	0.8198	0.8217	0.7612	0.7634
	20	0.7442	0.7457	0.6522	0.6538
	40	0.6543	0.6551	0.5521	0.5528
	80	0.5630	0.5634	0.4599	0.4602
0.99	10	0.9068	0.9152	0.8697	0.8810
	20	0.8523	0.8577	0.7761	0.7829
	40	0.7748	0.7780	0.6733	0.6768
	80	0.6819	0.6835	0.5721	0.5738

TABLE 9.23. Containment probability values for a bivariate $SK(3)$ distribution with Fisher (F) and Jeyaratnam (J) $1 - \alpha$ correlation confidence intervals for $\rho = 0.0$ and $\rho = 0.4$.

$1 - \alpha$	n	$\rho = 0.0$		$\rho = 0.4$	
		F	J	F	J
0.90	10	0.9007	0.8985	0.8707	0.8707
	20	0.9009	0.9002	0.8508	0.8499
	40	0.9015	0.9012	0.8284	0.8280
	80	0.9016	0.9015	0.8022	0.8021
0.95	10	0.9474	0.9485	0.9248	0.9262
	20	0.9479	0.9486	0.9095	0.9105
	40	0.9482	0.9485	0.8920	0.8925
	80	0.9490	0.9491	0.8697	0.8700
0.99	10	0.9863	0.9888	0.9758	0.9796
	20	0.9869	0.9881	0.9682	0.9705
	40	0.9873	0.9879	0.9588	0.9601
	80	0.9878	0.9880	0.9455	0.9462

TABLE 9.24. Containment probability values for a bivariate $SK(3)$ distribution with Fisher (F) and Jeyaratnam (J) $1 - \alpha$ correlation confidence intervals for $\rho = 0.6$ and $\rho = 0.8$.

		$\rho = 0.6$		$\rho = 0.8$	
$1 - \alpha$	n	F	J	F	J
0.90	10	0.8451	0.8424	0.8145	0.8117
	20	0.8068	0.8060	0.7575	0.7566
	40	0.7670	0.7667	0.7027	0.7023
	80	0.7246	0.7245	0.6490	0.6488
0.95	10	0.9052	0.9067	0.8810	0.8827
	20	0.8751	0.8762	0.8306	0.8318
	40	0.8382	0.8388	0.7803	0.7810
	80	0.8010	0.8013	0.7275	0.7279
0.99	10	0.9660	0.9708	0.9536	0.9596
	20	0.9488	0.9518	0.9217	0.9257
	40	0.9256	0.9275	0.8825	0.8849
	80	0.8968	0.8980	0.8387	0.8401

TABLE 9.25. Containment probability values for a bivariate $SK(25)$ distribution with Fisher (F) and Jeyaratnam (J) $1 - \alpha$ correlation confidence intervals for $\rho = 0.0$ and $\rho = 0.4$.

		$\rho = 0.0$		$\rho = 0.4$	
$1 - \alpha$	n	F	J	F	J
0.90	10	0.9009	0.8988	0.9134	0.9114
	20	0.9010	0.9003	0.9151	0.9145
	40	0.9006	0.9004	0.9159	0.9157
	80	0.9005	0.9004	0.9157	0.9156
0.95	10	0.9476	0.9487	0.9551	0.9561
	20	0.9489	0.9496	0.9577	0.9583
	40	0.9496	0.9496	0.9592	0.9595
	80	0.9494	0.9496	0.9599	0.9600
0.99	10	0.9862	0.9888	0.9889	0.9910
	20	0.9881	0.9892	0.9911	0.9921
	40	0.9891	0.9897	0.9923	0.9927
	80	0.9896	0.9898	0.9925	0.9928

TABLE 9.26. Containment probability values for a bivariate $SK(25)$ distribution with Fisher (F) and Jeyaratnam (J) $1 - \alpha$ correlation confidence intervals for $\rho = 0.6$ and $\rho = 0.8$.

$1 - \alpha$	n	$\rho = 0.6$		$\rho = 0.8$	
		F	J	F	J
0.90	10	0.9288	0.9270	0.9485	0.9471
	20	0.9322	0.9317	0.9556	0.9552
	40	0.9340	0.9338	0.9590	0.9589
	80	0.9347	0.9346	0.9605	0.9604
0.95	10	0.9648	0.9657	0.9759	0.9765
	20	0.9691	0.9696	0.9817	0.9821
	40	0.9704	0.9707	0.9844	0.9845
	80	0.9716	0.9717	0.9853	0.9854
0.99	10	0.9919	0.9935	0.9950	0.9960
	20	0.9943	0.9950	0.9973	0.9976
	40	0.9951	0.9954	0.9981	0.9982
	80	0.9959	0.9960	0.9985	0.9986

$1 - \alpha$ (0.90, 0.95, 0.99), ρ (0.0, 0.4, 0.6, 0.8), and n (10, 20, 40, 80) for the Fisher (F) and Jeyaratnam (J) confidence intervals. In each table, the Monte Carlo containment probability values for a $1 - \alpha$ confidence interval based on the Fisher Z transform and a $1-\alpha$ confidence interval based on the Jeyaratnam technique have been obtained from the same 1,000,000 bivariate random samples of size n drawn with replacement from the designated bivariate distribution characterized by the specified population correlation ρ. If the Fisher (1921) and Jeyaratnam (1992) techniques are appropriate, the containment probabilities should agree with the nominal $1 - \alpha$ values.

Some general observations can be made about the Monte Carlo results contained in Tables 9.13 through 9.26. First, in each of the tables there is little difference between the Fisher and Jeyaratnam Monte Carlo containment probability values, and both techniques provide values close to the nominal $1 - \alpha$ values for the $N(0, 1)$ distribution analyzed in Tables 9.13 and 9.14 with any value of ρ and for any of the other distributions analyzed in Tables 9.13 through 9.26 when $\rho = 0.0$. Second, for the skewed and heavy-tailed distributions, i.e., $GL(0.1)$, $GL(0.01)$, $SK(2)$, and $SK(3)$, with n held constant, the differences between the Monte Carlo containment probability values and the nominal $1 - \alpha$ values become greater as $|\rho|$ increases. Third, except for distributions $N(0, 1)$ and $SK(25)$, the differences between the Monte Carlo containment probability values and the nominal $1 - \alpha$ values increase with increasing n and $|\rho| > 0.0$ for the skewed and heavy-tailed distributions, i.e., $GL(0.1)$, $GL(0.01)$, $SK(2)$, and $SK(3)$.

9.2.3 Hypothesis Testing

In this section, Monte Carlo tests of hypotheses are based on the seven distributions: $N(0,1)$, $GL(1)$, $GL(0.1)$, $GL(0.01)$, $SK(2)$, $SK(3)$, and $SK(25)$. Each simulation is based on 1,000,000 bivariate random samples of size $n = 20$ and $n = 80$ for $\rho = 0.0$ and $\rho = 0.6$ and compared to nominal upper-tail values of $P = 0.99$, 0.90, 0.75, 0.50, 0.25, 0.10, and 0.01. Two tests of $\rho \neq 0.0$ are considered. The first test is based on the Fisher Z transform and uses the standardized test statistic (T) given by

$$ T = \frac{Z - \mu_Z}{\sigma_Z}, $$

where $Z = \tanh^{-1}(r)$, $\mu_Z = \tanh^{-1}(\rho)$, and $\sigma_Z = 1/\sqrt{n-3}$. The second test is based on corrected values proposed by Gayen (1951) where $Z = \tanh^{-1}(r)$,

$$ \mu_Z = \tanh^{-1}(\rho) + \frac{\rho}{2(n-1)}\left[1 + \frac{5 - \rho^2}{4(n-1)}\right], $$

and

$$ \sigma_Z = \left\{\frac{1}{n-1}\left[1 + \frac{4 - \rho^2}{2(n-1)} + \frac{22 - 6\rho^2 - 3\rho^4}{6(n-1)^2}\right]\right\}^{1/2}. $$

Incidentally, the value "16" in Equation (11) for σ_Z^2 on page 132 in Volume 3 of the *Encyclopedia of Statistical Sciences* (Kotz and Johnson, 1983) is in error and should be replaced with the value "6."

The results of the Monte Carlo analyses are summarized in Tables 9.27 through 9.40, which contain simulated upper-tail P-values for the seven distributions with specified nominal values of P (0.99, 0.95, 0.75, 0.50, 0.25, 0.10, 0.01), ρ (0.0, 0.6), and n (20, 80) for the Fisher (F) and Gayen (G) test statistics. In each table, the Monte Carlo upper-tail P-values for tests of hypotheses based on the Fisher and Gayen approaches have been obtained from the same 1,000,000 bivariate random samples of size n drawn with replacement from the designated bivariate distribution characterized by the specified population correlation, ρ. If the Fisher (1921) and Gayen (1951) techniques are appropriate, the upper-tail P-values should agree with the nominal upper-tail values, P, in Tables 9.27 through 9.40.

Considered as a set, some general statements can be made about the Monte Carlo results contained in Tables 9.27 through 9.40. First, both the Fisher Z transform and the Gayen correction provide very satisfactory results for the $N(0,1)$ distribution analyzed in Tables 9.27 and 9.28 with any value of ρ and for any of the other distributions analyzed in Tables 9.29 through 9.40 when $\rho = 0.0$. Second, in general, the Monte Carlo upper-tail P-values obtained with the Gayen correction are better than those obtained with the Fisher Z transform, especially near $P = 0.50$. Where differences

TABLE 9.27. Upper-tail P-values compared with nominal values (P) for a bivariate $N(0, 1)$ distribution with Fisher (F) and Gayen (G) tests of hypotheses on ρ for $n = 20$.

P	$\rho = 0.0$		$\rho = 0.6$	
	F	G	F	G
0.99	0.9894	0.9893	0.9915	0.9895
0.90	0.9016	0.9014	0.9147	0.9022
0.75	0.7531	0.7529	0.7754	0.7525
0.50	0.5001	0.5001	0.5281	0.4997
0.25	0.2464	0.2466	0.2685	0.2471
0.10	0.0983	0.0985	0.1098	0.0986
0.01	0.0108	0.0108	0.0126	0.0110

TABLE 9.28. Upper-tail P-values compared with nominal values (P) for a bivariate $N(0, 1)$ distribution with Fisher (F) and Gayen (G) tests of hypotheses on ρ for $n = 80$.

P	$\rho = 0.0$		$\rho = 0.6$	
	F	G	F	G
0.99	0.9898	0.9898	0.9908	0.9899
0.90	0.9009	0.9009	0.9065	0.9005
0.75	0.7514	0.7514	0.7622	0.7512
0.50	0.5008	0.5008	0.5141	0.5006
0.25	0.2495	0.2496	0.2601	0.2494
0.10	0.0999	0.1000	0.1054	0.0995
0.01	0.0102	0.0102	0.0110	0.0101

TABLE 9.29. Upper-tail P-values compared with nominal values (P) for a bivariate $GL(1)$ distribution with Fisher (F) and Gayen (G) tests of hypotheses on ρ for $n = 20$.

P	$\rho = 0.0$		$\rho = 0.6$	
	F	G	F	G
0.99	0.9892	0.9891	0.9878	0.9853
0.90	0.9019	0.9016	0.9020	0.8888
0.75	0.7539	0.7537	0.7638	0.7419
0.50	0.4999	0.4999	0.5324	0.5060
0.25	0.2457	0.2460	0.2895	0.2688
0.10	0.0981	0.0983	0.1314	0.1197
0.01	0.0109	0.0109	0.0195	0.0173

TABLE 9.30. Upper-tail P-values compared with nominal values (P) for a bivariate $GL(1)$ distribution with Fisher (F) and Gayen (G) tests of hypotheses on ρ for $n = 80$.

	$\rho = 0.0$		$\rho = 0.6$	
P	F	G	F	G
0.99	0.9897	0.9897	0.9851	0.9838
0.90	0.9011	0.9011	0.8880	0.8817
0.75	0.7518	0.7518	0.7451	0.7348
0.50	0.5004	0.5004	0.5158	0.5037
0.25	0.2495	0.2495	0.2815	0.2715
0.10	0.1000	0.1000	0.1290	0.1228
0.01	0.0102	0.0102	0.0190	0.0177

TABLE 9.31. Upper-tail P-values compared with nominal values (P) for a bivariate $GL(0.1)$ distribution with Fisher (F) and Gayen (G) tests of hypotheses on ρ for $n = 20$.

	$\rho = 0.0$		$\rho = 0.6$	
P	F	G	F	G
0.99	0.9918	0.9918	0.9869	0.9841
0.90	0.9059	0.9056	0.8954	0.8818
0.75	0.7502	0.7499	0.7560	0.7342
0.50	0.2436	0.4908	0.5297	0.5045
0.25	0.1016	0.2438	0.2982	0.2784
0.10	0.0137	0.1018	0.1441	0.1323
0.01	0.0000	0.0138	0.0257	0.0231

TABLE 9.32. Upper-tail P-values compared with nominal values (P) for a bivariate $GL(0.1)$ distribution with Fisher (F) and Gayen (G) tests of hypotheses on ρ for $n = 80$.

	$n = 20$			
	$\rho = 0.0$		$\rho = 0.6$	
P	F	G	F	G
0.99	0.9916	0.9916	0.9819	0.9802
0.90	0.9026	0.9026	0.8774	0.8710
0.75	0.7484	0.7484	0.7347	0.7247
0.50	0.4937	0.4937	0.5144	0.5027
0.25	0.2470	0.2470	0.2921	0.2824
0.10	0.1016	0.1016	0.1435	0.1373
0.01	0.0122	0.0122	0.0265	0.0250

TABLE 9.33. Upper-tail P-values compared with nominal values (P) for a bivariate $GL(0.01)$ distribution with Fisher (F) and Gayen (G) tests of hypotheses on ρ for $n = 20$.

P	$\rho = 0.0$		$\rho = 0.6$	
	F	G	F	G
0.99	0.9924	0.9923	0.9865	0.9837
0.90	0.9060	0.9058	0.8940	0.8803
0.75	0.7491	0.7488	0.7544	0.7329
0.50	0.4893	0.4893	0.5301	0.5054
0.25	0.2429	0.2431	0.3010	0.2810
0.10	0.1019	0.1021	0.1476	0.1357
0.01	0.0141	0.0142	0.0279	0.0250

TABLE 9.34. Upper-tail P-values compared with nominal values (P) for a bivariate $GL(0.01)$ distribution with Fisher (F) and Gayen (G) tests of hypotheses on ρ for $n = 80$.

P	$\rho = 0.0$		$\rho = 0.6$	
	F	G	F	G
0.99	0.9920	0.9920	0.9890	0.9792
0.90	0.9030	0.9030	0.8740	0.8675
0.75	0.7481	0.7481	0.7311	0.7210
0.50	0.4921	0.4921	0.5135	0.5018
0.25	0.2469	0.2469	0.2947	0.2850
0.10	0.1019	0.1019	0.1476	0.1416
0.01	0.0128	0.0128	0.0285	0.0268

TABLE 9.35. Upper-tail P-values compared with nominal values (P) for a bivariate $SK(2)$ distribution with Fisher (F) and Gayen (G) tests of hypotheses on ρ for $n = 20$.

P	$\rho = 0.0$		$\rho = 0.6$	
	F	G	F	G
0.99	0.9842	0.9841	0.9487	0.9423
0.90	0.9096	0.9094	0.8159	0.8016
0.75	0.7739	0.7737	0.6918	0.6750
0.50	0.5001	0.5001	0.5327	0.5163
0.25	0.2263	0.2265	0.3797	0.3662
0.10	0.0905	0.0907	0.2650	0.2548
0.01	0.0159	0.0160	0.1333	0.1284

TABLE 9.36. Upper-tail P-values compared with nominal values (P) for a bivariate $SK(2)$ distribution with Fisher (F) and Gayen (G) tests of hypotheses on ρ for $n = 80$.

P	$\rho = 0.0$		$\rho = 0.6$	
	F	G	F	G
0.99	0.9852	0.9852	0.8480	0.8442
0.90	0.9167	0.9167	0.7162	0.7111
0.75	0.7838	0.7837	0.6221	0.6165
0.50	0.5002	0.5002	0.5121	0.5064
0.25	0.2172	0.2172	0.4060	0.4011
0.10	0.0834	0.0834	0.3224	0.3182
0.01	0.0151	0.0151	0.2099	0.2071

TABLE 9.37. Upper-tail P-values compared with nominal values (P) for a bivariate $SK(3)$ distribution with Fisher (F) and Gayen (G) tests of hypotheses on ρ for $n = 20$.

P	$\rho = 0.0$		$\rho = 0.6$	
	F	G	F	G
0.99	0.9883	0.9883	0.9766	0.9726
0.90	0.9034	0.9032	0.8731	0.8595
0.75	0.7559	0.7557	0.7394	0.7192
0.50	0.4998	0.4998	0.5348	0.5119
0.25	0.2440	0.2442	0.3249	0.3067
0.10	0.0967	0.0970	0.1790	0.1672
0.01	0.0118	0.0119	0.0506	0.0471

TABLE 9.38. Upper-tail P-values compared with nominal values (P) for a bivariate $SK(3)$ distribution with Fisher (F) and Gayen (G) tests of hypotheses on ρ for $n = 80$.

P	$\rho = 0.0$		$\rho = 0.6$	
	F	G	F	G
0.99	0.9887	0.9887	0.9463	0.9437
0.90	0.9031	0.9031	0.8215	0.8152
0.75	0.7553	0.7553	0.6941	0.6854
0.50	0.4998	0.4998	0.5169	0.5076
0.25	0.2450	0.2451	0.3394	0.3315
0.10	0.0973	0.0973	0.2107	0.2051
0.01	0.0112	0.0112	0.0807	0.0783

TABLE 9.39. Upper-tail P-values compared with nominal values (P) for a bivariate $SK(25)$ distribution with Fisher (F) and Gayen (G) tests of hypotheses on ρ for $n = 20$.

	$\rho = 0.0$		$\rho = 0.6$	
P	F	G	F	G
0.99	0.9890	0.9889	0.9955	0.9943
0.90	0.9014	0.9017	0.9337	0.9217
0.75	0.7538	0.7536	0.7928	0.7679
0.50	0.5005	0.5005	0.5179	0.4861
0.25	0.2463	0.2465	0.2354	0.2133
0.10	0.0975	0.0978	0.0830	0.0734
0.01	0.0111	0.0112	0.0072	0.0062

TABLE 9.40. Upper-tail P-values compared with nominal values (P) for a bivariate $SK(25)$ distribution with Fisher (F) and Gayen (G) tests of hypotheses on ρ for $n = 80$.

	$\rho = 0.0$		$\rho = 0.6$	
P	F	G	F	G
0.99	0.9899	0.9899	0.9958	0.9953
0.90	0.9006	0.9006	0.9292	0.9237
0.75	0.7512	0.7512	0.7831	0.7714
0.50	0.5004	0.5004	0.5076	0.4924
0.25	0.2493	0.2493	0.2295	0.2184
0.10	0.0999	0.0999	0.0785	0.0734
0.01	0.0103	0.0103	0.0054	0.0049

exist, the Fisher Z transform is somewhat better than the Gayen correction when $P \geq 0.75$ and the Gayen correction is better when $P \leq 0.50$. Third, discrepancies between the Monte Carlo upper-tail P-values and the nominal values (P) are noticeably larger for $n = 80$ than for $n = 20$ and for $\rho = 0.6$ than for $\rho = 0.0$, especially for the skewed and heavy-tailed distributions, i.e., $GL(0.1)$, $GL(0.01)$, $SK(2)$, and $SK(3)$. Fourth, the Monte Carlo upper-tail P-values in Tables 9.29 through 9.40 are consistently closer to the nominal values for $\rho = 0.0$ than for $\rho = 0.6$.

To illustrate the differences in results among the seven distributions, consider the first and last values in the last column in each table, i.e., the two Gayen values corresponding to $P = 0.99$ and $P = 0.01$ for $n = 80$, and $\rho = 0.6$ in Tables 9.27 to 9.40, inclusive. If an investigator were to test the null hypothesis $H_0 : \rho = 0.6$ with a two-tailed test at $\alpha = 0.02$, then given the $N(0,1)$ distribution analyzed in Tables 9.27 and 9.28, the investigator would reject $H_0 : \rho = 0.6$ about 0.0202 of the time (i.e., $1.0000 - 0.9899 + 0.0101 = 0.0202$), which is ever so close to $\alpha = 0.02$. For the light-tailed $GL(1)$ or logistic distribution analyzed in Tables 9.29 and 9.30, the investigator would reject $H_0 : \rho = 0.6$ about $1.0000 - 0.9838 + 0.0177 = 0.0339$ of the time, compared with the specified $\alpha = 0.02$. For the skewed $GL(0.1)$ distribution analyzed in Tables 9.31 and 9.32, the investigator would reject $H_0 : \rho = 0.6$ about 0.0446 of the time and for the $GL(0.01)$ distribution analyzed in Tables 9.33 and 9.34, which has a more pronounced skewness than $GL(0.1)$, the rejection rate is 0.0476, compared to $\alpha = 0.02$. The heavy-tailed distributions $SK(2)$ and $SK(3)$ analyzed in Tables 9.35 through 9.38 yield rejection rates of 0.3629 and 0.1346, respectively, which are not the least bit close to $\alpha = 0.02$. Finally, the very light-tailed $SK(25)$ distribution analyzed in Tables 9.39 and 9.40 yields a reversal with a very conservative rejection rate of 0.0096, compared to $\alpha = 0.02$.

9.2.4 Discussion

The Fisher Z transform of the sample correlation coefficient r is widely used for both estimating population ρ values and for testing hypothesized values of $\rho \neq 0.0$. The Fisher Z transform is presented in most statistics textbooks and is a standard feature of many statistical software packages. The assumptions underling the use of the Fisher Z transform are (1) a simple random sample drawn with replacement from (2) a bivariate normal distribution. It is commonly believed that the Fisher Z transform is robust to nonnormality. For example, Pearson (1929, p. 357) observed that "the normal bivariate surface can be mutilated and distorted to a remarkable degree without affecting the frequency distribution of r in samples as small as 20." Given correlated nonnormal bivariate distributions, these Monte Carlo analyses show that the Fisher Z transform is not robust.

In general, while the Fisher Z transform and the alternative techniques proposed by Gayen (1951) and Jeyaratnam (1992) provide accurate results for a bivariate normal distribution with any value of ρ and for nonnormal bivariate distributions when $\rho = 0.0$, serious problems appear with nonnormal bivariate distributions when $|\rho| > 0.0$. The results for the light-tailed $SK(25)$ distribution are, in general, slightly conservative when $|\rho| > 0.0$ (cf. Liu et al., 1996, p. 508). This is usually not seen as a serious problem in practice, as conservative results imply possible failure to reject the null hypothesis and a potential increase in type II error. In comparison, the results for the heavy-tailed distributions $SK(2)$ and $SK(3)$ and the skewed distributions $GL(0.1)$ and $GL(0.01)$ are quite liberal when $|\rho| > 0.0$. Also, $GL(1)$, a heavier-tailed distribution than $N(0,1)$, yields slightly liberal results. Liberal results are much more serious than conservative results, because they imply possible rejection of the null hypothesis and a potential increase in type I error.

Most surprisingly, for the heavy-tailed and skewed distributions, small samples provide better estimates than large samples. Tables 9.41 and 9.42 extend the analyses of Tables 9.17 through 9.24 to larger sample sizes.

TABLE 9.41. Containment P-values for the bivariate $GL(0.1)$ and $GL(0.01)$ distributions with Fisher (F) $1 - \alpha$ correlation confidence intervals.

		$GL(0.1)$		$GL(0.01)$	
$1 - \alpha$	n	$\rho = 0.0$	$\rho = 0.6$	$\rho = 0.0$	$\rho = 0.6$
0.90	10	0.9016	0.8729	0.9019	0.8693
	20	0.9013	0.8593	0.9015	0.8545
	40	0.9010	0.8510	0.9012	0.8454
	80	0.9006	0.8459	0.9002	0.8394
	160	0.9004	0.8431	0.9004	0.8366
	320	0.9003	0.8405	0.9003	0.8338
	640	0.9002	0.8400	0.9001	0.8332
0.95	10	0.9486	0.9281	0.9485	0.9255
	20	0.9495	0.9197	0.9496	0.9160
	40	0.9495	0.9136	0.9495	0.9092
	80	0.9498	0.9100	0.9500	0.9055
	160	0.9504	0.9075	0.9503	0.9025
	320	0.9500	0.9063	0.9500	0.9011
	640	0.9498	0.9053	0.9499	0.9001
0.99	10	0.9871	0.9793	0.9869	0.9872
	20	0.9882	0.9770	0.9881	0.9752
	40	0.9890	0.9752	0.9889	0.9732
	80	0.9895	0.9737	0.9897	0.9712
	160	0.9896	0.9726	0.9896	0.9702
	320	0.9899	0.9721	0.9899	0.9697
	640	0.9900	0.9721	0.9899	0.9696

In Tables 9.41 and 9.42, the investigation is limited to Monte Carlo containment probability values obtained from the Fisher Z transform for the skewed bivariate distributions based on $GL(0.1)$ and $GL(0.01)$ and for the heavy-tailed bivariate distributions based on $SK(2)$, and $SK(3)$, with $\rho = 0.0$ and $\rho = 0.6$ and for $n = 10, 20, 40, 80, 160, 320,$ and 640. Inspection of Tables 9.41 and 9.42 confirms that the trend observed in Tables 9.15 through 9.24 continues with larger sample sizes, producing increasingly smaller containment probability values with increasing n for $|\rho| > 0.0$, where $\rho = 0.6$ is considered representative of larger $|\rho|$ values. The impact of large sample sizes is most pronounced in the heavy-tailed bivariate distribution based on $SK(2)$ and the skewed bivariate distribution based on $GL(0.01)$ where, with $\rho = 0.6$, the divergence between the containment probability values and the nominal $1 - \alpha$ values for $n = 10$ and $n = 640$ is quite extreme. For example, $SK(2)$ with $1 - \alpha = 0.90$, $\rho = 0.6$ and $n = 10$ yields a containment probability value of 0.7487, whereas $n = 640$ for this case yields a containment probability value of 0.2677, compared with 0.90.

TABLE 9.42. Containment P-values for the bivariate $SK(2)$ and $SK(3)$ distributions with Fisher (F) $1 - \alpha$ correlation confidence intervals.

$1 - \alpha$	n	$SK(2)$ $\rho = 0.0$	$\rho = 0.6$	$SK(3)$ $\rho = 0.0$	$\rho = 0.6$
0.90	10	0.8961	0.7487	0.9007	0.8451
	20	0.9002	0.6650	0.9009	0.8068
	40	0.9050	0.5755	0.9015	0.7670
	80	0.9097	0.4884	0.9016	0.7246
	160	0.9138	0.4060	0.9021	0.6822
	320	0.9173	0.3314	0.9025	0.6369
	640	0.9204	0.2677	0.9016	0.5934
0.95	10	0.9403	0.8217	0.9474	0.9052
	20	0.9415	0.7457	0.9479	0.8751
	40	0.9436	0.6551	0.9482	0.8382
	80	0.9461	0.5634	0.9490	0.8010
	160	0.9490	0.4714	0.9495	0.7590
	320	0.9514	0.3889	0.9497	0.7164
	640	0.9535	0.3147	0.9500	0.6714
0.99	10	0.9797	0.9152	0.9863	0.9660
	20	0.9789	0.8577	0.9869	0.9488
	40	0.9788	0.7780	0.9873	0.9256
	80	0.9794	0.6835	0.9878	0.8968
	160	0.9802	0.5854	0.9877	0.8639
	320	0.9811	0.4901	0.9883	0.8272
	640	0.9817	0.4020	0.9885	0.7877

Obviously, large samples have a greater chance of selecting extreme values than small samples. Consequently, the Monte Carlo containment probabilities become worse with increasing sample size when heavy-tailed distributions are encountered.

It is clear that the Fisher Z transform provides very good results for the bivariate normal distribution and any of the other distributions when $\rho = 0.0$. However, if a distribution is not bivariate normal and $|\rho| > 0.0$, then the Fisher Z random variable does not follow a normal distribution. Geary (1947, p. 241) admonished: "Normality is a myth; there never was, and never will be, a normal distribution." In the absence of bivariate normality and in presence of correlated heavy-tailed bivariate distributions, such as those contaminated by extreme values, or correlated skewed bivariate distributions, the Fisher Z transform and related techniques can yield inaccurate results and probably should not be used.

Given that normal populations are rarely encountered in actual research situations (Geary, 1947; Micceri, 1989), and that both heavy-tailed symmetric distributions and heavy-tailed skewed distributions are prevalent in, for example, psychological research (Micceri, 1989), considerable caution should be exercised when using the Fisher Z transform or related techniques such as those proposed by Gayen (1951) and Jeyaratnam (1992), as these methods clearly are not robust to deviations from normality when $|\rho| \neq 0.0$. The question remains as to just how a researcher can know if the data have been drawn from a population that is not bivariate normal and $\rho \neq 0.0$. In general, there is no easy answer to this question. However, a researcher cannot simply ignore a problem just because it is annoying. Unfortunately, given a nonnormal population with $\rho \neq 0.0$, there appears to be no published alternative tests of significance nor viable options for the construction of confidence intervals.

9.3   Multivariate Similarity Between Two Samples

It is sometimes necessary to assess the similarity between multivariate measurements of corresponding unordered disjoint categories from two populations. For example, it may be of interest to compare two samples on an array of psychological tests, e.g., female and male children on a battery of tests for depression: self esteem, anxiety, social introversion, pessimism, and defiance(Mielke and Berry, 2007).[4]

9.3.1   Methodology

Consider two samples consisting of M and N objects in g unordered disjoint categories in which $m_i > 0$ and $n_i > 0$ are the number of objects in the ith of the g categories for $i = 1, ..., g$. Thus,

$$M = \sum_{i=1}^{g} m_i$$

and

$$N = \sum_{i=1}^{g} n_i.$$

Also, suppose that r distinct multivariate measurements are associated with each object. Let $\mathbf{x}_I = (x_{I1}, ..., x_{Ir})$ denote the row vector of r measurements for the Ith of M objects in Sample 1. Also, let $\mathbf{y}_J = (y_{J1}, ..., y_{Jr})$ denote the row vector of r measurements for the Jth of N objects in Sample 2. Assume that the observed M and N objects in Samples 1 and 2,

---

[4]Adapted and reprinted with permission of Psychological Reports from P.W. Mielke, Jr. and K.J. Berry. Two-sample multivariate similarity permutation comparison. *Psychological Reports*, 2007, 100, 257–262. Copyright © 2007 by Psychological Reports.

respectively, are ordered so that the objects occur in the g categories according to the respective ordered category size structures $(m_1, ..., m_g)$ and $(n_1, ..., n_g)$. Let

$$s_i = \sum_{j=1}^{i} m_j$$

and

$$t_i = \sum_{j=1}^{i} n_j$$

for $i = 1, ..., g$. Also, let $s_0 = t_0 = 0$ and note as well that $s_g = M$ and $t_g = N$. If Δ_{IJ} is the r-dimensional Euclidean distance between the Ith and Jth objects in Samples 1 and 2, respectively, then

$$\Delta_{IJ} = \left[\sum_{k=1}^{r} \left(x_{Ik} - y_{Jk} \right)^2 \right]^{1/2}.$$

The average Euclidean distance between Sample 1 and Sample 2 objects in the ith category is given by

$$d_i = \frac{1}{m_i n_i} \sum_{I=s_{i-1}+1}^{s_i} \sum_{J=t_{i-1}+1}^{t_i} \Delta_{IJ}$$

for $i = 1, ..., g$. Then the two-sample multivariate permutation similarity comparison statistic is given by

$$W = \sum_{i=1}^{g} C_i d_i,$$

where $C_i > 0$ for $i = 1, ..., g$ and

$$\sum_{i=1}^{g} C_i = 1.$$

Whereas the present choice for C_i is

$$C_i = \frac{(m_i n_i)^{1/2}}{\sum_{j=1}^{g} (m_j n_j)^{1/2}},$$

alternative choices for C_i include

$$C_i = \frac{m_i n_i}{\sum_{j=1}^{g} m_j n_j},$$

$$C_i = \frac{m_i + n_i}{M + N},$$

and

$$C_i = \frac{1}{g}$$

for $i = 1, ..., g$. The present choice of

$$C_i = \frac{(m_i n_i)^{1/2}}{\sum_{j=1}^{g} (m_j n_j)^{1/2}},$$

while seemingly arbitrary, is based on empirically minimizing the variance of W. As with MRPP, the intuitive choice of Δ_{IJ} being Euclidean distance is also arbitrary since any other symmetric distance function could be used. Note that statistic W conceptually corresponds to the MRPP statistic δ in that all paired-object between-sample distance functions of W being confined to g specific categories is analogous to all paired-object distance functions of δ being confined to g specific groups. Statistic W takes on smaller values when the between-category variability is large relative to the within-category variability. Under H_0, each of the $M!N!$ possible orderings of the M and N objects is equally likely. If Samples 1 and 2 are similar, then the anticipated observed values of W will be smaller than expected under H_0.

The exact mean of W under H_0 is given by

$$E[W] = \frac{1}{MN} \sum_{I=1}^{M} \sum_{J=1}^{N} \Delta_{IJ}.$$

If W_o is the observed value of W, then the exact P-value under H_0 is

$$P\left(W \leq W_o \mid H_0\right).$$

An observed chance-corrected measure of similarity ($\Re_o$), a specific agreement measure and effect size, is given by

$$\Re_o = 1 - \frac{W_o}{E[W]}.$$

If a random sample of L values of W is denoted by $W_1, ..., W_L$, then the nonasymptotic approximate resampling P-value (P_r) associated with W_o is given by

$$P_r = \frac{1}{L} \sum_{i=1}^{L} \Psi_i,$$

where

$$\Psi_i = \begin{cases} 1 & \text{if } W_i \leq W_o, \\ 0 & \text{otherwise.} \end{cases}$$

If the P-value is very small, then a value L may not be large enough to provide an estimate of the P-value other than 0. However, this concern is addressed since the distribution of W under H_0 appears to be approximately normal when both M and N are large. An estimate of the standard deviation of W (σ_W) obtained from the resampling of the L values of W under H_0 ($\hat{\sigma}_W$) is given by

$$\hat{\sigma}_W = \left[\frac{1}{L} \sum_{i=1}^{L} \left(W_i - E[W] \right)^2 \right]^{1/2},$$

and an alternative asymptotic approximate normal P-value is given by $P\left(Z \leq Z_o\right)$, where

$$Z_o = \frac{W_o - E[W]}{\hat{\sigma}_W},$$

and Z is a $N(0,1)$ random variable.

9.3.2 Examples

Two examples are provided. The first example compares two samples of subjects on a univariate response variable, i.e., $r = 1$, and the second example compares two samples of subjects on a multivariate response variable, i.e., $r = 4$. For presentation purposes, both examples analyze artificially small data sets.

Example 1

Consider a comparison between two samples of 10th grade students drawn from $g = 5$ high schools in a local school district. One sample consists of $M = 19$ female students and the second sample consists of $N = 28$ male students. The students are scored on the Spielberger State–Trait Anxiety Inventory (STAI). The Spielberger State–Trait Anxiety Inventory is a self-report inventory consisting of 20 items to assess state anxiety, i.e., feelings of tension, apprehension, worry, and nervousness, and another 20 items to assess trait anxiety, i.e., viewing the world as threatening or dangerous (Spielberger, 1972, 1983). The data are listed in Table 9.43 where the scores are from the combined state/trait anxiety inventories, i.e., an overall measure of anxiety.

For the data in Table 9.43, $M = 19$, $N = 28$, $g = 5$, $r = 1$,

$$C_i = \frac{\left(m_i n_i\right)^{1/2}}{\sum\limits_{j=1}^{g} \left(m_j n_j\right)^{1/2}}$$

for $i = 1, ..., g = 5$, $W_o = 19.6630$, $\Re_o = 0.1265$, and the nonasymptotic approximate resampling P-value based on $L = 1{,}000{,}000$ is 0.0195.

TABLE 9.43. Univariate state/trait anxiety inventory scores from $g = 5$ high schools for $M = 19$ female students and $N = 28$ male students.

	High school				
Gender	A	B	C	D	E
Females	14	17	12	16	12
	18	27	13	20	70
	21	47	30	57	70
	37		45	62	
	44				
Males	13	19	13	15	13
	19	28	14	22	28
	22	36	31	57	37
	36	42	46	63	71
	41	46	54		71
	45		63		76
	50				

TABLE 9.44. Multivariate Louisiana educational assessment program scores in English language arts (ELA), social studies (SOC), mathematics (MAT), and science (SCI) for $g = 5$ elementary schools on $M = 12$ students in 2002 and $N = 14$ students in 2004.

	Elementary school				
Year	A	B	C	D	E
2002	$(1,2,2,4)^*$	$(1,1,5,3)$	$(1,5,1,5)$	$(3,1,2,4)$	$(3,2,2,2)$
	$(5,2,3,4)$	$(2,1,3,5)$	$(1,2,3,4)$	$(4,3,2,1)$	$(5,5,4,4)$
	$(1,2,4,3)$		$(5,4,2,1)$		
2004	$(1,2,4,3)$	$(3,1,5,4)$	$(1,5,1,5)$	$(4,1,2,5)$	$(1,1,1,5)$
	$(1,2,2,5)$	$(2,1,5,3)$	$(5,4,2,1)$	$(3,1,2,4)$	$(1,1,3,5)$
		$(2,2,1,2)$	$(1,2,3,4)$	$(4,2,1,1)$	
			$(4,3,1,2)$		

*The four scores in parentheses represent ELA, SOC, MAT, and SCI, respectively, where 5 is Advanced, 4 is Proficient, 3 is Basic, 2 is Approaching Basic, and 1 is Unsatisfactory.

For comparison, $E[W] = 22.5094$, $\hat{\sigma}_W = 1.3156$, $Z_0 = -2.1636$, and the asymptotic approximate normal P-value is 0.0152.

Example 2

The Louisiana Educational Assessment Program (LEAP) is a series of standardized tests that evaluate the progress of 4th and 8th grade students during the course of their studies. The four LEAP tests are in English language arts (ELA), social studies (SOC), mathematics (MAT), and science (SCI). Consider a comparison of 4th grade scores from nine elementary schools in a local school district. Each student is scored on the four LEAP tests on a scale from 5 to 1 representing Advanced, Proficient, Basic, Approaching Basic, and Unsatisfactory, respectively. The results for a sample of $M = 12$ students in 2002 and a sample of $N = 14$ students in 2004 are listed in Table 9.44.

For the data in Table 9.44, $M = 12$, $N = 14$, $g = 5$, $r = 4$,

$$C_i = \frac{(m_i n_i)^{1/2}}{\sum\limits_{j=1}^{g} (m_j n_j)^{1/2}}$$

for $i = 1, ..., g = 5$, $W_o = 3.1624$, $\Re_o = 0.1277$, and the nonasymptotic approximate resampling P-value based on $L = 1{,}000{,}000$ is 0.0205. For comparison, $E[W] = 3.6254$, $\hat{\sigma}_W = 0.2169$, $Z_o = -2.1346$, and the asymptotic approximate normal P-value is 0.0164.

Appendix A
Computer Programs

Appendix A contains a listing of the computer programs used in the book, organized by chapter. The programs are written in FORTRAN–77 and are available at the following Web site:

$$\text{http://www.stat.colostate.edu/permute}$$

A.1 Chapter 2

Programs MRPP, EMRPP, and RMRPP are the basic programs for analyzing multivariate completely randomized designs. Specifically, MRPP, EMRPP, and RMRPP all generate the MRPP statistic, δ, an associated P-value, and the chance-corrected measure of agreement, $\Re$. Each of the three programs allows for input of either Euclidean or Hotelling commensuration, choices of the distance function value v, the number of groups g, the group sizes n_i for $i = 1, ..., g$, the number of dimensions r, the truncation constant B, the group weighting constant C_i for $i = 1, ..., g$, and options for inclusion of an excess group and/or a tie-adjusted rank transformation of the response measurements. Program MRPP computes an approximate P-value based on three exact moments of the Pearson type III distribution. Program EMRPP computes an exact P-value based on the proportion of M δ values as extreme or more extreme than the observed value of δ (Berry, 1982). Program RMRPP computes an approximate resampling P-value based on the proportion of L δ values as extreme or more extreme than the observed value of δ, where a value for L is input by the user. The classical Bartlett–Nanda–Pillai test with $g = 2$ is equivalent to the two-sample Hotelling T^2 test and the results in Section 2.11 are obtained with program HOT2. Programs ETSLT and RTSLT are efficient exact and resampling $v = 2$ P-value programs, respectively, for the two-sample Fisher–Pitman test and numerous linear rank tests as an option. Programs EGSLT and RGSLT are efficient exact and resampling $v = 2$ programs, respectively, for the g-sample Fisher–Pitman test and numerous rank tests as an option.

Program RMEDQ obtains the r-dimensional median for an r-dimensional data set when $r \geq 2$ and computes selected quantile distances from the median. Program RMEDQ1 computes selected univariate ($r = 1$) quantile values for a univariate data set and then yields selected quantile distances from the median.

A.2   Chapter 3

In Chapter 3, the autoregressive analyses are accomplished with three programs. Programs MRSP, EMRSP, and RMRSP all generate the δ statistic and an associated P-value. Program MRSP computes an approximate P-value based on three exact moments of the Pearson type III distribution. Program EMRSP computes an exact P-value based on the proportion of δ values as extreme or more extreme than the observed value of δ. Program RMRSP computes an approximate resampling P-value based on the proportion of L δ values as extreme or more extreme than the observed value of δ.

The asymmetric contingency table analyses, including the Goodman and Kruskal t_a and t_b statistics, are computed with four programs. Program RCEG computes either t_a or t_b, the approximate Pearson type III P-value, and allows for the inclusion of an excess group. Program RCPT computes t_a, t_b, and the approximate Pearson type III P-values, but does not allow for an excess group. Program EMRPP computes either t_a or t_b, and the exact P-value. Program RMRPP computes either t_a or t_b, and the approximate resampling P-value.

The analyses of generalized runs are computed from four programs. Program WWRUN provides the Wald–Wolfowitz test statistic and the exact P-value. Program GRUN computes the generalized runs test statistic and the approximate Pearson type III P-value. Program EGRUN obtains the generalized runs test statistic and the exact P-value. Program RGRUN yields the generalized runs test statistic and the approximate resampling P-value.

A.3   Chapter 4

Programs MRBP, EMRBPb ($b = 2, ..., 12$), and RMRBP are the basic programs for analyzing balanced multivariate randomized block designs. Specifically, MRBP, EMRBPb, and RMRBP all generate the MRBP statistic, δ, an associated P-value, and the chance-corrected measure of agreement, $\Re$. Programs MRBP, EMRBPb, and RMRBP allow for input of Euclidean commensuration, choices of the distance function value v, the number of groups g, the number of blocks b, the number of dimensions r, and an option for alignment. For rank data, each of the programs provides tie-adjusted rank tests, including Friedman's two-way analysis of variance, which is equivalent to Kendall's coefficient of concordance, Spearman's rank-order correlation coefficient, and Spearman's footrule. Program MRBP computes an approximate Pearson type III P-value, program EMRBPb computes the exact P-value with b blocks ($b = 2, ..., 12$), and program RMRBP computes an approximate resampling P-value. Only $(g!)^{b-1}$ permutations are used in program EMRBPb since all possible relative orderings in question consist of the orderings of $b-1$ blocks relative to a fixed ordering of one specified block. Two special programs for $b = 2$ when g is large are provided. Program MRBPW2B computes an approximate Pearson type III P-value and program RMRBPW2B computes an approximate resampling P-value.

Cochran's Q test, including McNemar's test, is computed with program QTEST. The matrix occupancy problem, including the committee problem, is computed with program ASTHMA. EOSMP and ROSMP are efficient exact and resampling $v = 2$ programs, respectively, for one-sample and matched-pairs Fisher–Pitman tests and the power of ranks test as an option.

Univariate matched pairs permutation tests are provided by two programs. Program PTMP computes both the exact P-value and an approximate Pearson type III P-value. Program RPTMP computes an approximate resampling P-value. Multivariate matched-pairs permutation tests are provided by three programs. Program MVPTMP computes an approximate Pearson type III P-value, program EMVPTMP computes the exact P-value, and program RMVPTMP computes an approximate resampling P-value. Hotelling's one-sample and two-sample matched-pairs T^2 tests are computed by two programs. Program HOSMP computes the T^2 test statistic and yields a P-value under the usual normal assumptions. Program EHOSMP computes the T^2 test statistic and the exact P-value under the permutation model.

Programs AGREECI and AGREEPV yield the quantiles and P-value, respectively, for the simple agreement measure in the special case of MRBP where $v = 1$, $b = 2$, and $r = 1$. Program AGREE1 computes the $\Re$ measure of agreement and an approximate Pearson type III P-value for multiple raters and multiple dimensions. Program AGREE2 computes an approximate Pearson type III P-value for the difference between two independent $\Re$ values. Program AGREE3 computes the $\Re$ measure of agreement and an approximate Pearson type III P-value for multiple raters and a standard. In addition, programs E2KAP2 and E3KAP2 provide exact analyses for chance-corrected weighted kappa statistics for 2×2 and 3×3 tables, respectively. Also, programs RKAP2, RKAP3, VARKAP2, and VARKAP3 yield approximate two- and three-dimensional resampling and normal analyses for the chance-corrected weighted kappa statistic, respectively.

A.4   Chapter 5

Program REGRES computes the LAD coefficients for the MRPP regression analysis and an approximate Pearson type III P-value given that the residuals among groups are exchangeable random variables. Program EREGRES computes the LAD coefficients for the MRPP regression analysis and the exact P-value. Program SREGRES computes the LAD coefficients for the MRPP regression analysis and an approximate resampling P-value. Programs MREG, EMREG, and SMREG are the multivariate extensions of programs REGRES, EREGRES, and SREGRES, respectively. Program OLSREG computes the OLS coefficients for the classical OLS regression analysis and a P-value based on the usual normal assumptions. Program CRLAD computes the LAD coefficients for the Cade–Richards LAD regression analysis and the associated P-value. Program CROLS computes the OLS coefficients for the Cade–Richards OLS regression analysis and the associated P-value. Program LADRHO computes the LAD regression coefficients, measures of agreement and correlation between the observed and predicted values, and an approximate Pearson type III P-value. In addition, program LADRHO also computes a drop-one cross-validation agreement measure, autoregressive P-values for the observed ordering of both the response variables and the residuals. Program RLADRHO provides the same output as program LADRHO, but with approximate resampling P-values instead of the approximate Pearson type III P-values. Programs MLAD and RMLAD are the multivariate extensions of programs LADRHO and RLADRHO, respectively, without the drop-one cross-validation agreement measure.

A.5   Chapter 6

Program EXGF computes a P-value for Fisher's exact discrete goodness-of-fit test for k categories ($k = 2, ..., 6$). Program GF computes approximate Pearson type III P-values for the Pearson χ^2 and Zelterman discrete goodness-of-fit tests for k categories ($k = 2, ..., 50$). Program RGF computes approximate resampling P-values for Fisher's exact, Pearson's χ^2, Zelterman, and likelihood-ratio discrete goodness-of-fit tests for k categories $(k = 2, ..., 50)$. Programs M2 through M20 compute exact P-values for Fisher's exact, Pearson's χ^2, Zelterman, and likelihood-ratio discrete goodness-of-fit tests for k categories $(k = 2, ..., 20)$, respectively. If the k category probabilities are equal, then program EBGF uses Euler partitions to efficiently obtain Fisher's exact, exact Pearson χ^2, exact Zelterman, exact likelihood-ratio, exact Freeman–Tukey, and exact Cressie–Read P-values. Program PTN compares the number of distinct Euler partitions of n for a multinomial with n equal probabilities with the number of distinct partitions for a multinomial with n unequal probabilities.

Program KOLM computes an approximate resampling P-value for the Kolmogorov goodness-of-fit test. Program KOLMASYM computes an approximate P-value for the Kolmogorov test based on an adjustment to Kolmogorov's asymptotic solution (Conover, 1999). Program VCGF computes an approximate resampling P-value for an extended goodness-of-fit test based on coverages involving any positive power $(v > 0)$, including the Kendall–Sherman $(v = 1)$ and Greenwood–Moran $(v = 2)$ goodness-of-fit coverage tests. Program KSGF computes the exact P-value for the Kendall–Sherman goodness-of-fit coverage test. Programs GMGF and XKSGF compute approximate Pearson type III P-values for the Greenwood–Moran and Kendall–Sherman goodness-of-fit coverage tests, respectively. Program FPROPT computes exact P-values for Fisher's maximum coverage test.

A.6 Chapter 7

Program RXC computes approximate Pearson type III P-values for the Pearson χ^2 and Zelterman tests for $r \times c$ contingency tables with $r = 2, ..., 20$ and $c = 2, ..., 20$. Program RWAY computes approximate Pearson type III P-values for the Pearson χ^2 and Zelterman tests for r-way contingency tables with $2 \leq r \leq 10$ and up to 20 categories in each of the r dimensions. Program ERWAY computes the exact P-value for Fisher's exact test for $2 \times 2, ..., 2 \times 6$, 3×3, and $2 \times 2 \times 2$ contingency tables. Programs F2X2,...,F2X16, F2X2X2, F3X3,...,F3X10, F4X4,...,F4X9, F5X5,..., F5X8, F6X6, and F6X7 compute exact P-values for Fisher's exact, Pearson χ^2, Zelterman, and likelihood-ratio tests for the corresponding contingency tables. Program GMA yields the Gail and Mantel (1977) approximation for the number of reference tables associated with an $r \times c$ contingency table. Program SRXC computes the Patefield (1981) approximate resampling Fisher's exact, Pearson's χ^2, Zelterman, and likelihood-ratio test P-values for an $r \times c$ contingency table. Programs S2W, S3W, and S4W are alternative resampling programs to obtain two-way, three-way, and four-way contingency table P-values for the Fisher exact, Pearson χ^2, Zelterman, and likelihood-ratio tests. Thus, the only advantage for the algorithm of program S2W over the usually more efficient algorithm of program SRXC (Patefield, 1981) is the feature of conceptually simple extensions to any r-way contingency table with $r > 2$. Since exact analyses are essentially impossible for most independence analyses of r-way contingency table categories, program XrW ($r = 2, ..., 6$) provides comparisons of nonasymptotic resampling, nonasymptotic Pearson type III, and asymptotic χ^2 P-values. Programs Y2X3, Y3X5, and YSRXC are modifications of programs F2X3, F3X5, and SRXC to include the Goodman and Kruskal t_a and t_b statistics. Any of the F*X* programs may be analogously modified to a Y*X* program for this purpose. Also for $r \times c$ contingency tables, program RXC computes (1) approximate Pearson type III P-values for the Pearson χ^2 and Zelterman tests and (2) approximate asymptotic P-values based on the χ^2 distribution with $(r - 1)(c - 1)$ df for the Pearson χ^2, Zelterman, and likelihood-ratio tests. Program EI222 computes exact P-values for the three first-order interactions and one second-order interaction for $2 \times 2 \times 2$ contingency tables. Program EI2222 computes exact P-values for the six first-order interactions, four second-order interactions, and one third-order interaction for $2 \times 2 \times 2 \times 2$ contingency tables. Program RCPT computes an approximate Pearson type III P-value for Goodman and Kruskal's t_a and t_b statistics for $r \times c$ contingency tables.

A.7   Chapter 8

Program RCPT computes an approximate Pearson type III P-value for Goodman and Kruskal's t_a and t_b statistics for $r \times c$ contingency tables. Program KOLM computes an approximate resampling P-value for the two-sample Kolmogorov–Smirnov test. Program KOLMASYM computes an approximate P-value for the Kolmogorov–Smirnov test based on an adjustment to Kolmogorov's asymptotic solution (Conover, 1999). Program GSECT computes approximate resampling and Pearson type III P-values and program EGSECT computes exact P-values for the g-sample empirical coverage test involving any positive power ($v > 0$). Program WWRUN computes the exact P-value for the Wald–Wolfowitz two-sample runs test. Program GRUN computes an approximate Pearson type III P-value for the generalized runs test, program EGRUN computes the exact P-value for the generalized runs test, and program RGRUN computes an approximate resampling P-value for the generalized runs test. Programs MRPP and RMRPP compute approximate Pearson type III and resampling P-values, respectively, for the comparisons of the various tests discussed in Section 8.2.4.

A.8   Chapter 9

Program FCPV computes the classical Fisher continuous method for combining P-values. Program EDCPV provides a general exact discrete method for combining P-values when no restrictions are made on the point probabilities. Program FECPV is a special case of program EDCPV to obtain exact combined P-values for the multinomial models associated with the log-linear analyses in Chapter 7 that utilize the partitioning method of Euler when the point probabilities are equal. Programs EC1TPV and EC2TPV are special cases of program EDCPV that provide exact combined P-values for Fisher–Pitman variations of the matched-pairs and two-sample t tests, respectively, where the point probabilities are again equal. Other modifications of program EDCPV are anticipated for various independent experiments that might be encountered. Program RMRPC implements a resampling permutation comparison between two samples for multivariate similarity among g unordered disjoint categories. Finally, program MRPC yields an approximate normal distribution P-value based on the exact mean and variance of the multivariate similarity statistic W.

References

Agresti A. Measures of nominal-ordinal association. *Journal of the American Statistical Association*; 1981; 76: 524–529.

Agresti A. *Categorical Data Analysis*. New York: Wiley; 1990.

Agresti A; B Finlay. *Statistical Methods for the Social Sciences* (3rd ed.). Upper Saddle River, NJ: Prentice–Hall; 1997.

Agresti A; D Wackerly. Some exact conditional tests of independence for $R \times C$ cross-classification tables. *Psychometrika*; 1977; 42: 111–125.

Agresti A; I Liu. Modeling a categorical variable allowing arbitrarily many category choices. *Biometrics*; 1999; 55: 936–943.

Agresti A; I Liu. Strategies for modeling a categorical variable allowing multiple category choices. *Sociological Methods & Research*; 2001; 29: 403–434.

Anderson DR; DJ Sweeney; TA Williams. *Introduction to Statistics: Concepts and Applications*. New York: West; 1994.

Anderson MJ; P Legendre. An empirical comparison of permutation methods for tests of partial regression coefficients in a linear model. *Journal of Statistical Computation and Simulation*; 1999; 62: 271–303.

Anderson TW. *An Introduction to Multivariate Statistical Analysis*. New York: Wiley; 1958.

Anderson TW. *An Introduction to Multivariate Statistical Analysis* (2nd ed.). New York: Wiley; 1984.

Ansari AR; RA Bradley. Rank-sum tests for dispersion. *Annals of Mathematical Statistics*; 1960; 31: 1174–1189.

Appelbaum MI; EM Cramer. Some problems in the nonorthogonal analysis of variance. *Psychological Bulletin*; 1974; 81: 335–343.

Armitage P; LM Blendis; HC Smyllie. The measurement of observer disagreement in the recording of signs. *Journal of the Royal Statistical Society, Series A*; 1966; 129: 98–109.

Babbie E. *The Practice of Social Research* (9th ed.). Belmont, CA: Wadsworth; 2001.

Badescu V. Use of Wilmott's index of agreement to the validation of meteorological models. *The Meteorological Magazine*; 1993; 122: 282–286.

Bakeman R; BF Robinson; V Quera. Testing sequential association: Estimating exact *p* values using sampled permutations. *Psychological Methods*; 1996; 1: 4–15.

Barnard GA. A new test for 2×2 tables. *Nature*; 1945; 156: 177.

Barnard GA. Significance tests for 2×2 tables. *Biometrika*; 1947a; 34: 123–138.

Barnard GA. A note on E. S. Pearson's paper. *Biometrika*; 1947b; 34: 168–169.

Barnston AG; HM van den Dool. A degeneracy in cross-validated skill in regression-based forecasts. *Journal of Climate*; 1993; 6: 963–977.

Barrodale I; FDK Roberts. An improved algorithm for discrete ℓ_1 linear approximation. *Society for Industrial and Applied Mathematics Journal on Numerical Analysis*; 1973; 10: 839–848.

Barrodale I; FDK Roberts. Solution of an overdetermined system of equations in the ℓ_1 norm. *Communications of the Association for Computing Machinery*; 1974; 17: 319–320.

Bartko JJ. The intraclass correlation coefficient as a measure of reliability. *Psychological Reports*; 1966; 19: 3–11.

Bartko JJ. On various intraclass correlation reliability coefficients. *Psychological Bulletin*; 1976; 83: 762–765.

Bartko JJ; WT Carpenter. On the methods and theory of reliability. *The Journal of Nervous and Mental Disease*; 1976; 163: 307–317.

Bartlett MS. Contingency table interactions. *Journal of the Royal Statistical Society Supplement*; 1935; 2: 248–252.

Bartlett MS. Properties of sufficiency and statistical tests. *Proceedings of the Royal Society, Series A*; 1937; 160: 268–282.

Bartlett MS. A note on tests of significance in multivariate analysis. *Proceedings of the Cambridge Philosophical Society*; 1939; 34: 33–40.

Bearer CF. The special and unique vulnerability of children to environmental hazards. *Neurotoxicology*; 2000; 21: 925–934.

Berkson J. In dispraise of the exact test. *Journal of Statistical Planning and Inference*; 1978; 2: 27–42.

Berry KJ. Algorithm AS 179: Enumeration of all permutations of multi-sets with fixed repetition numbers. *Applied Statistics*; 1982; 31: 169–173.

Berry KJ; JE Johnston; PW Mielke. Permutation methods for the analysis of matched-pairs experimental designs. *Psychological Reports*; 2003; 92: 1141–1150.

Berry KJ; JE Johnston; PW Mielke. Exact goodness-of-fit tests for unordered equiprobable categories. *Perceptual and Motor Skills*; 2004; 98: 909–919.

Berry KJ; JE Johnston; PW Mielke. Exact and resampling probability values for weighted kappa. *Psychological Reports*; 2005; 96: 243–252.

Berry KJ; KL Kvamme; PW Mielke. Improvements in the permutation test for the spatial analysis of artifacts into classes. *American Antiquity*; 1983; 48: 547–553.

Berry KJ; PW Mielke. Computation of finite population parameters and approximate probability values for multi-response permutation procedures (MRPP). *Communications in Statistics—Simulation and Computation*; 1983a; 12: 83–107.

Berry KJ; PW Mielke. Moment approximations as an alternative to the F test in analysis of variance. *British Journal of Mathematical and Statistical Psychology*; 1983b; 36: 202–206.

Berry KJ; PW Mielke. Computation of exact probability values for multi-response permutation procedures (MRPP). *Communications in Statistics—Simulation and Computation*; 1984; 13: 417–432.

Berry KJ; PW Mielke. Goodman and Kruskal's tau-b statistic: A nonasymptotic test of significance. *Sociological Methods & Research*; 1985a; 13: 543–550.

Berry KJ; PW Mielke. Subroutines for computing exact chi-square and Fisher's exact probability tests. *Educational and Psychological Measurement*; 1985b; 45: 153–159.

Berry KJ; PW Mielke. Goodman and Kruskal's tau-b statistic: A FORTRAN–77 subroutine. *Educational and Psychological Measurement*; 1986; 46: 645–649.

Berry KJ; PW Mielke. Exact chi-square and Fisher's exact probability test for 3 by 2 cross-classification tables. *Educational and Psychological Measurement*; 1987; 47: 631–636.

Berry KJ; PW Mielke. Simulated power comparisons of the asymptotic and nonasymptotic Goodman and Kruskal tau tests for sparse R by C tables. *Probability and Statistics: Essays in Honor of Franklin A. Graybill*. JN Srivastava, editor. Amsterdam: North–Holland; 1988a: 9–19.

Berry KJ; PW Mielke. A generalization of Cohen's kappa agreement measure to interval measurement and multiple raters. *Educational and Psychological Measurement*; 1988b; 48: 921–933.

Berry KJ; PW Mielke. Monte Carlo comparisons of the asymptotic chi-square and likelihood-ratio tests with the nonasymptotic chi-square test for sparse $r \times c$ tables. *Psychological Bulletin*; 1988c; 103: 256–264.

Berry KJ; PW Mielke. Analyzing independence in r-way contingency tables. *Educational and Psychological Measurement*; 1989; 49: 605–607.

Berry KJ; PW Mielke. A generalized agreement measure. *Educational and Psychological Measurement*; 1990; 50: 123–125.

Berry KJ; PW Mielke. A family of multivariate measures of association for nominal independent variables. *Educational and Psychological Measurement*; 1992; 52: 41–55.

Berry KJ; PW Mielke. Nonasymptotic goodness-of-fit tests for categorical data. *Educational and Psychological Measurement*; 1994; 54: 676–679.

Berry KJ; PW Mielke. Agreement measure comparisons between two independent sets of raters. *Educational and Psychological Measurement*; 1997a; 57: 360–364.

Berry KJ; PW Mielke. Measuring the joint agreement between multiple raters and a standard. *Educational and Psychological Measurement*; 1997b; 57: 527–530.

Berry KJ; PW Mielke. Spearman's footrule as a measure of agreement. *Psychological Reports*; 1997c; 80: 839–846.

Berry KJ; PW Mielke. Extension of Spearman's footrule to multiple rankings. *Psychological Reports*; 1998a; 82: 376–378.

Berry KJ; PW Mielke. Least sum of absolute deviations regression: Distance, leverage and influence. *Perceptual and Motor Skills*; 1998b; 86: 1063–1070.

Berry KJ; PW Mielke. A FORTRAN program for permutation covariate analyses of residuals based on Euclidean distance. *Psychological Reports*; 1998c; 82: 371–375.

Berry KJ; PW Mielke. Least absolute regression residuals: Analyses of block designs. *Psychological Reports*; 1998d; 83: 923–929.

Berry KJ; PW Mielke. Least absolute regression residuals: Analyses of randomized designs. *Psychological Reports*; 1999a; 84: 947–954.

Berry KJ; PW Mielke. Least absolute regression residuals: Analyses of split-plot designs. *Psychological Reports*; 1999b; 85: 445–453.

Berry KJ; PW Mielke. An asymmetric test of homogeneity of proportions. *Psychological Reports*; 2000a; 87: 259–265.

Berry KJ; PW Mielke. A Monte Carlo investigation of the Fisher Z transformation for normal and nonnormal distributions. *Psychological Reports*; 2000b; 87: 1101–1114.

Berry KJ; PW Mielke. Least sum of Euclidean regression residuals: Estimation of effect size. *Psychological Reports*; 2002; 91: 955–962.

Berry KJ; PW Mielke. Permutation analysis of data with multiple binary category choices. *Psychological Reports*; 2003a; 92: 91–98.

Berry KJ; PW Mielke. Longitudinal analysis of data with multiple binary category choices. *Psychological Reports*; 2003b; 94: 127–131.

Berry KJ; PW Mielke; HK Iyer. Factorial designs and dummy coding. *Perceptual and Motor Skills*; 1998; 87: 919–927.

Berry KJ; PW Mielke; KL Kvamme. Efficient permutation procedures for analysis of artifact distributions. *Intrasite Spatial Analysis in Archaeology*. HJ Hietala, editor. Cambridge, UK: Cambridge University Press; 1984: 54–74.

Berry KJ; PW Mielke; HW Mielke. The Fisher–Pitman test: An attractive alternative to the F test. *Psychological Reports*; 2002; 90: 495–502.

Berry KJ; PW Mielke; RKW Wong. Approximate MRPP P-values obtained from four exact moments. *Communications in Statistics—Simulation and Computation*; 1986; 15: 581–589.

Bhapkar VP; GG Koch. On the hypothesis of 'no interaction' in contingency tables. *Biometrika*; 1968; 24: 567–594.

Bilder CR; TM Loughin. On the first-order Rao–Scott correction of the Umesh–Loughin–Scherer statistic. *Biometrics*; 2001; 57: 1253–1255.

Bilder CR; TM Loughin; D Nettleton. Multiple marginal independence testing for pick any/C variables. *Communications in Statistics—Simulation and Computation*; 2000; 29: 1285–1316.

Biondini ME; PW Mielke; KJ Berry. Data-dependent permutation techniques for the analysis of ecological data. *Vegetatio*; 1988a; 75: 161–168.

Biondini ME; PW Mielke; EF Redente. Permutation techniques based on Euclidean analysis spaces: A new and powerful statistical method for ecological research. *Coenoses*; 1988b; 3: 155–174.

Bishop YMM; SE Fienberg; PW Holland. *Discrete Multivariate Analysis: Theory and Practice*; Cambridge, MA: MIT Press; 1975.

Blattberg R; T Sargent. Regression with non-Gaussian stable disturbances: Some sampling results. *Econometrica*; 1971; 39: 501–510.

Bond CF; K Richardson. Seeing the Fisher Z-transformation. *Psychometrika*; 2004; 69: 291–303.

Booth JG; RW Butler. An importance sampling algorithm for exact conditional tests in log-linear models. *Biometrika*; 1999; 86: 321–332.

Bradley DR; TD Bradley; SG McGrath; SD Cutcomb. Type I error rate of the chi-square test of independence in $R \times C$ tables that have small expected frequencies. *Psychological Bulletin*; 1979; 86: 1290–1297.

Bradley DR; SD Cutcomb. Monte Carlo simulations and the chi-square test of independence. *Behavior Research Methods & Instrumentation*; 1977; 9: 193–201.

Bradley JV. *Distribution-Free Statistical Tests*. Englewood Cliffs, NJ: Prentice–Hall; 1968.

Brennan RL; DL Prediger. Coefficient kappa: Some uses, misuses, and alternatives. *Educational and Psychological Measurement*; 1981; 41: 687–699.

Brockwell PJ; PW Mielke. Asymptotic distributions of matched-pairs permutation statistics based on distance measures. *The Australian Journal of Statistics*; 1984; 26: 30–38.

Brockwell PJ; PW Mielke; J Robinson. On non-normal invariance principles for multi-response permutation procedures. *The Australian Journal of Statistics*; 1982; 24: 33–41.

Brown BM. Cramer–von Mises distributions and permutation tests. *Biometrika*; 1982; 69: 619–624.

Brown GW; AM Mood. On median tests for linear hypotheses. *Proceedings of the Second Berkeley Symposium on Mathematical Statistics and*

Probability. J Neyman, editor. Berkeley, CA: University of California Press; 1951; 1: 159–166.

Browne MW. A critical evaluation of some reduced-rank regression procedures. *Research Bulletin No. 70-21*; Princeton, NJ: Educational Testing Service; 1970.

Browne MW. Predictive validity of a linear regression equation. *British Journal of Mathematical and Statistical Psychology*; 1975a; 28: 79–87.

Browne MW. A comparison of single sample and cross-validation methods for estimating the mean squared error of prediction in multiple linear regression. *British Journal of Mathematical and Statistical Psychology*; 1975b; 28: 112–120.

Browne MW; R Cudeck. Single sample cross-validation indices for covariance structures. *Multivariate Behavioral Research*; 1989; 24: 445–455.

Browne MW; R Cudeck. Alternative ways of assessing model fit. *Sociological Methods and Research*; 1992; 21: 230–258.

Burrows PM. Selected percentage points of Greenwood's statistic. *Journal of the Royal Statistical Society, Series A*; 1979; 142: 256–258.

Butler RW; S Huzurbazar; JG Booth. Saddlepoint approximations for the Barlett–Nanda–Pillai trace statistic in multivariate analysis. *Biometrika*; 1992; 79: 705–715.

Cade BS; JD Richards. Permutation tests for least absolute deviation regression. *Biometrics*; 1996; 52: 886–902.

Cade BS; JD Richards. A permutation test for quantile regression. *Journal of Agricultural, Biological, and Environmental Statistics*; 2006; 11: 106–126.

Cade BS; JD Richards; PW Mielke. Rankscore and permutation testing alternatives for regression quantile estimates. *Journal of Statistical Computation and Simulation*; 2006; 76: 331–355.

Caffo BS; JG Booth. A Markov chain Monte Carlo algorithm for approximating exact conditional tests. *Journal of Computational Graphics and Statistics*; 2001; 10: 730–745.

Camilli G; KD Hopkins. Applicability of chi-square to 2×2 contingency tables with small expected cell frequencies. *Psychological Bulletin*; 1978; 85: 163–167.

Camilli G; KD Hopkins. Testing for association in 2×2 contingency tables with very small sample sizes. *Psychological Bulletin*; 1979; 86: 1011–1014.

Camstra A; A Boomsma. Cross-validation in regression and covariance structure analysis. *Sociological Methods and Research*; 1992; 21: 89–115.

Carlson JE; NH Timm. Analysis of nonorthogonal fixed-effects designs. *Psychological Bulletin*; 1974; 81: 563–570.

Castellan, NJ. Shuffling arrays: Appearances may be deceiving. *Behavior Research Methods, Instruments, & Computers*; 1992; 24: 72–77.

Changnon SA. Hail measurement techniques for evaluating suppression projects. *Journal of Applied Meteorology*; 1969; 8: 596–603.

Changnon SA. The climatology of hail in North America. Hail: A Review of Hail Science and Hail Suppression. *Meteorology Monographs, No. 38.* American Meteorological Society; 1977: 107–128.

Changnon SA. Temporal and spatial variations in hail in the upper Great Plains and Midwest. *Journal of Climate and Applied Meteorology;* 1984; 23: 1531–1541.

Changnon SA. Use of crop-hail data in hail suppression evaluation. *Proceedings of the Fourth WMO Scientific Conference on Weather Modification, Volume II.* Geneva: WMO; 1985: 563–567.

Chen RS; WP Dunlap. SAS procedures for approximate randomization tests. *Behavior Research Methods, Instruments, & Computers;* 1993; 25: 406–409.

CHIAA Staff. *Crop–Hail Insurance Statistics.* Chicago: Crop–Hail Insurance Actuarial Association; 1978.

Cicchetti DV; R Heavens. A computer program for determining the significance of the difference between pairs of independently derived values of kappa or weighted kappa. *Educational and Psychological Measurement;* 1981; 41: 189–193.

Cicchetti DV; D Showalter; PJ Tyrer. The effect of number rating scale categories on levels of interrater reliability: A Monte Carlo investigation. *Applied Psychological Measurement;* 1985; 9: 31–36.

Cochran WG. The comparison of percentages in matched samples. *Biometrika;* 1950; 37: 256–266.

Cohen J. A coefficient of agreement for nominal scales. *Educational and Psychological Measurement;* 1960; 20: 37–46.

Cohen J; P Cohen. *Applied Regression/Correlation Analysis for the Behavioral Sciences.* Hillsdale, NJ: Lawrence Erlbaum; 1975.

Cohen Hubal EA; LS Sheldon; JM Burke; TR McCurdy; MR Berry; ML Rigas; VG Zartarian; NCG Freeman. Children's exposure assessment: A review of factors in. inluencing children's exposure, and the data available to characterize and assess that exposure. *Environmental Health Perspectives;* 2000; 108: 475–486.

Commenges D. Transformations which preserve exchangeability and application to permutation tests. *Nonparametric Statistics;* 2003; 15: 171–185.

Conger AJ. Integration and generalization of kappas for multiple raters. *Psychological Bulletin;* 1980; 88: 322–328.

Conger AJ. Kappa reliabilities for continuous behaviors and events. *Educational and Psychological Measurement;* 1985; 45: 861–868.

Conover WJ. *Practical Nonparametric Statistics* (3rd ed.). New York: Wiley; 1999.

Conti LH; RE Musty. The effects of delta-9-tetrahydrocannabinol injections to the nucleus accumbens on the locomotor activity of rats. *The Cannabinoids: Chemical, Pharmacologic, and Therapeutic Aspects.* S Arurell, WL Dewey, and RE Willette, editors. New York: Academic Press; 1984: 649–655.

Coombs CH. *A Theory of Data*. New York: Wiley; 1964.

Copas JB. Regression, prediction and shrinkage. *Journal of the Royal Statistical Society, Series B*; 1983; 45: 311–354.

Copenhaver TW; PW Mielke. Quantit analysis: A quantal assay refinement. *Biometrics*; 1977; 33: 175–186.

Costner HL. Criteria for measures of association. *American Sociological Review*; 1965; 30: 341–353.

Cotton WR; J Thompson; PW Mielke. Real-time mesoscale prediction on workstations. *Bulletin of the American Meteorological Society*; 1994; 75: 349–362.

Cramer EM; MI Appelbaum. Nonorthogonal analysis of variance—once again. *Psychological Bulletin*; 1980; 87: 51–57.

Cressie N; TRC Read. Multinomial goodness-of-fit tests. *Journal of the Royal Statistical Society, Series B*; 1984; 46: 440–464.

Crittenden KS; AC Montgomery. A system of paired asymmetric measures of association for use with ordinal dependent variables. *Social Forces*; 1980; 58: 1178–1194.

Crow EL; AB Long; JE Dye; AJ Heymsfield; PW Mielke. Results of a randomized hail suppression experiment in northeast Colorado, part II: Surface data base and primary statistical analysis. *Journal of Applied Meteorology*; 1979; 18: 1538–1558.

Cureton EE. Rank-biserial correlation. *Psychometrika*; 1956; 21: 287–290.

Cureton EE. Rank-biserial correlation—when ties are present. *Educational and Psychological Measurement*; 1968; 28: 77–79.

Cytel Software Corporation. *StatXact: Statistical Software for Exact Nonparametric Inferences* (Version 5). Cambridge, MA: Cytel Software Corporation; 2002.

D'Agostino RB; W Chase; A Belanger. The appropriateness of some common procedures for testing equality of two independent binomial proportions. *The American Statistician*; 1988; 42: 198–202.

Darroch JN. Interactions in multi-factor contingency tables. *Journal of the Royal Statistical Society, Series B*; 1962; 24: 251–263.

Darroch JN. Multiplicative and additive interaction in contingency tables. *Biometrika*; 1974; 61: 207–214.

David FN. *Tables of the Distribution of the Correlation Coefficient*. Cambridge, UK: Cambridge University Press; 1938.

Decady YJ; DR Thomas. A simple test of association for contingency tables with multiple column responses. *Biometrics*; 2000; 56: 893–896.

Delucchi KL. The use and misuse of chi-square: Lewis and Burke revisited. *Psychological Bulletin*; 1983; 94: 166–176.

Denker M; ML Puri. Asymptotic behavior of multi-response permutation procedures. *Advances in Applied Mathematics*; 1988; 9: 200–210.

Dennis AS. *Weather Modification by Cloud Seeding* (Volume 24). Cambridge, MA: Academic Press; 1980.

Dessens J. Hail in southwestern France, II: Results of a 30-year hail prevention project with silver iodide from the ground. *Journal of Climate and Applied Meteorology*; 1986; 25: 48–58.

Diaconis P; RL Graham. Spearman's footrule as a measure of disarray. *Journal of the Royal Statistical Society, Series B*; 1977; 39: 262–268.

Dielman TE. A comparison of forecasts from least absolute value and least squares regression. *Journal of Forecasting*; 1986; 5: 189–195.

Dielman TE. Corrections to a comparison of forecasts from least absolute and least squares regression. *Journal of Forecasting*; 1989; 8: 419–420.

Dielman TE; R Pfaffenberger. Least absolute regression: Necessary sample sizes to use normal theory inference procedures. *Decision Science*; 1988; 19: 734–743.

Dielman TE; EL Rose. Forecasting in least absolute value regression with autocorrelated errors: A small-sample study. *International Journal of Forecasting*; 1994; 10: 539–547.

Dineen LC; BC Blakesley. Letter to the editors: Definition of Spearman's footrule. *Applied Statistics*; 1982; 31: 66.

Draper D; JS Hodges; CL Mallows; D Pregibon. Exchangeability and data analysis. *Journal of the Royal Statistical Society, Series A*; 1993; 156: 9–37.

Duran BS; PW Mielke. Robustness of sum of squared ranks test. *Journal of the American Statistical Association*; 1968; 63: 338–344.

Durbin J; GS Watson. Testing for serial correlation in least squares regression. *Biometrika*; 1950; 37: 409–428.

Edgington ES. *Randomization Tests* (4th ed.). Boca Raton, FL: Chapman & Hall; 2007.

Edgington ES; O Haller. Combining probabilities from discrete probability distributions. *Educational and Psychological Measurement*; 1984; 44: 265–274.

Eicker PJ; MM Siddiqui; PW Mielke. A matrix occupancy problem. *Annals of Mathematical Statistics*; 1972; 43: 988–996.

Elsner JB; CP Schmertmann. Improving extended-range seasonal predictions of intense Atlantic hurricane activity. *Weather and Forecasting*; 1993; 8: 345–351.

Endler JA; PW Mielke. Comparing entire colour patterns as birds see them. *Biological Journal of the Linnean Society*; 2005; 86: 405–431.

Engebretson DC; ME Beck. On the shape of directional data. *Journal of Geophysical Research*; 1978; 83: 5979–5982.

Euler L. *Introduction to Analysis of the Infinite, Book 1*. JD Blanton, translator. New York; Springer–Verlag; 1748/1988.

Federer B; A Waldvogel; W Schmid; HH Schiesser; F Hampel; M Schweingruber; W Stahel; J Bader; JF Mezeix; N Doras; G Daubigny; G Dermegreditchian; D Vento. Main results of Grossversuch–IV. *Journal of Climate and Applied Meteorology*; 1986; 25: 917–957.

Ferguson, GA. *Statistical Analysis in Psychology and Education* (5th ed.). New York: McGraw–Hill; 1981.

Fisher RA. Frequency distribution of the values of the correlation coefficient in samples from an indefinitely large population. *Biometrika*; 1915; 10: 507–521.

Fisher RA. On the 'probable error' of a coefficient of correlation deduced from a small sample. *Metron*; 1921; 1: 3–32.

Fisher RA. On the interpretation of χ^2 from contingency tables, and on the calculation of p. *Journal of the Royal Statistical Society*; 1922; 85: 87–94.

Fisher RA. Tests of significance in harmonic analysis. *Proceedings of the Royal Society, Series A*; 1929; 125: 54–59.

Fisher RA. *Statistical Methods for Research Workers* (5th ed.). Edinburgh: Oliver & Boyd; 1934.

Fisher RA. *The Design of Experiments*. Edinburgh: Oliver & Boyd; 1935.

Fisher RA. Dispersion on a sphere. *Proceedings of the Royal Society of London, Series A*; 1953; 217: 295–305.

Fleiss JL. Measuring nominal scale agreement among many raters. *Psychological Bulletin*; 1971; 76: 378–382.

Fleiss JL; DV Cicchetti. Inference about weighted kappa in the non-null case. *Applied Psychological Measurement*; 1978; 2: 113–117.

Fleiss JL; J Cohen. The equivalence of weighted kappa and the intraclass correlation coefficient as measures of reliability. *Educational and Psychological Measurement*; 1973; 33: 613–619.

Fleiss JL; J Cohen; BS Everitt. Large sample standard errors of kappa and weighted kappa. *Psychological Bulletin*; 1969; 72: 323–327.

Franklin LA. Exact tables of Spearman's footrule for $N = 11(1)18$ with estimate of convergence and errors for the normal aproximation. *Statistics & Probability Letters*; 1988; 6: 399–406.

Freedman D; D Lane. A nonstochastic interpretation of reported significance levels. *Journal of Business & Economic Statistics*; 1983; 1: 292–298.

Freeman LC. *Elementary Applied Statistics*. New York: Wiley; 1965.

Freidlin B; JL Gastwirth. Should the median test be retired from general use? *The American Statistician*; 2000; 54: 161–164.

Friedman M. The use of ranks to avoid the assumption of normality implicit in the analysis of variance. *Journal of the American Statistical Association*; 1937; 32: 675–701.

Gail M; N Mantel. Counting the number of contingency tables with fixed marginals. *Journal of the American Statistical Association*; 1977; 72: 859–862.

Gato R; SR Jammalamadaka. A conditional saddlepoint approximation for testing problems. *Journal of the American Statistical Association*; 1999; 94: 533–541.

Gayen AK. The frequency distribution of the product-moment correlation coefficient in random samples of any size drawn from non-normal universes. *Biometrika*; 1951; 38: 219–247.

Geary RC. Testing for normality. *Biometrika*; 1947; 34: 1070–1100.

Geisser S. The predictive sample reuse method with applications. *Journal of the American Statistical Association*; 1975; 70: 320–328.

Gittelsohn AM. An occupancy problem. *The American Statistician*; 1969; 23: 11–12.

Glick N. Additive estimators for probabilities of correct classification. *Pattern Recognition*; 1978; 10: 211–222.

Good P. *Permutation Tests: A Practical Guide to Resampling Methods for Testing Hypotheses*. (2nd ed.). New York: Springer–Verlag; 2000.

Good P. Extensions of the concept of exchangeability and their applications. *Journal of Modern Applied Statistical Methods*; 2002; 1: 243–247.

Good PI. *Resampling Methods: A Practical Guide to Data Analysis*, (3rd ed.). Boston, MA: Birkhäuser; 2006.

Goodman LA. The multivariate analysis of qualitative data: Interactions among multiple classifications. *Journal of the American Statistical Association*; 1970; 65: 226–256.

Goodman LA; WH Kruskal. Measures of association for cross classifications. *Journal of the American Statistical Association*; 1954; 49: 732–764.

Goodman LA; WH Kruskal. Measures of association for cross classifications, III: Approximate sampling theory. *Journal of the American Statistical Association*; 1963; 58: 310–364.

Goodman LA; WH Kruskal. Measures of association for cross classifications, IV: Simplification of asymptotic variances. *Journal of the American Statistical Association*; 1972; 67: 415–421.

Gordon MH; EH Loveland; EE Cureton. An extended table of chi-squared for two degrees-of-freedom, for use in combining probabilities from independent samples. *Psychometrika*; 1952; 17: 311–316.

Grant LO; PW Mielke. A randomized cloud seeding experiment at Climax, Colorado, 1960–65. *Proceedings of the Fifth Berkeley Symposium on Mathematical Statistics and Probability*. L LeCam and J Neyman, editors. Berkeley, CA: University of California Press; 1967; 5: 115–131.

Gravetter FJ; LB Wallnau. *Statistics for the Behavioral Sciences* (6th ed.). Belmont, CA: Wadsworth; 2004.

Gray WM; CW Landsea; PW Mielke; KJ Berry. Predicting Atlantic seasonal hurricane activity 6–11 months in advance. *Weather and Forecasting*; 1992; 7: 440–455.

Greenland S. On the logical justification of conditional tests for two-by-two contingency tables. *The American Statistician*; 1991; 45: 248–251.

Greenwood M. The statistical study of infectious diseases. *Journal of the Royal Statistical Society*; 1946; 109: 85–110.

Grizzle JE. Continuity correction in the χ^2 test for 2×2 tables. *The American Statistician*; 1967; 21: 28–32.

Guetzkow H. Unitizing and categorizing problems in coding qualitative data. *Journal of Clinical Psychology*; 1950; 6: 47–58.

Haber M. Sample sizes for the exact test of 'no interaction' in 2×2×2 tables. *Biometrics*; 1983; 39: 493–498.

Haber M. A comparison of tests for the hypothesis of no three-factor interaction in 2×2×2 contingency tables. *Journal of Statistical Computing and Simulation*; 1984; 20: 205–215.

Haberman SJ. *Analysis of qualitative data, Volume I: Introductory Topics*. New York: Academic Press; 1978.

Haberman SJ. *Analysis of qualitative data, Volume II: New Developments*. New York: Academic Press; 1979.

Haberman SJ. Analysis of dispersion of multinomial responses. *Journal of the American Statistical Association*; 1982; 77: 568–580.

Haldane JBS. The mean and variance of χ^2, when used as a test of homogeneity, when expectations are small. *Biometrika*; 1940; 31: 346–355.

Hardy GH; S Ramanujan. Asymptotic formulae in combinatory analysis. *Proceedings of the London Mathematical Society*; 1918; 17: 75–115.

Harter S. *Manual for the Self-perception Profile for Children*. Denver, CO: University of Denver; 1985.

Haviland MG. Yates correction for continuity and the analysis of 2×2 contingency tables (with comments). *Statistics in Medicine*; 1990; 9: 363–383.

Hayes AF. Permustat: Randomization tests for the Macintosh. *Behavior Research Methods, Instruments, & Computers*; 1996a; 28: 473–475.

Hayes AF. Permutation test is not distribution-free: Testing H_0: $\rho = 0$. *Psychological Methods*; 1996b; 1: 184–198.

Hays WL. *Statistics* (4th ed.). New York: Holt, Rinehart, & Winston; 1988.

Hess JC; JB Elsner. Extended-range hindcasts of tropical-origin Atlantic hurricane activity. *Geophysical Research Letters*; 1994; 21: 365–368.

Hettmansperger TP; JW McKean. *Robust Nonparametric Methods*. London, UK: Arnold; 1998.

Holst L; JS Rao. Asymptotic theory for some families of two-sample nonparametric statistics. *Sankhyā*; 1980; A42: 19–52.

Holway AH; EG Boring. The apparent size of the moon as a function of the angle of regard: Further experiments. *American Journal of Psychology*; 1940a; 53: 537–553.

Holway AH; EG Boring. The moon illusion and the angle of regard. *American Journal of Psychology*; 1940b; 53; 109–116.

Horst P. *Psychological Measurement and Prediction*. Belmont, CA: Wads-worth; 1966.

Hotelling H. The generalization of Student's ratio. *Annals of Mathematical Statistics*; 1931; 2: 360–378.

Hotelling H. New light on the correlation coefficient and its transforms. *Journal of the Royal Statistical Society, Series B*; 1953; 15: 193–232.

Howell DC. *Statistical Methods for Psychology* (4th ed.). Belmont, CA: Duxbury; 1997.

Howell DC. *Statistical Methods for Psychology* (5th ed.). Belmont, CA: Duxbury; 2002.

Howell DC. *Statistical Methods for Psychology* (6th ed.). Belmont, CA: Duxbury; 2007.

Howell DC; SH McConaughy. Nonorthogonal analysis of variance: Putting the question before the answer. *Educational and Psychological Measurement*; 1982; 42: 9–24.

Hubert L. A note on Freeman's measure of association for relating an ordered to an unordered factor. *Psychometrika*; 1974; 39: 517–520.

Hubert L. Kappa revisited. *Psychological Bulletin*; 1977; 84: 289–297.

Hubert L. *Assignment Methods in Combinatorial Data Analysis*. New York: Marcel Dekker; 1987.

Huberty CJ; JM Wisenbaker; JC Smith. Assessing predictive accuracy in discriminant analysis. *Multivariate Behavioral Research*; 1987; 22: 307–329.

Huh M-H; M Jhun. Random permutation testing in multiple linear regression. *Communications in Statistics—Theory and Methods*; 2001; 30: 2023–2032.

Hunter AA. On the validity of measures of association: The nominal-nominal, two-by-two case. *American Journal of Sociology*; 1973; 79: 99–109.

Iachan R. Measures of agreement for incompletely ranked data. *Educational and Psychological Measurement*; 1984; 44: 823–830.

Irving, E. *Palaeomagnetism and Its Application to Geological and Geophysical Problems*. New York: Wiley; 1964.

Iyer HK; KJ Berry; PW Mielke. Computation of finite population parameters and approximate probability values for multi-response randomized block permutations (MRBP). *Communications in Statistics—Simulation and Computation*; 1983; 12: 479–499.

Iyer HK; DF Vecchia; PW Mielke. Higher order cumulants and Tchebyshev-Markov bounds for *P*-values in distribution-free matched-pairs tests. *Journal of Statistical Planning and Inference*; 2002; 116: 131–147.

Jammalamadaka SR; A Sengupta. *Topics in Circular Statistics*. River Edge, NJ: World Scientific; 2001.

Jammalamadaka SR; X Zhou. Bahadur efficiencies of spacings tests for goodness of fit. *Annals of the Institute of Statistical Mathematics*; 1989; 41: 541–553.

Jeyaratnam S. Confidence intervals for the correlation coefficient. *Statistics & Probability Letters*; 1992; 15: 389–393.

Johnston, JE; KJ Berry; PW Mielke. A measure of effect size for experimental designs with heterogeneous variances. *Perceptual and Motor Skills*; 2004; 98: 3–18.

Jonckheere AR. A distribution-free *k*-sample test against ordered alternatives. *Biometrika*; 1954; 41: 133–145.

Kahaner D; C Moler; S Nash. *Numerical Methods and Software*. Englewood Cliffs: Prentice–Hall; 1988.

Kaufman EH; GD Taylor; PW Mielke; KJ Berry. An algorithm and FORTRAN program for multivariate LAD (ℓ_1 of ℓ_2) regression. *Computing*; 2002; 68: 275–287.

Kaufman L; JH Kaufman. Explaining the moon illusion. *Proceedings of the National Academy of Sciences of the United States of America*; 2000; 97: 500–505.

Kaufman L; I Rock. The moon illusion: I. *Science*; 1962; 136: 953–961.

Kelley TL. An unbiased correlation ratio measure. *Proceedings of the National Academy of Sciences*; 1935; 21: 554–559.

Kelly FP; TH VonderHaar; PW Mielke. Imagery randomized block analysis (IRBA) applied to the verification of cloud edge detectors. *Journal of Atmospheric and Oceanic Technology*; 1989; 6: 671–679.

Kendall MG. Discussion on Professor Greenwood's paper on "The statistical study of infectious diseases." *Journal of the Royal Statistical Society*; 1946; 109: 103–105.

Kendall MG. *Rank Correlation Methods*. London: Charles Griffin & Company; 1948.

Kendall MG. *Rank Correlation Methods* (3rd ed.). London: Charles Griffin & Company; 1962.

Kendall MG; BB Smith. The problem of m rankings. *The Annals of Mathematical Statistics*; 1939; 10: 275–287.

Kennedy PE; BS Cade. Randomization tests for multiple regression. *Communications in Statistics—Simulation and Computation*; 1996; 25: 923–936.

Kennedy WJ; JE Gentle. *Statistical Computing*. New York: Marcel Dekker; 1980.

Keppel G. *Design and Analysis: A Researcher's Handbook* (2nd ed.). Englewood Cliffs, NJ: Prentice–Hall; 1982.

Keppel G; S Zedeck. *Data Analysis for Research Designs: Analysis of Variance and Multiple Regression/Correlation Approaches*. New York: Freeman; 1989.

Kiefer J. K-sample analogues of the Kolmogorov–Smirnov and Cramer–von Mises tests. *Annals of Mathematical Statistics*; 1959; 30: 420–447.

Kincaid WM. The combination of tests based on discrete distributions. *Journal of the American Statistical Association*; 1962; 57: 10–19.

Kolmogorov AN. Sulla determinazione empirica di una legge di distribuzione. *Giornale dell' Istituto Italiano degli Attuari*; 1933; 4: 83–91.

Kotz S; NL Johnson. *Encyclopedia of Statistical Sciences*. New York: Wiley; 1983.

Kovacs M; HS Akiskal; C Gatsonis; PL Parrone. Childhood-onset dysthymic disorder. *Archives of General Psychiatry*; 1994; 51: 365–374.

Kraemer HC. Improved approximation to the non-null distribution of the correlation coefficient. *Journal of the American Statistical Association*; 1973; 68: 1004–1008.

Krippendorff K. Bivariate agreement coefficients for reliability of data. *Sociological Methodology*. EG Borgatta, editor. San Francisco: Jossey–Bass; 1970a: 139–150.

Krippendorff K. Estimating the reliability, systematic error and random error of interval data. *Educational and Psychological Measurement*; 1970b; 30: 61–70.

Kruskal WB; WA Wallis. Use of ranks on one-criterion variance analysis. *Journal of The Statistical Association*; 1952; 47: 583–621. Addendum: 1953; 48: 907–911.

Lachenbruch PA. An almost unbiased method of obtaining confidence intervals for the probability of misclassification in discriminant analysis. *Biometrics*; 1967; 23: 639–645.

Lachenbruch PA; MR Mickey. Estimation of error rates in discriminant analysis. *Technometrics*; 1968; 10: 1–11.

Lamb PJ. Large-scale tropical Atlantic surface circulation patterns during recent sub-Saharan weather anomalies. *Tellus*; 1978; 30: 240–251.

Lancaster HO. The combination of probabilities arising from data in discrete distributions. *Biometrika*; 1949; 36: 370–382.

Landis JR; GG Koch. An application of hierarchical kappa-like statistics in the assessment of majority agreement among multiple observers. *Biometrics*; 1977; 33: 363–374.

Larochelle A. A re-examination of certain statistical methods in palaeomagnetism. *Geological Survey of Canada*; 1967a; paper 67–17.

Larochelle A. Further considerations on certain statistical methods in palaeomagnetism. *Geological Survey of Canada*; 1967b; paper 67–26.

Lee TJ; RA Pielke; PW Mielke. Modeling the clear-sky surface energy budget during FIFE 1987. *Journal of Geophysical Research*; 1995; 100: 25,585–25,593.

Lehmann EL. *Testing Statistical Hypotheses* (2nd ed.). New York: Wiley; 1986.

Levine JH. Joint-space analysis of "pick-any" data: Analysis of choices from an unconstrained set of alternatives. *Psychometrika*; 1979; 44: 85–92.

Lewis C; G Keren. You can't have your cake and eat it too: Some considerations of the error term. *Psychological Bulletin*; 1977; 84: 1150–1154.

Lewis T; IW Saunders; M Westcott. The moments of the Pearson chi-squared statistic and the minimum expected value in two-way tables. *Biometrika*; 1984; 71: 515–522. Correction: 1989; 76: 407.

Light RJ. Measures of response agreement for qualitative data: Some generalizations and alternatives. *Psychological Bulletin*; 1971; 76: 365–377.

Light RJ; BH Margolin. An analysis of variance for categorical data. *Journal of the American Statistical Association*; 1971; 66: 534–544.

Lindley DV; MR Novick. The role of exchangeability in inference. *Annals of Statistics*; 1981; 9: 45–58.

Littell RC; JL Folks. Asymptotic optimality of Fisher's method of combining independent tests. *Journal of the American Statistical Association*; 1971; 66: 802–806.

Littell RC; JL Folks. Asymptotic optimality of Fisher's method of combining independent tests: II. *Journal of the American Statistical Association*; 1973; 68: 193–194.

Liu WC; JA Woodward; DG Bonett. The generalized likelihood ratio test for the Pearson correlation. *Communications in Statistics—Simulation and Computation*; 1996; 25: 507–520.

Livezey RE; AG Barnston; BK Neumeister. Mixed analog/persistence prediction of seasonal mean temperatures for the USA. *International Journal of Climatology*; 1990; 10: 329–340.

Loughin TM; PN Scherer. Testing for association in contingency tables with multiple column responses. *Biometrics*; 1998; 54: 630–637.

Louisiana Department of Education. District Composite Report, Section 4. *Student Achievement for Saint Bernard, Jefferson, and Orleans Parishes (January 2001). LEAP 21 Test Results 1999–2000.* http://www.louisiana-schools.net/DOE/PDFs/DCR99/list.pdf [cited 24 January 2002].

Lovie AD. Who discovered Spearman's rank correlation? *British Journal of Mathematical and Statistical Psychology*; 1995; 48: 255–269.

Ludbrook J; H Dudley. Why permutation tests are superior to *t* and *F* tests in biomedical research. *The American Statistician*; 1998; 52: 127–132.

Lunneborg CE. *Data Analysis by Resampling: Concepts and Applications.* Pacific Grove, CA: Duxbury; 2000.

MacCallum RC; M Roznowski; CM Mar; JV Reith. Alternative strategies for cross-validation of covariance structure models. *Multivariate Behavioral Research*; 1994; 29: 1–32.

Magnus A; PW Mielke; TW Copenhaver. Closed expressions for the sum of an infinite series with application to quantal response assays. *Biometrics*; 1977; 33: 221–223.

Mahaffey KR; JL Annest; J Roberts; RS Murphy. National estimates of blood lead levels: United States, 1976–1980. *New England Journal of Medicine*; 1982; 307: 573–579.

Manly BFJ. *Randomization, Bootstrap and Monte Carlo Methods in Biology.* (2nd ed.). London, UK: Chapman & Hall; 1997.

Mann HB; DR Whitney. On a test of whether one of two random variables is stochastically larger than the other. *The Annals of Mathematical Statistics*; 1947; 18: 50–60.

Mantel N. Approaches to a health research occupancy problem. *Biometrics*; 1974; 30: 355–362.

Mantel N; BS Pasternack. A class of occupancy problems. *The American Statistician*; 1968; 22: 23–24.

Mantel N; RS Valand. A technique of nonparamertric multivariate analysis. *Biometrics*; 1970; 26: 547–558.

Marascuilo LA; M McSweeney. *Nonparametric and Distribution-Free Methods for the Social Sciences.* Monterey, CA: Brooks/Cole; 1977.

Mardia KV; PE Jupp. *Directional Statistics.* Chichester, NY: Wiley; 2000.

Margolin BH; RJ Light. An analysis of variance for categorical data, II: Small sample comparisons with chi square and other competitors. *Journal of the American Statistical Association*; 1974; 69: 755–764.

Markó T; F Söver; P Simeonov. On the damage reduction in Bulgarian and Hungarian hail suppression projects. *Journal of Weather Modification*; 1990; 22: 82–89.

Mathew T; K Nordström. Least squares and least absolute deviation procedures in approximately linear models. *Statistics & Probability Letters*; 1993; 16: 153–158.

Maxim PS. *Quantitative Research Methods in the Social Sciences.* New York: Oxford University Press; 1999.

May M. Disturbing behavior: Neurotoxic effects in children. *Environmental Health Perspectives*; 2000; 108: 262–267.

May RB; MA Hunter. Some advantages of permutation tests. *Canadian Psychology*; 1993; 34: 401–407.

May RB; MEJ Masson; MA Hunter. *Application of Statistics in Behavioral Research*; New York: Harper & Row; 1990.

McCabe GJ; DR Legates. General-circulation model simulations of winter and summer sea-level pressures over North America. *International Journal of Climatology*; 1992; 12: 815–827.

McKean JW; GL Sievers. Coefficients of determination for least absolute deviation analysis. *Statistics & Probability Letters*; 1987; 5: 49–54.

McNemar Q. Note on the sampling error of the differences between correlated proportions and percentages. *Psychometrika*; 1947; 12: 153–157.

Mehta CR; NR Patel. A network algorithm for performing Fisher's exact test in $r \times c$ contingency tables. *Journal of the American Statistical Association*; 1983; 78: 427–434.

Mehta CR; NR Patel. Algorithm 643: FEXACT: A FORTRAN subroutine for Fisher's exact test on unordered $r \times c$ contingency tables. *Association for Computing Machinery Transactions on Mathematical Software*; 1986a; 12: 154–161.

Mehta CR; NR Patel. A hybrid algorithm for Fisher's exact test in unordered $r \times c$ contingency tables. *Communications in Statistics—Theory and Methods*; 1986b; 15: 387–403.

Mesinger F; N Mesinger. Has hail suppression in eastern Yugoslavia led to a reduction in the frequency of hail? *Journal of Applied Meteorology*; 1992; 31: 104–111.

Micceri T. The unicorn, the normal curve, and other improbable creatures. *Psychological Bulletin*; 1989; 105: 156–166.

Michaelsen J. Cross-validation in statistical climate forecast models. *Journal of Climate and Applied Meteorology*; 1987; 26: 1589–1600.

Mielke HW. Lead in the inner cities. *American Scientist*; 1999; 87: 62–73.

Mielke HW; JC Anderson; KJ Berry; PW Mielke; RL Chaney; M Leech. Lead concentrations in inner-city soils as a factor in the child lead problem. *American Journal of Public Health*; 1983; 73: 1366–1369.

Mielke HW; KJ Berry; PW Mielke; ET Powell; CR Gonzales. Multiple metal accumulation as a factor in learning achievement within various New Orleans elementary school communities. *Environmental Research*; 2005a; 97: 67–75.

Mielke HW; CR Gonzales; MK Smith; PW Mielke. Quantities and associations of lead, zinc, cadmium, manganese, chromium, nickel, vanadium, and copper in fresh Mississippi delta alluvium and New Orleans alluvial soils. *Science of the Total Environment*; 2000; 246: 249–259.

Mielke PW. Asymptotic behavior of two-sample tests based on powers of ranks for detecting scale and location alternatives. *Journal of the American Statistical Association*; 1972; 67: 850–854.

Mielke PW. Another family of distributions for describing and analyzing precipitation data. *Journal of Applied Meteorology*; 1973; 12: 275–280. Corrigendum: 1974; 13: 516.

Mielke PW. Squared rank test appropriate to weather modification crossover design. *Technometrics*; 1974; 16: 13–16.

Mielke PW. Convenient beta distribution likelihood techniques for describing and comparing meteorological data. *Journal of Applied Meteorology*; 1975; 14: 985–990.

Mielke PW. Simple iterative procedures for two-parameter gamma distribution maximum likelihood estimates. *Journal of Applied Meteorology*; 1976; 15: 181–183.

Mielke PW. Clarification and appropriate inferences for Mantel and Valand's nonparametric multivariate analysis technique. *Biometrics*; 1978; 34: 277–282.

Mielke PW. On asymptotic non-normality of null distributions of MRPP statistics. *Communications in Statistics—Theory and Methods*; 1979; 8: 1541–1550. Errata: 1981; 10: 1795 and 1982; 11: 847.

Mielke PW. Meteorological applications of permutation techniques based on distance functions. *Handbook of Statistics Volume 4*. PR Krishnaiah and PK Sen, editors. Amsterdam: North–Holland; 1984: 813–830.

Mielke PW. Geometric concerns pertaining to applications of statistical tests in the atmospheric sciences. *Journal of the Atmospheric Sciences*; 1985; 42: 1209–1212.

Mielke PW. Non-metric statistical analyses: Some metric alternatives. *Journal of Statistical Planning and Inference*; 1986; 13: 377–387.

Mielke PW. L_1, L_2 and L_∞ regression models: Is there a difference? *Journal of Statistical Planning and Inference*; 1987; 16: 430.

Mielke PW. The application of multivariate permutation methods based on distance functions in the earth sciences. *Earth–Science Reviews*; 1991; 31: 55–71.

Mielke PW. Comments on the Climax I & II experiments including replies to Rangno & Hobbs. *Journal of Applied Meteorology*; 1995; 34: 1228–1232.

Mielke PW. Some exact and nonasymptotic analyses of discrete goodness-of-fit and r-way contingency tables. *Advances in the Theory and Practice of Statistics: A Volume in Honor of Samuel Kotz*. NL Johnson and N Balakrishnan, editors. New York: Wiley; 1997: 179–192.

Mielke PW; KJ Berry. An extended class of matched pairs tests based on powers of ranks. *Psychometrika*; 1976; 41: 89–100.

Mielke PW; KJ Berry. An extended class of permutation techniques for matched pairs. *Communications in Statistics—Theory and Methods*; 1982; 11: 1197–1207.

Mielke PW; KJ Berry. Asymptotic clarifications, generalizations, and concerns regarding an extended class of matched pairs tests based on powers of ranks. *Psychometrika*; 1983; 48: 483–485.

Mielke PW; KJ Berry. Non-asymptotic inferences based on the chi-square statistic for r by c contingency tables. *Journal of Statistical Planning and Inference*; 1985; 12: 41–45.

Mielke PW; KJ Berry. Cumulant methods for analyzing independence of r-way contingency tables and goodness-of-fit frequency data. *Biometrika*; 1988; 75: 790–793.

Mielke PW; KJ Berry. Fisher's exact probability test for cross-classification tables. *Educational and Psychological Measurement*; 1992; 52: 97–101.

Mielke PW; KJ Berry. Exact goodness-of-fit probability tests for analyzing categorical data. *Educational and Psychological Measurement*; 1993; 53: 707–710.

Mielke PW; KJ Berry. Permutation tests for common locations among samples with unequal variances. *Journal of Educational and Behavioral Statistics*; 1994; 19: 217–236.

Mielke PW; KJ Berry. Nonasymptotic inferences based on Cochran's Q test. *Perceptual and Motor Skills*; 1995; 81: 319–322.

Mielke PW; KJ Berry. An exact solution to an occupancy problem: A useful alternative to Cochran's Q test. *Perceptual and Motor Skills*; 1996a; 82: 91–95.

Mielke PW; KJ Berry. Exact probabilities for first-order and second-order interactions in $2 \times 2 \times 2$ contingency tables. *Educational and Psychological Measurement*; 1996b; 56: 843–847.

Mielke PW; KJ Berry. Permutation covariate analyses of residuals based on Euclidean distance. *Psychological Reports*; 1997a; 81: 795–802.

Mielke PW; KJ Berry. Permutation-based multivariate regression analysis: The case for least sum of absolute deviations regression. *Annals of Operations Research*; 1997b; 74: 259–268.

Mielke PW; KJ Berry. Exact probabilities for first-order, second-order, and third-order interactions in $2\times2\times2\times2$ contingency tables. *Perceptual and Motor Skills*; 1998; 86: 760–762.

Mielke PW; KJ Berry. Multivariate tests for correlated data in completely randomized designs. *Journal of Educational and Behavioral Statistics*; 1999; 24: 109–131.

Mielke PW; KJ Berry. Euclidean distance based permutation methods in atmospheric science. *Data Mining and Knowledge Discovery*; 2000a; 4: 7–28.

Mielke PW; KJ Berry. The Terpstra–Jonckheere test for ordered alternatives: Randomized probability values. *Perceptual and Motor Skills*; 2000b; 91: 447–450.

Mielke PW; KJ Berry. Multivariate multiple regression analyses: A permutation method for linear models. *Psychological Reports*; 2002a; 91: 3–9. Erratum: 91: 2.

Mielke PW; KJ Berry. Data dependent analyses in psychological research. *Psychological Reports*; 2002b; 91: 1225–1234.

Mielke PW; KJ Berry. Categorical independence tests for large sparse r-way contingency tables. *Perceptual and Motor Skills*; 2002c; 95: 606–610.

Mielke PW; KJ Berry. Multivariate multiple regression prediction models: A Euclidean distance approach. *Psychological Reports*; 2003; 92: 763–769.

Mielke PW; KJ Berry. Two-sample multivariate similarity permutation comparison. *Psychological Reports*; 2007; 100: 257–262.

Mielke PW; KJ Berry; GW Brier. Applications of multi-response permutation procedures for examining seasonal changes in monthly mean sea-level pressure patterns. *Monthly Weather Review*; 1981a; 109: 120–126.

Mielke PW; KJ Berry; PJ Brockwell; JS Williams. A class of nonparametric tests based on multiresponse permutation procedures. *Biometrika*; 1981b; 68: 720–724.

Mielke PW; KJ Berry; JL Eighmy. A permutation procedure for comparing archaeomagnetic polar directions. *Archaeomagnetic Dating*. JL Eighmy and RS Sternberg, editors. Tucson: University of Arizona Press; 1991: 102–108.

Mielke PW; KJ Berry; ES Johnson. Multi-response permutation procedures for a priori classifications. *Communications in Statistics—Theory and Methods*; 1976; 5: 1409–1424.

Mielke PW; KJ Berry; JE Johnston. Asymptotic log-linear analysis: Some cautions concerning sparse contingency tables. *Psychological Reports*; 2004a; 94: 19–32.

Mielke PW; KJ Berry; JE Johnston. Comparisons of continuous and discrete methods for combining probability values associated with matched-pairs t test data. *Perceptual and Motor Skills*; 2005b; 100: 799–805.

Mielke PW; KJ Berry; JE Johnston. A FORTRAN program for computing the exact variance of weighted kappa. *Perceptual and Motor Skills*; 2005c; 101: 468–472.

Mielke PW; KJ Berry; CW Landsea; WM Gray. Artificial skill and validation in meteorological forecasting. *Weather and Forecasting*; 1996a; 11: 153–169.

Mielke PW; KJ Berry; CW Landsea; WM Gray. A single-sample estimate of shrinkage in meteorological forecasting. *Weather and Forecasting*; 1997; 12: 847–858.

Mielke PW; KJ Berry; JG Medina. Climax I and II: Distortion resistant residual analyses. *Journal of Applied Meteorology*; 1982; 21: 788–792.

Mielke PW; KJ Berry; CO Neidt. A permutation test for multivariate matched-pair analyses: Comparisons with Hotelling's multivariate matched-pair T^2 test. *Psychological Reports*; 1996b; 78: 1003–1008.

Mielke PW; KJ Berry; D Zelterman. Fisher's exact test of mutual independence for 2×2×2 cross-classification tables. *Educational and Psychological Measurement*; 1994; 54: 110–114.

Mielke PW; GM Brier; LO Grant; GJ Mulvey; PN Rosenzweig. A statistical reanalysis of the replicated Climax I and II wintertime orographic cloud seeding experiments. *Journal of Applied Meteorology*; 1981c; 20: 643–659.

Mielke PW; CF Chappell; LO Grant. On precipitation sensor network densities for evaluating wintertime orographic cloud seeding experiments. *Water Resources Bulletin*; 1972; 8: 1219–1224.

Mielke PW; LO Grant; CF Chappell. Elevation and spatial variation effects of wintertime orographic cloud seeding. *Journal of Applied Meteorology*; 1970; 9: 476–488. Corrigenda: 1971; 10: 442 and 1976; 15: 801.

Mielke PW; LO Grant; CF Chappell. An independent replication of the Climax wintertime orographic cloud seeding experiment. *Journal of Applied Meteorology*; 1971; 10: 1198–1212. Corrigendum: 1976; 15: 801.

Mielke PW; H Iyer. Permutation techniques for analyzing multiresponse data from randomized block experiments. *Communications in Statistics—Theory and Methods*; 1982; 11: 1427–1437.

Mielke PW; ES Johnson. Three-parameter kappa distribution maximum likelihood estimates and likelihood ratio tests. *Monthly Weather Review*; 1973; 101: 701–707.

Mielke PW; ES Johnson. Some generalized beta distributions of the second kind having desirable application features in hydrology and meteorology. *Water Resources Research*; 1974; 10: 223–226.

Mielke PW; JE Johnston; KJ Berry. Combining probability values from independent permutation tests: A discrete analog of Fisher's classical method. *Psychological Reports*; 2004b; 95: 449–458.

Mielke PW; JG Medina. A new covariate ratio procedure for estimating treatment differences with applications to Climax I and II experiments. *Journal of Climate and Applied Meteorology*; 1983; 22: 1290–1295.

Mielke PW; PK Sen. On asymptotic non-normal null distributions for locally most powerful rank test statistics. *Communications in Statistics—Theory and Methods*; 1981; 10: 1079–1094.

Mielke PW; MM Siddiqui. A combinatorial test for independence of dichotomous responses. *Journal of the American Statistical Association*; 1965; 60: 437–441.

Mielke PW; YC Yao. A class of multiple sample tests based on empirical coverages. *Annals of the Institute of Statistical Mathematics*; 1988; 40: 165–178.

Mielke PW; YC Yao. On g-sample empirical coverage tests: Exact and simulated null distributions of test statistics with small and moderate sample sizes. *Journal of Statistical Computation and Simulation*; 1990; 35: 31–39.

Miller JR; EI Boyd; RA Schleusener; AS Dennis. Hail suppression data from western North Dakota, 1969–1972. *Journal of Applied Meteorology*; 1975; 14: 755–762.

Miller, JR; MJ Fuhs. Results of hail suppression efforts in North Dakota as shown by crop hail insurance data. *Journal of Weather Modification*; 1987; 19: 45–49.

Minkowski H. Über die positiven quadratishen formen und über kettenbruchähnliche algorithmen. *Journal für die reine und angewandte Mathematic*; 1891; 107: 278–297.

Mondimore FM; *Adolescent Depression: A Guide for Parents*. Baltimore, MD: Johns Hopkins University Press; 2002.

Mood AM. On the asymptotic efficiency of certain nonparametric two-sample tests. *The Annals of Mathematical Statistics*; 1954; 25: 514–522.

Moran PAP. The random division of an interval. *Journal of the Royal Statistical Society, Series B*; 1947; 9: 92–98. Corrigendum: *Journal of the Royal Statistical Society, Series A*; 1981; 144: 388.

Mosier CI. Symposium: The need and means of cross-validation, I: Problems and designs of cross-validation. *Educational and Psychological Measurement*; 1951; 11: 5–11.

Mosteller F; JW Tukey. *Data Analysis and Regression*. Reading, MA: Addison–Wesley; 1977.

Mudholkar GS; YP Chaubey. On the distribution of Fisher's transformation of the correlation coefficient. *Communications in Statistics—Simulation and Computation*; 1976; 5: 163–172.

Murphy AH; RL Winkler. Probability forecasting in meteorology. *Journal of the American Statistical Association*; 1984; 79: 489–500.

Myers JL; AD Well. *Research Design & Statistical Analysis*. New York: HarperCollins; 1991.

Nanda DN. Distribution of the sum of roots of a determinantal equation. *Annals of Mathematical Statistics*; 1950; 21: 432–439.

Nicholls N. Predictability of interannual variations of Australian seasonal tropical cyclone activity. *Monthly Weather Review*; 1985; 113: 1144–1149.

O'Brien RG. Comment on "Some problems in the nonorthogonal analysis of variance." *Psychological Bulletin*; 1976; 83: 72–74.

O'Neill ME. A comparison of the additive and multiplicative definitions of second-order interaction in $2 \times 2 \times 2$ contingency tables. *Journal of Statistical Computing and Simulation*; 1982; 15: 33–50.

O'Reilly FJ; PW Mielke. Asymptotic normality of MRPP statistics from invariance principles of U-statistics. *Communications in Statistics—Theory and Methods*; 1980; 9: 629–637.

Odoroff CL. A comparision of minimum logit chi-square estimation and maximum likelihood estimation in 2×2×2 and 3×2×2 contingency tables. *Journal of the American Statistical Association*; 1970; 65: 1617–1631.

Onstott TC. Application of the Bingham distribution function in paleomagnetic studies. *Journal of Geophysical Research*; 1980; 85: 1500–1510.

Orlowski LA; WD Grundy; PW Mielke; SA Schumm. Geological applications of multi-response permutation procedures. *Mathematical Geology*; 1993; 25: 483–500.

Orlowski LA; SA Schumm; PW Mielke. Reach classifications of the lower Mississippi river. *Geomorphology*; 1995; 14: 221–234.

Osgood CE; GJ Suci; PH Tannenbaum. *The Measurement of Meaning*. Urbana, IL: University of Illinois Press; 1957.

Overall JE; DM Lee; CW Hornick. Comparison of two strategies for analysis of variance in nonorthogonal designs. *Psychological Bulletin*; 1981; 90: 367–375.

Overall JE; DK Spiegel. Concerning least squares analysis of experimental data. *Psychological Bulletin*; 1969; 72: 311–322.

Overall JE; DK Spiegel; J Cohen. Equivalence of orthogonal and nonorthogonal analysis of variance. *Psychological Bulletin*; 1975; 82: 182–186.

Patefield WM. Algorithm AS 159: An efficient method of generating random $R \times C$ tables with given row and column totals. *Applied Statistics*; 1981; 30: 91–97.

Pearson ES. Some notes on sampling with two variables. *Biometrika*; 1929; 21: 337–360.

Pearson ES. The choice of statistical tests illustrated on the interpretation of data classes in a 2×2 table. *Biometrika*; 1947; 34: 139–167.

Pearson ES. On questions raised by the combination of tests based on discontinuous distributions. *Biometrika*; 1950; 37: 383–398.

Pearson ES; HO Hartley. *Biometrika Tables for Statisticians, Vol. II*. Cambridge, UK: Cambridge University Press; 1972.

Pearson K. On the criterion that a given system of deviations from the probable in the case of a correlated system of variables is such that it can reasonably supposed to have arisen from random sampling. *Philosophy Magazine*; 1900; 50: 157–172.

Pearson K. *Mathematical Contributions to the Theory of Evolution: XVI. On Further Methods of Determining Correlation*. Drapers' Company Research Memoirs Biometric Series IV. London: Dulau; 1907.

Pellicane PJ; RS Potter; PW Mielke. Permutation procedures as a statistical tool in wood related applications. *Wood Science and Technology;* 1989; 23: 193–204.

Pesarin F. *Multivariate Permutation Tests: With Applications in Biostatistics.* Chichester, UK: Wiley; 2001.

Pfaffenberger R; J Dinkel. Absolute deviations curve-fitting: An alternative to least squares. *Contributions to Survey Sampling and Applied Statistics.* HA David, editor. New York: Academic Press; 1978: 279–294.

Picard RR; KN Berk. Data splitting. *The American Statistician;* 1990; 44: 140–147.

Picard RR; RD Cook. Cross-validation of regression models. *Journal of the American Statistical Association;* 1984; 79: 575–583.

Piccarreta R. A new measure of nominal-ordinal association. *Journal of Applied Statistics;* 2001; 28: 107–120.

Piers EV. *Piers–Harris Children's Self-Concept Scale: Revised Manual.* Los Angeles, CA: Western Psychological Services; 1984.

Pillai KCS. Confidence interval for the correlation coefficient. *Sankhyā;* 1946; 7: 415–422.

Pillai KCS. Some new test criteria in multivariate analysis. *Annals of Mathematical Statistics;* 1955; 26: 117–121.

Pitman EJG. Significance tests which may be applied to samples from any populations. *Supplement to the Journal of the Royal Statistical Society;* 1937a; 4: 119–130.

Pitman EJG. Significance tests which may be applied to samples from any populations, II. The correlation coefficient test. *Supplement to the Journal of the Royal Statistical Society;* 1937b; 4: 225–232.

Pitman EJG. Significance tests which may be applied to samples from any populations, III. The analysis of variance test. *Biometrika;* 1938; 29: 322–335.

Plackett RL. A note on interactions in contingency tables. *Journal of the Royal Statistical Society, Series B;* 1962; 24: 162–166.

Pomar MI. Demystifying loglinear analysis: Four ways to assess interaction in a $2 \times 2 \times 2$ table. *Sociological Perspectives;* 1984; 27: 111–135.

Portnoy S; R Koenker. The Gaussian hare and the Laplacian tortoise: Computability of squared-error versus absolute-error estimators. *Statistical Science;* 1997; 12: 279–300.

Quetelet MA. *Letters Addressed to H. R. H. the Grand Duke of Saxe Coburg and Gotha on the Theory of Probabilities as Applied to the Moral and Political Sciences.* OG Downes, translator. London, UK: Charles & Edwin Layton; 1849.

Race RR; R Sanger. *Blood Groups in Man* (6th ed.). Oxford: Blackwell Scientific Publishers; 1975.

Rademacher H. On the partition function $p(n)$. *Proceedings of the London Mathematical Society;* 1937; 43: 241–254.

Radlow R; EF Alf. An alternate multinomial assessment of the accuracy of the χ^2 test of goodness-of-fit. *Journal of the American Statistical Association*; 1975; 80: 811–813.

Rao JS. Some tests based on arc lengths for the circle. *Sankhyā*, Series B; 1976; 38: 329–338.

Rao JS; VK Murthy. A two-sample nonparametric test based on spacing-frequencies. *Proceedings of the International Statistical Institute: Contributed Papers Volume*; 1981; 43rd Session: 223–227.

Rawlings RR. Note on nonorthogonal analysis of variance. *Psychological Bulletin*; 1972; 77: 373–374.

Rawlings RR. Comments on the Overall and Spiegel paper. *Psychological Bulletin*; 1973; 79: 168–169.

Reich RM; PW Mielke; FG Hawksworth. Spatial analysis of ponderosa pine trees infected with dwarf mistletoe. *Canadian Journal of Forest Research*; 1991; 21: 1808–1815.

Restle F. Moon illusion explained on the basis of relative size. *Science*; 1970; 167: 1092–1096.

Reynolds HT. *The Analysis of Cross-Classifications*. New York: Free Press; 1977.

Robinson J. Approximations to some test statistics for permutation tests in a completely randomized design. *The Australian Journal of Statistics*; 1983; 25: 358–369.

Rock I; L Kaufman. The moon illusion: II. *Science*; 1962; 136: 1023–1031.

Rolfe T. Randomized shuffling. *Dr. Dobb's Journal*; 2000; 25: 113–114.

Roscoe JT; JA Byars. An investigation of the restraints with respect to sample size commonly imposed on the use of the chi-square statistics. *Journal of the American Statistical Association*; 1971; 66: 755–759.

Rose RL; TC Jameson. Evaluation studies of longterm hail damage reduction programs in North Dakota. *Journal of Weather Modification*; 1986; 18: 17–20.

Ross HE; C Plug. *The Mystery of the Moon Illusion: Exploring Size Perception*. Oxford, UK: Oxford University Press; 2002.

Rousseeuw PJ. Least median of squares regression. *Journal of the American Statistical Association*; 1984; 79: 871–880.

Ruben H. Some new results on the distribution of the sample correlation coefficient. *Journal of the Royal Statistical Society*; 1966; 28: 514–525.

Rudolf RC; CM Sackiw; GT Riley. Statistical evaluation of the 1984–88 seeding experiment in northern Greece. *Journal of Weather Modification*; 1994; 26: 53–60.

Russell GS; DJ Levitin. An expanded table of probability values for Rao's spacing test. *Communications in Statistics—Simulation and Computation*; 1997; 24: 879–888.

Salama IA; D Quade. A note on Spearman's footrule. *Communications in Statistics—Simulation and Computation*; 1990; 19: 591–601.

Samiuddin M. On a test for an assigned value of correlation in a bivariate normal distribution. *Biometrika*; 1970; 57: 461–464.

Särndal CE. A comparative study of association measures. *Psychometrika*; 1974; 39: 165–187.

Schoener TW. An empirically based estimate of home range. *Theoretical Population Biology*; 1981; 20: 281–325.

Scott WA. Reliability of content analysis: The case of nominal scale coding. *Public Opinion Quarterly*; 1955; 19: 321–325.

Sethuraman J; JS Rao. Pitman efficiencies of tests based on spacings. *Nonparametric Techniques in Statistical Inference*. ML Puri, editor. Cambridge, UK: Cambridge University Press; 1970; 405–416.

Sherman B. A random variable related to the spacing of sample values. *Annals of Mathematical Statistics*; 1950; 21: 339–361.

Sheynin OB. R.J. Boscovich's work on probability. *Archive for History of Exact Sciences*; 1973; 9: 306–324.

Siddiqui MM. The consistency of a matching test. *Journal of Statistical Planning and Inference*; 1982; 6: 227–233.

Siegel S; NJ Castellan. *Nonparametric Statistics for the Behavioral Sciences* (2nd ed.). New York: McGraw–Hill; 1988.

Simeonov P. Comparative study of hail suppression efficiency in Bulgaria and France. *Atmospheric Research*; 1992; 28: 227–235.

Simpson EH. The interpretation of interaction in contingency tables. *Journal of the Royal Statistical Society, Series B*; 1951; 13: 238–241.

Slakter MJ. A comparison of the Pearson chi-square and Kolmogorov goodness-of-fit tests for small but equal expected frequencies. *Biometrika*; 1966; 53: 619–622.

Small CG. A survey of multidimensional medians. *International Statistical Review*; 1990; 58: 263–277.

Smirnov NV. Sur les écarts de la courbe de distribution empirique. *Matematičeskiĭ Sbornik*; 1939a; 6: 3–26.

Smirnov NV. On the estimation of the discrepancy between empirical curves of distribution for two independent samples. *Bulletin de l'Université de Moscov*; 1939b; 2: 3–16.

Smith PL; LR Johnson; DL Priegnitz; BA Boe; PW Mielke. An exploratory analysis of crop-hail insurance data for evidence of cloud-seeding effects in North Dakota. *Journal of Applied Meteorology*; 1997; 36: 463–473.

Snee RD. Validation of regression models: Methods and examples. *Technometrics*; 1977; 19: 415–428.

Solow AR. A randomization test for independence of animal locations. *Ecology*; 1989; 70: 1546–1549.

Spearman C. The proof and measurement of association between two things. *American Journal of Psychology*; 1904; 15: 72–101.

Spearman C. 'Footrule' for measuring correlation. *British Journal of Psychology*; 1906; 2: 89–108.

Spielberger CD. *Anxiety: Current Trends in Theory and Research.* New York: Academic Press; 1972.

Spielberger CD. *Manual for the State–Trait Anxiety Inventory.* Palo Alto, CA: Consulting Psychologists Press; 1983.

Sprott DA. A note on a class of occupancy problems. *The American Statistician*; 1969; 23: 12–13.

SPSS, Incorporated. *SPSS for Windows* (Release 11.5). Chicago, IL: SPSS, Incorporated; 2002.

Stark R; I Roberts. *Contemporary Social Research Methods.* Bellevue, WA: Micro–Case; 1996.

Stevens JP. *Intermediate Statistics: A Modern Approach.* Hillsdale, NJ: Erlbaum; 1990.

Stone M. Cross-validatory choice and assessment of statistical predictions. *Journal of the Royal Statistical Society, Series B*; 1974; 36: 111–147.

Stone M. Cross-validation: A review. *Mathematische Operationsforschung und Statistik*; 1978; 9: 127–139.

Stuart A. Spearman-like computation of Kendall's tau. *British Journal of Mathematical and Statistical Psychology*; 1977; 30: 104–112.

Subrahmanyam M. A property of simple least squares estimates. *Sankhyā*; 1972; 34B: 355–356.

Taha MAH. Rank test for scale parameter for asymmetrical one-sided distributions. *Publications de L'Institut de Statistiques de L'Université de Paris*; 1964; 13: 169–180.

Tate MW; LA Hyer. Inaccuracy of the χ^2 test of goodness-of-fit when expected frequencies are small. *Journal of the American Statistical Association*; 1973; 68: 836–841.

Taylor LD. Estimation by minimizing the sum of absolute errors. *Frontiers in Econometrics.* P Zamembka, editor. New York; Academic Press; 1974: 169–190.

Terpstra TJ. The asymptotic normality and consistency of Kendall's test against trend, when ties are present in one ranking. *Indagationes Mathematicae*; 1952; 14: 327–333.

Toussaint GT. Bibliography on estimation of misclassification. *IEEE Transactions on Information Theory*; 1974; 20: 472–479.

Trehub A; F Heilizer. Comments on the testing of combined results. *Journal of Clinical Psychology*; 1962; 18: 329–333.

Tucker DF; PW Mielke; ER Reiter. The verification of numerical models with multivariate randomized block permutation procedures. *Meteorology and Atmospheric Physics*; 1989; 40: 181–188.

Tukey JW. Discussion on symposium on statistics for the clinician. *Journal of Clinical Psychology*; 1950; 6: 61–74.

Umesh UN. Predicting nominal variable relationships with multiple response. *Journal of Forecasting*; 1995; 14: 585–596.

United States Census Bureau. *Geographical Areas Reference Manual.* Chapter 10: Census Tracts and Block Numbering Areas (2003). http://www.census.gov/geo/www/garm.html [Cited 6 March 2003].

Upton GJG. A comparison of alternative tests for the 2 × 2 comparative trial. *Journal of the Royal Statistical Society, Series A*; 1982; 145: 86–105.

Ury HK; DC Kleinecke. Tables of the distribution of Spearman's footrule. *Applied Statistics*; 1979; 28: 271–275.

Wald A; J Wolfowitz. On a test whether two samples are from the same population. *Annals of Mathematical Statistics*; 1940; 11: 147–162.

Walker DD; JC Loftis; PW Mielke. Permutation methods for determining the significance of spatial dependence. *Mathematical Geology*; 1997; 29: 1011–1024.

Wallis WA. The correlation ratio for ranked data. *Journal of the American Statistical Association*; 1939; 34: 533–538.

Wallis WA. Compounding probabilities from independent significance tests. *Econometrica*; 1942; 10: 229–248.

Watson GS. Analysis of dispersion on a sphere. *Monthly Notices of the Royal Astronomical Society, Geophysical Supplement*; 1956; 7: 153–159.

Watson GS; R Irving. Statistical methods in rock magnetism. *Monthly Notices of the Royal Astronomical Society, Geophysical Supplement*; 1957; 7: 289–300.

Watson GS; EJ Williams. On the construction of significance tests on the circle and sphere. *Biometrika*; 1956; 43: 344–352.

Watterson IG. Nondimensional measures of climate model performance. *International Journal of Climatology*; 1996; 16: 379–391.

Whaley FA. The equivalence of three independently derived permutation procedures for testing homogeneity of multidimensional samples. *Biometrics*; 1983; 39: 741–745.

White C. The committee problem. *American Statistician*; 1971; 25: 25–26.

Wilcoxon F. Individual comparisons by ranking methods. *Biometrics*; 1945; 1: 80–83.

Wilks SS. The likelihood test of independence in contingency tables. *The Annals of Mathematical Statistics*; 1935; 6: 190–196.

Wilks SS. The large-sample distribution of the likelihood ratio for testing composite hypotheses. *The Annals of Mathematical Statistics*; 1938; 9: 60–62.

Williams DA. Improved likelihood ratio test for complete contingency tables. *Biometrika*; 1976a; 63: 33–37.

Williams GW. Comparing the joint agreement of several raters with another rater. *Biometrics*; 1976b; 32: 619–627.

Willmott CJ. Some comments on the evaluation of model performance. *Bulletin of the American Meteorological Society*; 1982; 63: 1309–1313.

Willmott CJ; SG Ackleson; RE Davis; JJ Feddema; KM Klink; DR Legates; J O'Donnell; CM Rowe. Statistics for the evaluation and comparison of models. *Journal of Geophysical Research*; 1985; 90: 8995–9005.

Wilson HG. Least squares versus minimum absolute deviations estimation in linear models. *Decision Sciences*; 1978; 9: 322–325.

Wong RKW; N Chidambaram; PW Mielke. Application of multi-response permutation procedures and median regression for covariate analyses of possible weather modification effects on hail responses. *Atmosphere-Ocean*; 1983; 21: 1–13.

Yates, F. Tests of significance for 2×2 contingency tables (with discussion). *Journal of the Royal Statistical Society, Series A*; 1984; 147: 426–463.

Zachs S; H Solomon. On testing and estimating the interaction between treatments and environmental conditions in binomial experiments: The case of two stations. *Communications in Statistics—Theory and Methods*; 1976; 5: 197–223.

Zelterman D. Goodness-of-fit tests for large sparse multinomial distributions. *Journal of the American Statistical Association*; 1987; 82: 624–629.

Zelterman D; IS Chan; PW Mielke. Exact tests of significance in higher dimensional tables. *The American Statistician*; 1995; 49: 357–361.

Zimmerman GM; H Goetz; PW Mielke. Use of an improved statistical method for group comparisons to study effects of prairie fire. *Ecology*; 1985; 66: 606–611.

Author Index

Subject Index

Springer Series in Statistics *(continued from page ii)*

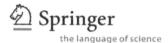

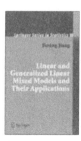

Linear and Generalized Linear Mixed Models and Their Applications

Jiming Jiang

This book covers two major classes of mixed effects models, linear mixed models and generalized linear mixed models, and it presents an up-to-date account of theory and methods in analysis of these models as well as their applications in various fields. The book offers a systematic approach to inference about non-Gaussian linear mixed models. Furthermore, it has included recently developed methods, such as mixed model diagnostics, mixed model selection, and jackknife method in the context of mixed models.

2007. 260 pp. (Springer Series in Statistics)
Hardcover ISBN 978-0-387-47941-5

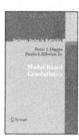

Model-based Geostatistics

Peter J. Diggle and Paulo Justiniano Ribeiro

Model-based geostatistics refers to the application of general statistical principles of modeling and inference to geostatistical problems. This volume is the first book-length treatment of model-based geostatistics. The book assumes a working knowledge of classical and Bayesian methods of inference, linear models, and generalized linear models, but does not require previous exposure to spatial statistical models or methods. The authors have used the material in MSc-level statistics courses.

2006. 230 pp. (Springer Series in Statistics) Hardcover
ISBN 978-0-387-32907-9

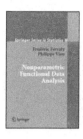

Nonparametric Functional Data Analysis

F. Ferraty and P. Vieu

This book links two fields of modern statistics by explaining how functional data can be studied through parameter-free statistical ideas. It starts from theoretical foundations including functional nonparametric modeling, description of the mathematical framework, construction of the statistical methods, and statements of their asymptotic behaviors. It proceeds to computational issues including R and S-PLUS routines.

2006. 296 pp. (Springer Series in Statistics) Hardcover
ISBN 978-0-387-30369-7

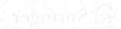